BRAIN AGING
MODELS, METHODS, AND MECHANISMS

FRONTIERS IN NEUROSCIENCE

Series Editors
Sidney A. Simon, Ph.D.
Miguel A.L. Nicolelis, M.D., Ph.D.

Published Titles

Apoptosis in Neurobiology
Yusuf A. Hannun, M.D., Professor of Biomedical Research and Chairman/Department
of Biochemistry and Molecular Biology, Medical University of South Carolina
Rose-Mary Boustany, M.D., tenured Associate Professor of Pediatrics and Neurobiology,
Duke University Medical Center

Methods for Neural Ensemble Recordings
Miguel A.L. Nicolelis, M.D., Ph.D., Professor of Neurobiology and Biomedical Engineering,
Duke University Medical Center

Methods of Behavioral Analysis in Neuroscience
Jerry J. Buccafusco, Ph.D., Alzheimer's Research Center, Professor of Pharmacology and
Toxicology, Professor of Psychiatry and Health Behavior, Medical College of Georgia

Neural Prostheses for Restoration of Sensory and Motor Function
John K. Chapin, Ph.D., Professor of Physiology and Pharmacology, State University of
New York Health Science Center
Karen A. Moxon, Ph.D., Assistant Professor/School of Biomedical Engineering, Science,
and Health Systems, Drexel University

Computational Neuroscience: Realistic Modeling for Experimentalists
Eric DeSchutter, M.D., Ph.D., Professor/Department of Medicine, University of Antwerp

Methods in Pain Research
Lawrence Kruger, Ph.D., Professor of Neurobiology (Emeritus), UCLA School of Medicine
and Brain Research Institute

Motor Neurobiology of the Spinal Cord
Timothy C. Cope, Ph.D., Professor of Physiology, Emory University School of Medicine

Nicotinic Receptors in the Nervous System
Edward D. Levin, Ph.D., Associate Professor/Department of Psychiatry and Pharmacology
and Molecular Cancer Biology and Department of Psychiatry and Behavioral
Sciences, Duke University School of Medicine

Methods in Genomic Neuroscience
Helmin R. Chin, Ph.D., Genetics Research Branch, NIMH, NIH
Steven O. Moldin, Ph.D, Genetics Research Branch, NIMH, NIH

Methods in Chemosensory Research
Sidney A. Simon, Ph.D., Professor of Neurobiology, Biomedical Engineering, and
Anesthesiology, Duke University
Miguel A.L. Nicolelis, M.D., Ph.D., Professor of Neurobiology and Biomedical Engineering,
Duke University

The Somatosensory System: Deciphering the Brain's Own Body Image
Randall J. Nelson, Ph.D., Professor of Anatomy and Neurobiology,
  University of Tennessee Health Sciences Center

The Superior Colliculus: New Approaches for Studying Sensorimotor Integration
William C. Hall, Ph.D., Department of Neuroscience, Duke University
Adonis Moschovakis, Ph.D., Institute of Applied and Computational Mathematics, Crete

New Concepts in Cerebral Ischemia
Rick C. S. Lin, Ph.D., Professor of Anatomy, University of Mississippi Medical Center

DNA Arrays: Technologies and Experimental Strategies
Elena Grigorenko, Ph.D., Technology Development Group, Millennium Pharmaceuticals

Methods for Alcohol-Related Neuroscience Research
Yuan Liu, Ph.D., National Institute of Neurological Disorders and Stroke, National Institutes
  of Health
David M. Lovinger, Ph.D., Laboratory of Integrative Neuroscience, NIAAA

In Vivo Optical Imaging of Brain Function
Ron Frostig, Ph.D., Associate Professor/Department of Psychobiology,
  University of California, Irvine

Primate Audition: Behavior and Neurobiology
Asif A. Ghazanfar, Ph.D., Primate Cognitive Neuroscience Lab, Harvard University

Methods in Drug Abuse Research: Cellular and Circuit Level Analyses
Dr. Barry D. Waterhouse, Ph.D., MCP-Hahnemann University

Functional and Neural Mechanisms of Interval Timing
Warren H. Meck, Ph.D., Professor of Psychology, Duke University

Biomedical Imaging in Experimental Neuroscience
Nick Van Bruggen, Ph.D., Department of Neuroscience Genentech, Inc., South San Francisco
Timothy P.L. Roberts, Ph.D., Associate Professor, University of Toronto

The Primate Visual System
John H. Kaas, Department of Psychology, Vanderbilt University
Christine Collins, Department of Psychology, Vanderbilt University

Neurosteroid Effects in the Central Nervous System
Sheryl S. Smith, Ph.D., Department of Physiology, SUNY Health Science Center

Modern Neurosurgery: Clinical Translation of Neuroscience Advances
Dennis A. Turner, Department of Surgery, Division of Neurosurgery, Duke University
  Medical Center

Sleep: Circuits and Functions
Pierre-Hervé Luoou, Université Claude Bernard Lyon I, Lyon, France

Methods in Insect Sensory Neuroscience
Thomas A. Christensen, Arizona Research Laboratories, Division of Neurobiology, University
  of Arizona, Tucson, AZ

Motor Cortex in Voluntary Movements
Alexa Riehle, INCM-CNRS, Marseille, France
Eilon Vaadia, The Hebrew University, Jeruselum, Israel

Neural Plasticity in Adult Somatic Sensory-Motor Systems
Ford F. Ebner, Vanderbilt University, Nashville, TN

Advances in Vagal Afferent Neurobiology
Bradley J. Undem, Johns Hopkins Asthma Center, Baltimore, MD
Daniel Weinreich, University of Maryland, Baltimore, MD

The Dynamic Synapse: Molecular Methods in Ionotropic Receptor Biology
Josef T. Kittler, University College, London
Stephen J. Moss, University of Pennsylvania

Animal Models of Cognitive Impairment
Edward D. Levin, Duke University Medical Center, Durham, NC
Jerry J. Buccafusco, Medical College of Georgia, Augusta, GA

The Role of the Nucleus of the Solitary Tract in Gustatory Processing
Robert M. Bradley, University of Michigan, Ann Arbor, MI

Brain Aging: Models, Methods, and Mechanisms
Frederico Bermudez-Rattoni, National University of Mexico, Mexico City, Mexico

Neural Plasticity and Memory: From Genes to Brain Imaging
Robert M. Bradley, University of Michigan, Ann Arbor, MI

BRAIN AGING
MODELS, METHODS, AND MECHANISMS

Edited by
David R. Riddle

Wake Forest University School of Medicine
Winston-Salem, NC

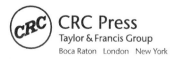

CRC Press
Taylor & Francis Group
Boca Raton London New York

CRC Press is an imprint of the
Taylor & Francis Group, an informa business

CRC Press
Taylor & Francis Group
6000 Broken Sound Parkway NW, Suite 300
Boca Raton, FL 33487-2742

© 2007 by Taylor & Francis Group, LLC
CRC Press is an imprint of Taylor & Francis Group, an Informa business

First issued in paperback 2019

No claim to original U.S. Government works

ISBN-13: 978-0-367-45310-7 (pbk)
ISBN-13: 978-0-8493-3818-2 (hbk)

Library of Congress Cataloging-in-Publication Data

Brain aging : models, methods, and mechanisms / [edited by] David R. Riddle.
    p. ; cm. -- (Frontiers in neuroscience)
"A CRC title."
Includes bibliographical references and index.
ISBN-13: 978-0-8493-3818-2 (hardcover : alk. paper)
ISBN-10: 0-8493-3818-2 (hardcover : alk. paper)
    1. Brain--Aging. I. Riddle, David R. II. Series: Frontiers in neuroscience (Boca Raton, Fla.)
    [DNLM: 1. Brain--physiopathology. 2. Aging--physiology. 3. Cognition--physiology. 4. Nerve Degeneration. WL 300 B81109 2007]

QP356.25.B728 2007
612.6'7--dc22
                                            2006036487

Visit the Taylor & Francis Web site at
http://www.taylorandfrancis.com

and the CRC Press Web site at
http://www.crcpress.com

Table of Contents

SECTION I   Assessing Cognitive Aging

Chapter 1

Elizabeth L. Glisky

Chapter 2

Mark B. Moss, Tara L. Moore, Stephen P. Schettler,
Ronald Killiany, and Douglas Rosene

Chapter 3

Joshua S. Rodefer and Mark G. Baxter

SECTION II   Quantifying Aging-Related Changes in the Brain

Chapter 4

Christoph Schmitz and Patrick R. Hof

Chapter 5

Alan Peters

SECTION III   Assessing Functional Changes in the Aging Nervous System

SECTION IV   Mechanisms Contributing to Brain Aging

Series Preface

Our goal in creating the *Frontiers in Neuroscience* series is to present the insights of experts on emerging fields and theoretical concepts that are, or will be, at the vanguard of neuroscience. Books in the series cover topics ranging from genetics, ion channels, apoptosis, electrodes, neural ensemble recordings in behaving animals, and even robotics. The series also covers new and exciting multidisciplinary areas of brain research, such as computational neuroscience and neuro-engineering, and describes breakthroughs in classical fields such as behavioral neuroscience. We want these books to be the books every neuroscientist will use to get acquainted with new ideas and frontiers in brain research. These books can be given to graduate students and postdoctoral fellows when they are looking for guidance to start a new line of research.

Each book is edited by an expert and consists of chapters written by the leaders in a particular field. Books are richly illustrated and contain comprehensive bibliographies. Chapters provide substantial background material relevant to the particular subject. We hope that as the volumes become available, the effort put in by us, the publisher, the book editors, and individual authors will contribute to the further development of brain research. The extent to which we achieve this goal will be determined by the utility of these books.

Preface

Studies of brain aging have certainly (dare we say it) come of age. The past two to three decades produced a striking increase in experimental investigations of the neurobiological basis of brain aging and of aging-related changes in neural and cognitive function. The public's interest in experimental gerontology has grown as the public has become more "gray," with both average age and life expectancy increasing in most developed countries. Driving the specific interest in the aging nervous system is the recognition that increased longevity has little appeal for most unless it is accompanied by maintenance of cognitive abilities. Indeed, if one searches the popular press or the Internet for information on aging, or for products that are purported to slow the aging process or limit its effects, one concludes that maintaining brain function may be the most important concern of older individuals. In recent years, neuroscientists with a variety of training and experimental approaches have joined established investigators of brain aging in developing increasingly powerful and quantitative methods. New animal model systems have been developed and old ones have become better characterized and standardized. In addition, advances in brain imaging techniques now permit investigations in aging humans with amazing resolution and sophistication, and also provide a bridge between human and animal studies. The (necessary and important) descriptive studies that dominated the field in earlier times increasingly are supplemented by more hypothesis-driven research, resulting in sophisticated investigations and models of the mechanisms of brain aging.

This volume provides an overview — an admittedly selective overview — of current research on brain aging. In presenting the most important and novel investigations in their areas of expertise, the contributors were asked to discuss not only data and mechanisms, but also the models and methods that are important in their work. The chapters do not include detailed experimental protocols, but each contains extensive references and highlights experimental concerns that are magnified or unique in studies of the aging brain. Readers will observe that many contributors note common challenges. Aging, some say, is not for wimps, and neither are aging studies. Investigating what happens to the brain in the latter part of the lifespan brings with it unique difficulties. For example, simply obtaining healthy individuals with known life histories at appropriate ages can be challenging (aging may be one of few areas of biomedical research in which good human subjects are arguably easier to obtain than appropriate experimental animals). It is critical to differentiate effects of aging from effects of aging-related disease; and even in the absence of ongoing disease, pathophysiological or developmental processes that occurred years or decades earlier may profoundly affect how an individual ages. This volume neither addresses all the critical experimental questions about the aging brain nor does it provide solutions to all the challenges inherent in such studies, but it should leave the reader with a broad and reasonably deep understanding of both recent progress and the future in this important field.

At this point I would like to express my sincere thanks to the many contributors to these chapters and to this volume. I have enjoyed excellent and friendly support from CRC Press staff, particularly David Fausel and Barbara Norwitz. Thanks to Series Editors Sidney Simon and Miguel Nicolelis for the invitation to undertake this project. Finally, I would like to thank Jesse Lichstein for her help in getting this book together for publication.

About the Editor

David R. Riddle, Ph.D., is an associate professor in the Department of Neurobiology and Anatomy and a member of the Interdisciplinary Program in Neuroscience, the Roena Kulynych Center for Memory and Cognition Research, and the Comprehensive Cancer Center at the Wake Forest University School of Medicine (WFUSM). He began his scientific training as a John Motley Morehead Foundation Scholar at the University of North Carolina, where he received his B.S. in zoology in 1984. Dr. Riddle completed his doctoral degree in the Neuroscience Program at the University of Michigan under the direction of Dr. Bruce Oakley, receiving his Ph.D. in 1990. He received postdoctoral training in developmental neurobiology in the Department of Neurobiology at the Duke University Medical Center, investigating activity- and trophic factor-dependent regulation of the development of the CNS in the laboratories of Dr. Dale Purves and Dr. Lawrence Katz.

Since joining the faculty at the WFUSM, Dr. Riddle's research has focused on the role of growth factors, particularly insulin-like growth factor-1 (IGF-1), in regulating neuronal structure and function in the developing, adult, and aging hippocampus and cerebral cortex. Currently, his laboratory focuses on IGF-1-dependent control of dendritic development, the regulation of neuronal and glial genesis in the adult and aging brain, and the impact of aging on the development of radiation-induced brain injury in cancer patients treated with whole brain irradiation. His studies are supported by grants from the National Institute of Neurological Disorders and Stroke and the National Institute on Aging. In addition to his research program, Dr. Riddle is active in graduate and medical education at the WFUSM, receiving the New Investigator in Basic Science Award in 2003 and the Award for Teaching Excellence in 2005.

Contributors

Michelle Adams, Ph.D.
Department of Neurobiology and
  Anatomy
Wake Forest University School of
  Medicine
Winston-Salem, North Carolina

Adam Bachstetter
Center of Excellence for Aging and
  Brain Repair
University of South Florida
Tampa, Florida

Mark G. Baxter, Ph.D.
Department of Experimental
  Psychology
Oxford University
Oxford, U.K.

Paula C. Bickford, Ph.D.
Center of Excellence for Aging and
  Brain Repair
University of South Florida
Tampa, Florida

Jennifer L. Bizon, Ph.D.
Department of Psychology and Faculty
  of Neuroscience
Texas A&M University
College Station, Texas

Judy K. Brunso-Bechtold, Ph.D.
Department of Neurobiology and
  Anatomy
Wake Forest University School of
  Medicine
Winston-Salem, North Carolina

Delrae M. Eckman, Ph.D.
Department of Pediatrics
Wake Forest University School of
  Medicine
Winston-Salem, North Carolina

Thomas C. Foster, Ph.D.
Department of Neuroscience
McKnight Brain Institute
University of Florida
Gainesville, Florida

Carmelina Gemma, Ph.D.
Center of Excellence for Aging and
  Brain Repair
University of South Florida
Tampa, Florida

Stephen D. Ginsberg, Ph.D.
Center for Dementia Research, Nathan
  Kline Institute
Departments of Psychiatry, Physiology,
  and Neuroscience
New York University School of
  Medicine
Orangeburg, New York

Elizabeth L. Glisky, Ph.D.
Department of Psychology
University of Arizona
Tucson, Arizona

Ki A. Goosens, Ph.D.
Brain and Cognitive Sciences
McGovern Institute for Brain Research
Massachusetts Institute of Technology
Cambridge, Massachusetts

Trey Hedden, Ph.D.
Department of Brain and Cognitive
  Sciences
Massachusetts Institute of Technology
Cambridge, Massachusetts

Patrick R. Hof, M.D.
Department of Neuroscience
Mount Sinai School of Medicine
New York, New York

Jeremy Ingraham
Program in Neuroscience
Wake Forest University School of
  Medicine
Winston-Salem, North Carolina

Ronald Killiany, Ph.D.
Department of Anatomy and
  Neurobiology
Boston University School of Medicine
Boston, Massachusetts

Ashok Kumar, Ph.D.
Department of Neuroscience
McKnight Brain Institute
University of Florida
Gainesville, Florida

Robin J. Lichtenwalner, Ph.D.
MedThink Communications
Raleigh, North Carolina

Tara L. Moore, Ph.D.
Department of Anatomy and
  Neurobiology
Boston University School of Medicine
Boston, Massachusetts

Mark B. Moss, Ph.D.
Department of Anatomy and
  Neurobiology
Boston University School of Medicine
Boston, Massachusetts

Michelle M. Nicolle, Ph.D.
Departments of Gerontology and
  Physiology/Pharmacology
Wake Forest University School of
  Medicine
Winston-Salem, North Carolina

Alan Peters, Ph.D.
Department of Anatomy and
  Neurobiology
Boston University School of
  Medicine
Boston, Massachusetts

David R. Riddle, Ph.D.
Department of Neurobiology and
  Anatomy
Wake Forest University School of
  Medicine
Winston-Salem, North Carolina

Joshua S. Rodefer, Ph.D.
Department of Psychology
University of Iowa
Iowa City, Iowa

Douglas Rosene, Ph.D.
Department of Anatomy and
  Neurobiology
Boston University School of
  Medicine
Boston, Massachusetts

Robert M. Sapolsky, Ph.D.
Department of Biological Sciences
Stanford University
Stanford, California

Stephen P. Schettler
Department of Anatomy and
  Neurobiology
Boston University School of
  Medicine
Boston, Massachusetts

Christoph Schmitz, M.D.
Department of Psychiatry and
  Neuropsychology
Division of Cellular Neuroscience
Maastricht University
Maastricht, The Netherlands

Lei Shi, M.D., Ph.D.
Department of Neurobiology and
  Anatomy
Wake Forest University School of
  Medicine
Winston-Salem, North Carolina

William E. Sonntag, Ph.D.
Department of
  Physiology/Pharmacology
Wake Forest University School of
  Medicine
Winston-Salem, North Carolina

Emil C. Toescu, M.D., Ph.D.
Department of Physiology, Division of
  Medical Sciences
University of Birmingham
Birmingham, U.K.

Jennifer Vila
Center of Excellence for Aging and
  Brain Repair
University of South Florida
Tampa, Florida

Hai-Yan Zhang, Ph.D.
Departments of Gerontology and
  Physiology/Pharmacology
Wake Forest University School of
  Medicine
Winston-Salem, North Carolina

Section I

Assessing Cognitive Aging

1 Changes in Cognitive Function in Human Aging

Elizabeth L. Glisky

CONTENTS

I.   INTRODUCTION: CHANGES IN COGNITIVE FUNCTION IN HUMAN AGING

As people age, they change in a myriad of ways — both biological and psychological. Some of these changes may be for the better, and others are not. This book primarily concerns the normally aging brain, the neuroanatomical and neurophysiological changes that occur with age, and the mechanisms that account for them. It is not primarily about the behavioral or cognitive concomitants of those changes. Nevertheless, there is ample evidence that alterations in brain structure and function are intimately tied to alterations in cognitive function. The complexity of both the neural and cognitive functions, however, makes exact mapping between brain and behavior extraordinarily difficult, and so these relations remain largely speculative, although ultimately testable. Establishing such links between brain and cognition is the principal goal of cognitive neuroscience.

The purpose of this chapter is to outline the changes in cognition that occur in normal human aging, in an effort to provide a backdrop against which neural changes can be interpreted (for review, see [1]). Although the relationship between brain and cognition is a dynamic one and may change across the lifespan, changes in these two domains will ultimately be related, and mechanisms underlying the changes will be discovered. Understanding age-related cognitive change will help focus and constrain neurobiological theories of aging in much the same way as theories of cognitive aging will be adapted to take account of new findings about the aging brain.

Just as age-related changes in brain structure and function are not uniform across the whole brain or across individuals, age-related changes in cognition are not uniform across all cognitive domains or across all older individuals. The basic cognitive functions most affected by age are attention and memory. Neither of these are unitary functions, however, and evidence suggests that some aspects of attention and memory hold up well with age while others show significant declines. Perception (although considered by many to be a precognitive function) also shows significant age-related declines attributable mainly to declining sensory capacities. Deficits at these early processing stages could affect cognitive functions later in the processing stream. Higher-level cognitive functions such as language processing and decision making may also be affected by age. These tasks naturally rely on more basic cognitive functions and will generally show deficits to the extent that those fundamental processes are impaired. Moreover, complex cognitive tasks may also depend on a set of executive functions, which manage and coordinate the various components of the tasks. Considerable evidence points to impairment of executive function as a key contributor to age-related declines in a range of cognitive tasks. Finally, although these cognitive functions will be reviewed separately below, it is abundantly clear that they overlap and interact in interesting and complex ways.

Although the overall picture might seem to be one of cognitive decline, enormous variability exists across individuals. Many older people out-perform young people, at least on some cognitive tasks, and others of the same age do at least as well as the young [2]. A question of great interest to aging researchers is what accounts for this variability. This chapter highlights the cognitive domains that show the greatest declines with age and are also the most variable. Areas of cognitive strength in normal aging are also discussed, because these may be recruited to compensate for areas of weakness. Theories of cognitive aging that have developed within each cognitive domain are outlined and brain regions hypothesized to underlie these functions are noted.

The next chapter section reviews some of the evidence for age-related impairments in basic cognitive functions, focusing primarily on attention and memory, and also discusses briefly the attentional and memory processes that show relative preservation with age.

II.   BASIC COGNITIVE FUNCTIONS

A.   ATTENTION

Attention is a basic but complex cognitive process that has multiple sub-processes specialized for different aspects of attentional processing. Some form of attention is involved in virtually all other cognitive domains, except when task performance has become habitual or automatic. Declines in attention can therefore have broad-reaching effects on one's ability to function adequately and efficiently in everyday life. The construct of attention defies simple definition, however, and it has been partitioned in a variety of ways by different researchers and theorists. The divisions used here are those that have been investigated most extensively in normal aging (for a comprehensive review of attention and aging, see [3]).

1.   Selective Attention

Selective attention refers to the ability to attend to some stimuli while disregarding others that are irrelevant to the task at hand. For example, in visual search tasks, people are asked to search a visual display for a target letter that is surrounded by other nontarget letters. The task can be made more difficult by increasing the similarity of targets and distractors (e.g., search for an F in a background of Es), or by increasing the number of relevant or irrelevant features that are part of the search criteria. In another task — the Stroop task — people are asked to name the color of ink in which an incongruent color word is printed, (e.g., the word "red" printed in green). Here, the word information tends to interfere with color naming, causing errors and an increase in response times. To perform well in these kinds of tasks, people have to select the relevant stimulus or dimensions for processing and ignore the irrelevant ones. Although findings are not entirely consistent across studies and may differ across tasks, in general older adults appear to be slower than younger adults in responding to the targets, but are not differentially affected by distraction [3, 4]. Thus, deficits found in many of these tasks can be largely attributed to a general slowing of information processing in older adults rather than to selective attention deficits per se.

2.   Divided Attention and Attention Switching

Divided attention has usually been associated with significant age-related declines in performance, particularly when tasks are complex. Divided attention tasks require the processing of two or more sources of information or the performance of two or more tasks at the same time. For example, people may have to monitor stimuli at two different spatial locations, or they may be asked to make semantic judgments about visually presented words while simultaneously monitoring for the occurrence of an auditorily presented digit [5]. The cost of dividing attention is assessed by comparing performance under dual task conditions to performance when the tasks are performed separately. Results suggest that older adults are more affected by the division of attention than young adults, particularly when the attentional demands of the two tasks are high. In addition, older adults seem less able to allocate resources appropriately when instructions are given to vary task priority [6]. These findings cannot be completely accounted for by a general slowing of information processing, but instead are usually explained in terms of declining processing resources associated with normal aging. Such limited resources are over-extended in older adults when attention must be divided between two or more sources. Similarly, the performance of older adults is slowed to a greater degree than that of young adults when attention must be switched from one task to another, requiring a change of mental set [4].

There is evidence that age deficits in divided attention and attention switching can be reduced by practice or extended training [7] and by aerobic exercise [8]. The exact mechanism of such improvements, however, is unclear. In the case of task-specific training, it is possible that some aspects of the tasks become automatic with practice, thus requiring fewer attentional resources. Alternatively, participants may develop strategies with extensive training that reduce the attentional demands of the tasks. It has been hypothesized that cardiovascular fitness may improve the efficiency of neural processes or may provide increased metabolic resources for task performance. Interestingly, the enhancement effects of aerobic exercise appear to be greatest on tasks involving executive control of attention [9], which depend largely on prefrontal cortex.

3.   Sustained Attention

Sustained attention refers to the ability to maintain concentration on a task over an extended period of time. Typically, vigilance tasks are used to measure sustained attention, in which people must monitor the environment for a relatively infrequent signal, such as a blip on a radar screen. In general, older adults are not impaired on vigilance tasks.

4.   Attention: Summary and Implications

Older adults show significant impairments on attentional tasks that require dividing or switching of attention among multiple inputs or tasks. They show relative preservation of performance on tasks that require selection of relevant stimuli; and although they are slower than young adults, they are not differentially impaired by distraction. They also are able to maintain concentration for an extended period of time. The tasks on which older adults show impairments tend to be those that require flexible control of attention, a cognitive function associated with the frontal lobes.

Importantly, these types of tasks appear to be amenable to training and show benefits of cardiovascular fitness.

Attentional deficits can have a significant impact on an older person's ability to function adequately and independently in everyday life. One important aspect of daily functioning affected by attentional problems is driving, an activity that, for many older people, is essential to independence. Driving requires a constant switching of attention in response to environmental contingencies. Attention must be divided between driving, monitoring the environment, and sorting out relevant from irrelevant stimuli in a cluttered visual array. Research has shown that divided attention impairments are significantly associated with increased automobile accidents in older adults [3, 10]. Given the previously noted findings of the effects of practice, extended training on driving simulators under divided attention conditions may be an important remedial activity for older people.

B.   WORKING MEMORY

Working memory is a multidimensional cognitive construct that has been hypothesized as the fundamental source of age-related deficits in a variety of cognitive tasks, including long-term memory, language, problem solving, and decision making. In fact, the majority of theories of cognitive aging seem to implicate working memory. Although there are several models of working memory, all agree that it is a limited capacity system that involves the active manipulation of information that is currently being maintained in focal attention (for reviews, see [11–13]). Short-term or primary memory, on the other hand, involves the simple maintenance of information over a short period of time. For example, one might maintain a phone number in short-term memory by simple rehearsal of the number. Older adults show minimal or no deficits in short-term memory and can typically hold about 7 ± 2 digits in mind as long as the digits are being rehearsed. Repeating the numbers backwards, however, requires an active reorganization or manipulation of the information held in short-term memory. This task thus requires working memory and shows impairments with age. In some sense, working memory is really a divided attention task — the contents of short-term memory must be maintained while simultaneously being manipulated or processed for some other purpose. Given the previously discussed findings of divided attention deficits with increased age, it is not surprising that older adults are impaired in working memory.

In the original working memory model of Baddeley and Hitch [14], the manipulation of information in short-term memory was handled by a central executive, and deficits in working memory were viewed as deficits in executive control, a function attributed primarily to prefrontal cortex. Recent neuroimaging research [15] has confirmed a role for dorsolateral prefrontal cortex (PFC) in the manipulation and updating of information in working memory, with left PFC involved more in verbal tasks and right PFC in visuospatial tasks. In recent years, however, the role of the central executive has been expanded to cover a range of executive control functions other than those associated strictly with working memory. These are elaborated in a later chapter section.

Although there is a general consensus that working memory is impaired in older adults, there is disagreement concerning the mechanisms involved, and much of the research has focused on testing a variety of theories. The next subsection outlines the main theories of working memory.

1.   Theories of Working Memory

Three theories of cognitive aging have been articulated within the context of working memory deficits, although they may apply more broadly across other cognitive domains: (1) one theory proposes a reduction of attentional resources, (2) one focuses on reduced speed of information processing, and (3) one ascribes problems to a failure of inhibitory control (for review, see [16]).

a.   *Attentional Resources*

Theories of age-related decline in working memory generally assume some reduction in processing resources. Craik and colleagues [17, 18] have suggested that the resource limitation is attentional and reflects a reduction in mental energy. Tasks with high attentional demands show impairments, whereas tasks requiring little or no attention (i.e., that are relatively automatic) are largely intact. Working memory tasks by their very nature involve divided attention and are therefore more likely to strain the limited resources of older adults. This theory is intuitively appealing, but it seems more descriptive than explanatory. The construct of attentional resources is poorly defined; and although neurophysiological correlates such as arousal or neural efficiency have been suggested [3], they have not been demonstrated empirically.

b.   *Speed of Information Processing*

Salthouse [19] has suggested that speed of processing might be considered a resource, and that age-related deficits in working memory and other cognitive tasks can be explained in terms of a general slowing of information processing. There is little disagreement that older adults are slower than younger adults and that slowing of fundamental cognitive processes may have detrimental effects on more complex tasks. Debate has focused, instead, on whether a generalized slowing can account for the bulk of the empirical findings or whether more process-specific components are also needed. Salthouse [20, 21] has demonstrated in numerous studies that slowing of information processing can account for a large proportion of the age-related variance in a variety of cognitive tasks, including working and long-term memory, and has argued that speed of processing is a cognitive primitive. Other investigators [22], however, have suggested that speed of processing and working memory provide independent contributions to higher-level cognition, and that working memory deficits must therefore be accounted for in terms of something other than speed. Finally, at some level, slowed processing, like attentional resources, is more a descriptor of aging cognition than an explanation for cognitive deficits and says nothing about what causes slowing with age. Here too, therefore, discovery of neurophysiological correlates may help to clarify mechanisms.

c. *Inhibitory Control*

Hasher, Zacks, and May [23, 24] proposed that a lack of inhibitory control might account for cognitive deficits associated with aging. Specifically, failure to suppress irrelevant information in working memory may effectively reduce its capacity, denying access to relevant information. For example, working memory span tasks involve the successive presentation across trials of increasingly long strings of digits or words. Age deficits could be attributable to the failure to delete from working memory digits or words from prior trials, thus reducing the "working space" for new stimuli [25]. Although considerable data suggest that older adults experience more interference from irrelevant information under some conditions [26], findings are mixed and other data fail to support an inhibitory deficit account [3]. It may be that there are different kinds of inhibition or that age-related effects are task- or paradigm-specific.

2. Working Memory: Summary and Implications

Older adults exhibit significant deficits in tasks that involve active manipulation, re-organization, or integration of the contents of working memory. Although the mechanisms underlying these age-related deficits are as yet poorly understood, the effects of such deficits are very likely far-reaching. Many complex everyday tasks such as decision-making, problem-solving, and the planning of goal-directed behaviors require the integration and reorganization of information from a variety of sources. It seems likely that attention, speed of information processing, and the ability to inhibit irrelevant information are all important functions for effective performance of these higher-level cognitive tasks. Whether these functions might be subsumed under a domain-general executive controller that is impaired by normal aging — something akin to the central executive in Baddeley's model of working memory — or whether there may be multiple control processes that are independently affected by aging, is currently an issue under investigation. The brain regions that are active during working memory tasks are also beginning to be identified in a variety of functional neuroimaging studies. Results suggest that different areas are activated in young and old adults, particularly within the prefrontal cortex, indicating that younger and older adults are performing these tasks differently [12]. An understanding of age-related neurophysiological changes may help to account for these differences.

C. LONG-TERM MEMORY

The cognitive domain that has probably received the most attention in normal aging is memory (for reviews, see [13, 27]). Many older adults complain of increased memory lapses as they age, and a major focus of research has been to try to distinguish memory declines attributable to normal aging from those that are indicative of pathological aging, particularly Alzheimer's disease. Like attention, memory is not a unitary construct; some kinds of memory remain relatively intact with age while others show significant declines. Long-term memory, unlike short-term and working memory, requires retrieval of information that is no longer present or being maintained in an active state. This information could have occurred a few minutes ago or been acquired many years ago. The next subsections review age-related changes in various kinds of long-term memory.

1.   Episodic Memory

Episodic memory refers to memory for personally experienced events that occurred in a particular place and at a particular time. This kind of memory allows one to think back through subjective time — what Tulving calls mental time travel [28] — and it usually evokes an "I remember" response. Episodic memory may be distinctly human; it is the most advanced form of memory and is ontogenetically the latest to develop. It also seems the most susceptible to brain damage and the most affected by normal aging.

The episodic memory problems experienced by older adults may involve deficient encoding, storage, or retrieval processes. At the input stage, older adults may encode new information less meaningfully or with less elaboration, so that memory traces are less distinctive, more similar to others in the memory system, and thereby more difficult to retrieve [29]. Alternatively, older people may attend to focal or salient information but fail to take account of peripheral detail, or they may fail to integrate contextual aspects of an experience with central content — what is sometimes referred to as a source memory problem [30]. Many of the common everyday memory lapses reported by normal older adults, such as forgetting where they parked their cars, likely involve poor encoding. These kinds of memory failures have generally been attributed to reduced use of effortful encoding strategies, which depend particularly on prefrontal brain regions. Another possibility is that noticing and integrating the various aspects of an experience involve divided attention and require working memory.

Older adults may also experience problems at the level of storage or consolidation. This aspect of episodic memory critically depends on medial temporal lobe structures, particularly the hippocampus. Consolidation is thought to involve the binding of various aspects of experience into a composite memory trace. What may be particularly critical for episodic memory and impaired in older adults is the extent to which an event is bound to its spatial and temporal context.

Finally, considerable evidence points to retrieval as a source of episodic memory problems in aging. Although it is clear that retrieval is at least partly dependent on encoding (i.e., well-encoded information is easier to retrieve), there are also effortful retrieval processes that appear to be impaired by aging. Older adults tend to show deficits on tests of free recall, to a somewhat lesser degree in cued recall, but minimally in recognition memory. Craik [18] has argued that the requirement to self-initiate strategic search processes in recall taxes the limited resources of older people. To the extent that environmental support can be provided at retrieval as well as at encoding (by providing good cues or using recognition tests, for example), the resource demands of encoding and retrieval are reduced and age differences are minimal. Similarly, Jennings and Jacoby [31] have demonstrated that recollection, which requires effortful retrieval of episodic detail, is impaired with age, whereas the more automatic judgments of familiarity are intact. Evidence from functional neuroimaging and neuropsychological studies suggests that these more strategic retrieval processes depend on the prefrontal cortex, as well as the hippocampus [32, 33].

2. Semantic Memory

Semantic memory refers to one's store of general knowledge about the world, including factual information such as "George Washington was the first president of the United States" and knowledge of words and concepts. Such information is not tied to the space or time of learning, and its retrieval is generally prefaced with "I know." Normally aging older adults do not have significant impairments in semantic memory. In fact, their knowledge of the world often exceeds that of young people. In addition, although access to information may be somewhat slower (particularly for words and names), the organization of the knowledge system seems unchanged with age (for review, see [34]). Semantic memories are believed to be stored in a variety of regions in posterior neocortex.

3. Autobiographical Memory

Autobiographical memory involves memory for one's personal past and includes memories that are both episodic and semantic in nature. The bulk of the evidence suggests that recent memories are easiest to retrieve, those from early childhood are most difficult to retrieve, and there is a monotonic decrease in retention from the present to the most remote past, with one exception. Events that occurred between the ages of 15 and 25 are recalled at a higher rate — what is referred to as the reminiscence bump — a finding that has usually been attributed to the greater salience or emotionality of the memories during this time period. This general pattern holds across all ages, suggesting that autobiographical memory is largely preserved with age (for review, see [35]). More detailed analyses of the nature of the autobiographical information retrieved, however, has suggested that although memory for personal semantics is intact in old age, memory for specific episodic or contextual details about one's personal past may be impaired. In a recent study, Levine et al. [36] observed that although older adults reported the gist of autobiographical event memories as well as young people, they reported fewer details. There may be exceptions to this finding, however. Recent studies of flashbulb memory have demonstrated that older adults remember as much as young adults about the details and circumstances surrounding highly emotional public events such as the death of Princess Diana or the 9/11 attack on the World Trade Center in New York City [37, 38].

4. Procedural Memory

Procedural memory refers to knowledge of skills and procedures such as riding a bicycle, playing the piano, or reading a book. These highly skilled activities are acquired more slowly than episodic memories through extensive practice. Once acquired, procedural memories are expressed rather automatically in performance and are not amenable to description (i.e., it is not easy to say "how" one reads).

When talking about procedural memory or knowledge, one is likely to say, "I know how to." In general, older adults show normal acquisition of procedural skills in both motor and cognitive domains and retain them across the lifespan. With high levels of expertise, there is often little slowing of skilled performance with age (at least until the very oldest ages), although some individual components of the skill may decline. So, for example, although the finger movements of a skilled typist slow down with age, overall typing speed is maintained because other aspects of the skill adjust (e.g., scanning further ahead in the text to be typed) [39]. Procedural memory depends on several brain regions, including the basal ganglia and the cerebellum.

5.   Implicit Memory

Implicit memory refers to a change in behavior that occurs as a result of prior experience, although one has no conscious or explicit recollection of that prior experience. For example, laboratory experiments have shown that it is easier to identify a degraded stimulus (e.g., from a brief exposure or partial information) if the stimulus was seen previously, even if one does not remember the prior occurrence. This "priming" probably occurs ubiquitously in everyday life and appears relatively intact in normal aging, although there are some inconsistencies in the literature (for review, see [40]). The most extensively studied form of implicit memory is perceptual priming, which occurs in response to a perceptual cue. Perceptual priming is modality specific and depends on sensory processing areas of the brain (e.g., in the visual domain, priming involves extra-striate regions of the visual cortex). Conceptual priming, which requires semantic processing and is observed in response to a conceptual cue, is also preserved in many older adults, and has been associated with left frontal and left temporal cortical regions.

6.   Prospective Memory

Much of what we have to remember in everyday life involves prospective memory — remembering to do things in the future, such as keep appointments, return a book to the library, or pay bills on time (for review, see [41]). Older adults do quite well on these daily tasks, using a variety of external aids such as calendars and appointment books to remind themselves of these activities. Certain habitual tasks such as taking medications at the appropriate times each day, however, may create difficulties for older people. For these tasks, there often are no salient reminders or cues in the environment, and so the tasks require the kinds of self-initiated activities that seem to be particularly problematic for older adults. Prospective memory may also rely on some aspect of working memory to maintain future intentions over time and likely also involves divided attention, both functions that show age-related deficits. Prospective memory and episodic memory tend not to be correlated and probably depend on different regions of the prefrontal cortex.

7.   Long-Term Memory: Summary and Implications

Aging principally affects episodic memory, namely memory for specific events or experiences that occurred in the past. Although many older adults believe that their memories for remote events are better than their memories for recent events, it is likely that older memories have become more semantic or gistlike, retaining the general core information but lacking details, particularly spatial and temporal context. These older memories have often joined the realm of things that we now "know." More problematic for older adults is remembering context or source information: where or when something was heard or read, or even whether something actually happened or was just thought about, what has been called "reality monitoring" [4?] Encoding and retrieval of these kinds of specific or peripheral details about a prior event may be particularly demanding of attentional resources, and good cues for the retrieval of such information may often be lacking. Although semantic memory is largely preserved in old age, the fact that what is retrieved from semantic memory is general knowledge, not specific detail, may contribute to the absence of age differences. The exception to this pattern might be the retrieval of a person's name or a specific word for a specific context, both of which show deficits in normal aging. The specificity of the information to be retrieved may therefore be a critical determinant of age differences [43]. There is some suggestion that age-related deficits in memory may be reduced for emotionally arousing events or materials [38], and so emotional or personal investment in an experience may be an important variable in episodic memory in older adults. High levels of emotion or stress, however, generally have negative effects on memory.

D.   PERCEPTION

Most people view perception as a set of processes that occurs prior to cognition. However, the boundaries between perception and cognition are unclear, and much evidence suggests that these domains are interactive with top-down cognitive processes affecting perception and perceptual processing having a clear impact on cognition. Evidence indicates that perceptual function is reduced in most older adults and is not always correctable by external aids (for review, see [44]). This suggests, at the very least, that researchers should pay careful attention to and control for sensory and perceptual deficits when conducting cognitive experiments. Evidence from a range of large-scale aging studies has demonstrated that a significant proportion of the age-related variance in several cognitive tasks can be accounted for by hearing and vision loss and that once these sensory differences are statistically controlled, there are no longer age differences in cognitive functioning [45]. Baltes and Lindenberger [45] proposed that overall neural degeneration may account for both sensory and cognitive deficits — what has been called the common cause hypothesis. Alternative explanations have also been proposed, however. For example, Schneider and Pichora-Fuller [44] suggested that perception and cognition are part of a highly integrated system and draw on a common pool of attentional resources. When parts of this system are stressed, such as when auditory or visual acuity are compromised and are essential to a task, other parts of the system will be negatively affected.

Declining sensory and perceptual abilities have important implications for the everyday lives of older adults. Hearing loss can isolate older people, preventing them from engaging in conversation and other social interactions. Visual impairments can limit mobility and interact with attentional deficits to make driving a particularly hazardous activity. As older people develop strategies to compensate for declining sensory abilities, the ways in which they perform other cognitive tasks may also be altered and may be less efficient. Retraining and practice on these tasks may help the adjustment and improve performance.

III. HIGHER-LEVEL COGNITIVE FUNCTIONS

A. SPEECH AND LANGUAGE

Speech and language processing are largely intact in older adults under normal conditions, although processing time may be somewhat slower than in young adults. In fact, there is evidence that discourse skills actually improve with age. Older people often tell well-structured elaborate narratives that are judged by others to be more interesting than those told by young [46]. They usually have more extensive vocabularies; and although they exhibit the occasional word-finding difficulty, older adults are easily able to provide circumlocutions to mask the problem. They are skilled conversationalists and appear to have few difficulties in processing ongoing speech. As noted above, however, some older adults have hearing loss and so, in conversational settings, may be required to interpret a weak or distorted acoustic signal. Even under these conditions, older people seem able to maintain good levels of comprehension by effectively using context to interpret the message [47]. Nevertheless, this compensatory top-down processing may have negative consequences for other cognitive operations and may be at least partly responsible for reducing the functional capacity of working memory. The converse relation has also been proposed, however, namely that the well-documented reduced working memory capacity in older adults limits the comprehension of syntactically complex text. The fact that comprehension of text is often measured by recall, a cognitive function known to be impaired in aging, complicates still further the interpretation of comprehension deficits. Older adults also experience problems with comprehension when individual words are presented at a very rapid rate, but they show sharply reduced impairments when such words form meaningful sentences. Here also, older people seem able to engage intact top-down processes to bolster deficiencies in bottom-up processing. They thus appear to retain good language skills well into older age. Deficits that occur under difficult processing conditions seem primarily attributable to sensory loss or working memory limitations, not to impairments in basic language capacities per se (for a comprehensive review, see [48]).

B. DECISION MAKING

Relatively little research has been done on the effects of aging on decision-making. Most of the work has highlighted the potential impact of attentional and working memory limitations on the ability to make decisions, but also has incorporated ideas involving motivation, relevance, emotional investment, and prior knowledge as important moderators of those effects, particularly in real-life contexts. Decision-making seems to be a domain that makes clear demands on processing resources, but in everyday life those demands may be reduced by life-relevant knowledge or expertise in the problem-solving domain. For example, research has shown that when making decisions about healthcare alternatives, buying a car, or buying insurance, older adults often come to the same kinds of decisions as younger adults but reach their conclusions in a different way. They tend to rely more on prior knowledge about the problem domain and less on new information, whereas young people, who likely have less knowledge about these issues, tend to sample and evaluate more current information and consider more alternatives before making their decisions (for review, see [49]).

Older adults, again possibly because of working memory limitations, tend to rely on expert opinion to a greater degree than young adults. Although this strategy may work reasonably well when the expert is well-qualified (e.g., a physician for medical decisions), it may leave older people susceptible to things such as investment scams. Poor decision-making may also be a result of episodic memory decline, particularly the loss of memory for details or source. For example, remembering that "Stock ABC is a good investment," without remembering where one heard such information, could lead to a bad decision.

C.   EXECUTIVE CONTROL

In the past decade, there has been an increasing focus on executive control as a primary contributor to cognitive decline with age. Executive control is a multi-component construct that consists of a range of different processes that are involved in the planning, organization, coordination, implementation, and evaluation of many of our nonroutine activities. This so-called central executive [14, 50] plays a key role in virtually all aspects of cognition, allocating attentional resources among stimuli or tasks, inhibiting distracting or irrelevant information in working memory, formulating strategies for encoding and retrieval, and directing all manner of problem-solving, decision-making, and other goal-directed activities. Executive control is particularly important for novel tasks for which a set of habitual processes is not readily available. Executive function depends critically on prefrontal cortex, which exerts its broad-reaching controlling influence via extensive reciprocal connections with posterior cortical regions. A parsimonious explanation of cognitive aging ascribes a causal role to executive control deficits — what has been called the frontal lobe hypothesis of aging [51]. In support of this hypothesis, both structural and functional neuroimaging studies have revealed a preferential decline in older adults in volume and function of prefrontal brain regions [52].

IV.   INTER-INDIVIDUAL VARIABILITY IN COGNITIVE FUNCTION

Although there are clear generalities and common principles that can be demonstrated in cognitive aging, what is perhaps most compelling about age-related cognitive change is its variability. Cognitive decline is not inevitable. Some older adults retain excellent cognitive function well into their 70s and 80s and perform as well or better than younger adults. Others, although within the normal range, show signs of decline by age 60. In addition, decline is not uniform across cognitive domains. For example, some older adults have excellent episodic memory function but impaired executive function, and vice versa [53]. So, although there are clear interactions among cognitive domains, it seems evident that they also have some degree of independence and may be more or less susceptible to aging in different individuals. What accounts for this variability is of considerable interest to researchers and to the increasing numbers of older people who want to ensure that their cognitive functioning remains intact well into their later years.

Inter-individual variability is likely attributable to a range of factors and mechanisms — biological, psychological, health-related, environmental, and lifestyle. One possibility is that variability is related to differential internal compensatory mechanisms. A number of recent functional neuroimaging studies have found different patterns of brain activation in older and younger adults while performing identical memory or working memory tasks. One such pattern involves greater bilateral activation in older adults for tasks that activate only unilateral brain regions in young adults [54, 55]. This increased activation has been observed particularly in a sub-group of high-functioning older people [56], and has been interpreted by many as compensatory activity, representing perhaps some reorganization of the aging brain. Others have suggested, however, that bilateral activation represents inefficient or less selective cognitive processing in older adults [57]. Another possibility is that such changes relate to declining sensory and perceptual abilities [44], which older people compensate for in a variety of different ways (for discussion, see [58]).

Lifestyle variables have also been the focus of much recent research on factors related to differential cognitive aging. Active lifestyles are generally associated with better outcomes, and aerobic exercise in particular has been shown to produce substantial benefits to cognitive function, particularly on those tasks requiring executive control [9]. Performance on these same kinds of non-automatic tasks is also particularly sensitive to circadian rhythms. For example, older people perform better at their peak time of day, usually in the morning, on tasks requiring inhibitory control [24]. Interestingly, stimulants such as caffeine have been found to reduce the time-of-day effects on strategic memory tasks, by enhancing performance during non-peak times of day [59].

V. SUMMARY

Age-related changes in cognitive function vary considerably across individuals and across cognitive domains, with some cognitive functions appearing more susceptible than others to the effects of aging. Much of the basic research in cognitive aging has focused on attention and memory, and indeed it may be that deficits in these fundamental processes can account for much of the variance observed in higher-level cognitive processes. The mapping of cognitive processes onto neural structures constitutes a relatively recent research enterprise driven largely by advances in neuroimaging technology (see Chapter 12, this volume). Early work in this area focused on establishing brain regions associated with different kinds of cognitive performance and revealed that normally aging older adults often appear to activate different brain structures than young people when performing cognitive tasks. The reasons for these differences are a matter of considerable debate. Ultimately, the understanding of age-related changes in cognition will require a parallel understanding of the age-related changes in the brain and the underlying mechanisms responsible for those changes. This volume explores the current state of research on the aging brain, providing some initial hypotheses concerning how changes in the nervous system may be related to the kinds of age-related cognitive changes that are outlined in this chapter.

ACKNOWLEDGMENTS

Preparation of this chapter was supported by The National Institute on Aging, Grant No. R01AG14792.

REFERENCES

1. Craik, F.I.M. and Salthouse, T.A., Eds., *The Handbook of Aging and Cognition,* Erlbaum, Mahwah, NJ, 2000.
2. Craik, F.I.M. and Jennings, J.M., Human memory, in *The Handbook of Aging and Cognition,* Craik, F.I.M. and Salthouse, T.A., Eds., Erlbaum, Hillsdale, NJ, 1992, 51.
3. McDowd, J.M. and Shaw, R.J., Attention and aging: a functional perspective, in *The Handbook of Aging and Cognition,* 2nd ed., Craik, F.I.M. and Salthouse, T.A., Eds., Erlbaum, Mahwah, NJ, 2000, 221.
4. Verhaeghen, P. and Cerella, J., Aging, executive control, and attention: a review of meta-analyses, *Neurosci. Behav. Rev.,* 26, 849, 2002.
5. McDowd, J.M. and Craik, F.I.M., Effects of aging and task difficulty on divided attention performance, *J. Exp. Psychol. Hum. Perc. Perf.,* 14, 267, 1988.
6. Tsang, P.S. and Shaner, T.L., Age, attention, expertise, and time-sharing performance, *Psychol. Aging,* 13, 323, 1998.
7. Kramer, A.F. et al., Training for executive control: task coordination strategies and aging, in *Attention and Performance XVII,* Gopher, D. and Koriat, A., Eds., MIT Press, Cambridge, MA, 1999, 617.
8. Hawkins, H.L., Kramer, A.F., and Capaldi, D., Aging, exercise, and attention, *Psychol. Aging,* 7, 643, 1992.
9. Colcombe, S. and Kramer, A.F., Fitness effects on the cognitive function of older adults: a meta-analytic study., *Psychol. Sci.,* 14, 125, 2003.
10. Park, D.C. and Gutchess, A.H., Cognitive aging and everyday life, in *Cognitive Aging: A Primer,* Park, D. and Schwarz, N., Eds., Psychology Press, Philadelphia, PA, 2000, 217.
11. Park, D.C. and Hedden, T., Working memory and aging, in *Perspectives on Human Memory and Cognitive Aging: Essays in Honour of Fergus Craik,* Naveh-Benjamin, M., Moscovitch, M., and Roediger III, H.L., Eds., Psychology Press, New York, 2001, 148.
12. Reuter-Lorenz, P.A. and Sylvester, C.-Y.C., The cognitive neuroscience of working memory and aging, in *Cognitive Neuroscience of Aging,* Cabeza, R., Nyberg, L., and Park, D., Eds., Oxford University Press, Oxford, 2005, 186.

13. Zacks, R.T., Hasher, L., and Li, K.Z.H., Human memory, in *The Handbook of Aging and Cognition*, 2nd ed., Craik, F.I.M., and Salthouse, T.A., Eds., Erlbaum, Mahwah, NJ, 2000, 293.

14. Baddeley, A.D. and Hitch, G.J., Working memory, in *The Psychology of Learning and Motivation*, Vol. 8, Bower, G.A., Ed., Academic Press, New York, 1974, 47.

15. Wager, T.D. and Smith, E.E., Neuroimaging studies of working memory: a meta-analysis, *Cogn. Affec. Behav. Neurosci.*, 3, 255, 2003.

16. Park, D., The basic mechanisms accounting for age-related decline in cognitive function, in *Cognitive Aging: A Primer*, Park, D. and Schwarz, N., Eds., Psychology Press, Philadelphia, PA, 2000, 3.

17. Craik, F.I.M. and Byrd, M., Aging and cognitive deficits: the role of attentional resources, in *Aging and Cognitive Processes*, Craik, F.I.M. and Trehub, S., Eds., Plenum, New York, 1982, 191.

18. Craik, F.I.M., A functional account of age differences in memory, in *Human Memory and Cognitive Capabilities, Mechanisms and Performances*, Klix, F. and Hagendorf, H., Eds., Elsevier, Amsterdam, 1986, 409.

19. Salthouse, T.A., Processing capacity and its role on the relations between age and memory, in *Memory Performance and Competencies: Issues in Growth and Development*, Weinert, F.E. and Schneider, W., Eds., Erlbaum, Hillsdale, NJ, 1995, 111.

20. Salthouse, T.A., The aging of working memory, *Neuropsychology*, 8, 535, 1994.

21. Salthouse, T.A., The processing-speed theory of adult age differences in cognition, *Psychol. Rev.*, 103, 403, 1996.

22. Park, D.C. et al., Mediators of long-term memory performance across the life span, *Psychol. Aging*, 11, 621, 1996.

23. Hasher, L. and Zacks, R.T., Working memory, comprehension, and aging: a review and a new view, in *The Psychology of Learning and Motivation*, Vol. 22, Bower, G.H., Ed., Academic Press, New York, 1988, 193.

24. Hasher, L., Zacks, R.T., and May, C.P., Inhibitory control, circadian arousal, and age, in *Attention and Performance XVII*, Gopher, D. and Koriat, A., Eds., MIT Press, Cambridge, MA, 1999, 653.

25. May, C.P., Hasher, L., and Kane, M.J., The role of interference in memory span, *Mem. Cognit.*, 27, 759, 1999.

26. Hedden, T. and Park, D.C., Aging and interference in verbal working memory, *Psychol. Aging*, 16, 666, 2001.

27. Kester, J.D. et al., Memory in elderly people, in *The Handbook of Memory Disorders*, 2nd ed., Baddeley, A.D., Kopelman, M.D., and Wilson, B.A., Eds., Wiley, West Sussex, U.K., 2002, 543.

28. Tulving, E., Episodic memory: from mind to brain, *Annu. Rev. Psychol.*, 53, 1, 2002.

29. Craik, F.I.M., On the transfer of information from temporary to permanent memory, *Philos. Trans. Roy. Soc. London*, B 302, 341, 1983.

30. Glisky, E.L., Rubin, S.R., and Davidson, P.S.R., Source memory in older adults: an encoding or retrieval problem?, *J. Exp. Psychol. Learn. Mem Cognit.*, 27, 1131, 2001.

31. Jennings, J.M. and Jacoby, L.L., An opposition procedure for detecting age-related deficits in recollection: telling effects of repetition, *Psychol. Aging*, 12, 352, 1997.

32. Davidson, P.S.R. and Glisky, E.L., Neuropsychological correlates of recollection and familiarity in normal aging, *Cogn. Affec. Behav. Neurosci*, 2, 174, 2002.

33. Nolde, S.F., Johnson, M.K., and D'Esposito, M., Left prefrontal activation during episodic remembering: an event-related fMRI study, *NeuroReport*, 9, 3509, 1998.

34. Light, L.L., The organization of memory in old age, in *The Handbook of Aging and Cognition*, Craik, F.I.M. and Salthouse, T.A., Eds., Erlbaum, Hillsdale, NJ, 1992, 111.

35. Rubin, D.C., Autobiographical memory and aging, in *Cognitive Aging: A Primer*, Park, D. and Schwarz, N., Eds., Psychology Press, Philadelphia, PA, 2000, 131.

36. Levine, B. et al., Aging and autobiographical memory: dissociating episodic from semantic retrieval, *Psychol. Aging*, 17, 677, 2002.

37. Davidson, P.S.R. and Glisky, E.L., Is flashbulb memory a special instance of source memory? Evidence from older adults, *Memory*, 10, 99, 2002.

38. Davidson, P.S.R., Cook, A.P., and Glisky, E.L., Flashbulb memories for September 11th are preserved in older adults, *Aging, Neuropsychology, and Cognition*, 13, 196, 2006.

39. Salthouse, T.A., Effects of age and skill in typing, J. Exp. Psychol. Gen., 113, 345, 1984.

40. Prull, M.W., Gabrieli, J.D.E., and Bunge, S.A., Age-related changes in memory: a cognitive neuroscience perspective, in *The Handbook of Aging and Cognition*, 2nd ed., Craik, F.I.M. and Salthouse, T.A., Eds., Erlbaum, Mahwah, NJ, 2000, 91.

41. West, R., The neural basis of age-related declines in prospective memory, in *Cognitive Neuroscience of Aging*, Cabeza, R., Nyberg, L., and Park, D., Eds., Oxford University Press, Oxford, 2005, 246.

42. Johnson, M.K., Hashtroudi, S., and Lindsay, D.S., Source monitoring, *Psychol. Bull.*, 114, 3, 1993.

43. Craik, F.I.M., Levels of processing: past, present ... and future? *Memory*, 10, 305, 2002.

44. Schneider, B.A. and Pichora-Fuller, M.K., Implications of perceptual deterioration for cognitive aging research, in *The Handbook of Aging and Cognition*, 2nd ed., Craik, F.I.M., and Salthouse, T.A., Eds., Erlbaum, Mahwah NJ, 2000, 155.

45. Baltes, P.B. and Lindenberger, U., Emergence of a powerful connection between sensory and cognitive functions across the adult lifespan: a new window to the study of cognitive aging? *Psychol. Aging*, 12, 12, 1997.

46. Kemper, S. and Kemtes, K., Aging and message production and comprehension, in *Cognitive Aging: A Primer*, Park, D. and Schwarz, N., Eds., Psychology Press, Philadelphia, PA, 2000, 197.

47. Wingfield, A., Speech perception and the comprehension of spoken language in adult aging, in *Cognitive Aging: A Primer*, Park, D. and Schwarz, N., Eds., Psychology Press, Philadelphia, PA, 2000, 175.

48. Wingfield, A. and Stine-Morrow, E.A.L., Language and speech, in *The Handbook of Aging and Cognition*, 2nd ed., Craik, F.I.M. and Salthouse, T.A., Eds., Erlbaum, Mahwah, NJ, 2000, 359.

49. Sanfey, A.G. and Hastie, R., Judgment and decision making across the adult life span: a tutorial review of psychological research, in *Cognitive Aging: A Primer*, Park, D. and Schwarz, N., Eds., Psychology Press, Philadelphia, PA, 2000, 253.

50. Baddeley, A.D., Fractionating the central executive, in *Principles of Frontal Lobe Function*, Stuss, D.T. and Knight, R.T., Eds., Oxford University Press, Oxford, 2002, 246.

51. West, R.L., An application of prefrontal cortex function theory to cognitive aging, *Psychol. Bull.*, 120, 272, 1996.

52. Raz, N., Aging of the brain and its impact on cognitive performance: integration of structural and functional findings, in *The Handbook of Aging and Cognition*, 2nd ed., Craik, F.I.M. and Salthouse, T.A., Eds., Erlbaum, Mahwah, NJ, 2000, 1.

53. Glisky, E.L., Polster, M.R., and Routhieaux, B.C., Double dissociation between item and source memory, *Neuropsychology*, 9, 229, 1995.

54. Grady, C.L. et al., The effects of encoding task on age-related differences in the functional neuroanatomy of face memory, *Psychol. Aging*, 17, 7, 2002.
55. Reuter-Lorenz, P.A. et al., Age differences in the frontal lateralization of verbal and spatial working memory revealed by PET, *J. Cognit. Neurosci.*, 12, 174, 2000.
56. Cabeza, R. et al., Aging gracefully: compensatory brain activity in high-performing older adults, *NeuroImage*, 17, 1394, 2002.
57. Logan, J.M. et al., Under-recruitment and non-selective recruitment: dissociable neural mechanisms associated with aging, *Neuron*, 33, 827, 2002.
58. Daselaar, S. and Cabeza, R., Age-related changes in hemispheric organization, in *Cognitive Neuroscience of Aging*, Cabeza, R., Nyberg, L., and Park, D., Eds., Oxford University Press, Oxford, 2005, 186.
59. Ryan, L., Hatfield, C., and Hofstetter, M., Caffeine reduces time-of-day effects on memory performance in older adults, *Psycho. Sci.*, 13, 68, 2002.

2 Successful vs. Unsuccessful Aging in the Rhesus Monkey

Mark B. Moss, Tara L. Moore, Stephen P. Schettler, Ronald Killiany, and Douglas Rosene

CONTENTS

I. INTRODUCTION

It is now well known that one generally experiences relatively mild changes in cognitive abilities with age, particularly with abilities such as short-term memory, executive functions, and confrontation naming [1]. However, a select group of these "successfully" aged individuals evidence virtually no change in their cognitive abilities with age, even into the eleventh decade of life [2]. Such individuals have often been referred to as examples of "pristine" successful aging. At the other end of the continuum, a large percentage of people are known to develop marked cognitive decline with age, characterized by a dementia state, with a majority of those developing Alzheimer's disease (AD). These individuals fall into the category of "unsuccessful" aging. In recent years, however, clinical researchers have characterized a group as individuals who, with advancing age, show a moderate impairment in one or more cognitive domains that affects the ability to carry out activities of daily living but does not reach the threshold of a dementia state. This category, classified by many as "mild cognitive impairment" (MCI), reasonably can be regarded as a second general category of "unsuccessful" aging. Although many consider MCI as the earliest stage of Alzheimer's disease, evidence suggests that MCI represents a separate static and chronic state of normal aging. The etiology of MCI is unknown, but stroke and heart disease risk factors, genetics, and education have all been raised as possible contributors.

While nongenetically altered laboratory animals do not evidence the brain changes seen in AD [3], they have reliably demonstrated age-related changes in cognitive function. Evidence from a wide range of studies in rodents, dogs, and nonhuman primates have shown as a group that aged subjects are significantly impaired relative to young controls on cognitive tasks that assess functions such as working memory, declarative memory, and executive function: the same functions that evidence impairment in human aging [4–16]. However, on close inspection of the data, the degree of impairment within the aged group is anything but uniform and, in fact, is often dichotomous. While the overall group effect yields an impairment in the given function, it is clear that individuals within the aged group evidence only mild or, in some cases, no impairment on the task while others demonstrate severe impairment.

The finding of individual differences, emphasized in the rodent literature (see [17]), has not been addressed previously in studies of nonhuman primates. This is due in part to the small number of studies in aging primates as well as the relatively small sample sizes of aged groups available within studies. This chapter presents data that we have collected over the past 15 years as part of an ongoing study using the rhesus monkey as a model of normal human aging. During this period, more than 125 rhesus monkeys ranging in age from 5 to 31 years of age have been assessed on multiple tests of recognition memory and executive function. In this chapter we present the data from these animals and discuss their varying levels of impairments and how this relates to clinical findings in human studies.

II.   NONHUMAN PRIMATES AS SUITABLE ANIMAL MODELS OF AGING

Several hypotheses have been advanced to account for the neural bases that underlie the cognitive decline that occurs in normal, disease-free aging, but the processes underlying such decline are still not well understood. This is in large part due to our inability to concurrently collect behavioral, physiological, and pathological data within a short interval of time in human studies. Additional limitations are encountered by problems related to inadequate preservation of tissue, as well as the usual problems of control over extraneous variables. Given these limitations, it is essential to use a suitable animal model of normal human aging to address some of these questions. In a recent symposium on aging and Alzheimer's disease, a number of investigators reiterated the value of non-human primates as an animal model of human aging (Assessing Cognition for Emerging Therapeutics in AD, Johns Hopkins School of Medicine, September 2004). Rhesus monkeys have a rich and well-studied behavioral repertoire that is well suited for these types of investigations of normal aging, as they do not develop Alzheimer's disease. In addition, with this animal model, not only is it possible to collect a wide range of behavioral, morphological, biochemical, and molecular data within a short period of time, but opportunities are also provided for the exploration of treatment modes and interventions to arrest or reverse age-related cognitive decline.

III.   COGNITIVE ASSESSMENT OF THE AGED NONHUMAN PRIMATE

As discussed above, monkeys have a rich behavioral repertoire that lends itself suitably to translational studies of human cognition. Indeed, several behavioral tasks developed in the human neuropsychological domain have now been successfully adapted to the nonhuman primate. In some instances, tasks developed for non-human primate studies have been incorporated into both research and clinical test batteries for human studies. This has occurred primarily in the domains of memory, executive function, and attention. The following subsections outline each of these domains as they relate to nonhuman primates.

A.   MEMORY

Perhaps the best-characterized change that occurs in normal aging is a decline in short-term memory function. The literature on memory dysfunction in human aging is voluminous and several reviews and books have been devoted to the subject (e.g., [18–21]). They show that changes in memory begin as early at the fifth decade of life, that is, middle age. This is supported by recent data from our long-standing study of normal aging in the rhesus monkey that indicates that memory changes also occur in early middle age in the monkey. Another characteristic of memory function that is impaired in normal human aging is the recall of information. The impairment in recall is greater than that observed in recognition memory, and this relationship appears to be independent of the type of stimulus material used [22–25].

Rabinowitz [26] reported a threefold impairment in recall relative to recognition even under conditions of cueing. Of interest, the rate of forgetting, often accelerated in many neurodegenerative disorders, does not appear to change with age [27, 28]. However, there is some evidence that older individuals show some degradation in recall when memory is assessed over very long delay intervals [29]. Deficits on tasks with increasing delays imposed between stimulus presentation and response trials have also been observed in aged monkeys. Using a delayed response procedure, several investigators [14, 30–33] have shown reduced memory by monkeys 18 years of age or older relative to young adult monkeys. Further, the degree of impairment appears related to the length of delay.

Since the seminal studies by Bartus and colleagues [14], evidence has accumulated from several laboratories demonstrating impairment in recognition memory in aged monkeys [4, 10, 11, 33–39]. A related series of studies has suggested that spatial memory appears adversely affected by the aging process, whereas object recognition is only mildly affected [4, 10, 11, 33–40]. In another study, we extended this finding by administering a spatial and a non-spatial form of the delayed recognition span test, a test of memory span, to groups of young adult and early senescent rhesus monkeys. The results of this study showed that aged animals were more impaired on the spatial than on the nonspatial stimulus conditions [35].

B.   EXECUTIVE FUNCTION

While there exists an impressive literature on age-related decline in memory with normal aging and age-related disease, the number of studies aimed at the assessment of executive function is more limited. *Executive function* is the term applied to such abilities as set-shifting, abstraction, and response suppression. Set-shifting refers to the capacity to keep track or correctly identify correct response-reward associations in the face of frequently changing contingencies. Abstraction refers to the capacity to identify a common element among stimuli that differ along several dimensions. Response inhibition refers to the ability to suppress previous response patterns to permit testing of new ones. Deficits in executive function have been attributed for the most part to dorsolateral prefrontal dysfunction [41–43].

In nonhuman primates, studies of frontal lobe function, the area of the cortex involved in mediating executive function and working memory, date back to the 1930s with Jacobsen's classical studies of the delayed response task in the chimpanzee [44]. Over the past 50 years, several investigators have confirmed and extended these early findings in a variety of species, including the monkey [45–49], and have demonstrated impairments on a variety of tasks with damage in various areas of the frontal lobe [47, 50–52].

More recently, in an attempt to closely approximate clinical studies of normal human aging with our nonhuman primate model, we have adapted a well-established human test of executive function, the Wisconsin Card Sorting Test (WCST) [53, 54] for use with nonhuman primates. Similar efforts to develop tests for monkeys that use the conceptual framework of those used with humans have been advanced by other laboratories. Dias and colleagues [55] assessed attentional set-shifting in primates with frontal lobe lesions as part of their CANTAB program software for testing both humans and monkeys. Our test, the Conceptual Set Shifting Task (CSST), more closely resembles the human WCST by using the color and shape stimuli and learning criteria of the WCST and requires the monkey to establish a pattern of responding to a concept based on a reward contingency, maintain responding to that concept for a period of time, and then shift to a different concept as the reward contingency changes [5, 56]. It thus assesses both abstraction and set-shifting in a way exactly analogous to the WCST. Moreover, the CSST has been shown to be sensitive to damage to the dorsolateral prefrontal cortex [43].

In normal aged humans, a variety of studies have reported impairments on tasks of executive function [1, 57–63], including specific age-related deficits in abstraction [64, 65] and set-shifting [63]. Caution in interpreting some of these results has been raised by some investigators [66] who suggest that deficits in abstraction may be exacerbated by tasks that make heavy demands on memory and attention. This concern was addressed in a later study that revealed impairments on tasks of abstraction and set shifting that had low memory and attentional demands in optimally healthy aged subjects [63].

IV. STUDIES ON SPECIFIC TASKS OF MEMORY AND EXECUTIVE FUNCTION

The behavioral tasks used in our studies were derived from two sources. The first source was a battery of learning, memory, and cognitive flexibility tasks that have been used as "benchmark" tests of function in monkeys with selective limbic system and frontal cortical lesions. Some of these tasks were subsequently adapted for use with normal aged humans and to patients with Alzheimer's disease, frontal lobe dementia, and a variety of amnestic disorders [67, 68]. The second source of tests came from those used in standard human neuropsychological testing that have been modified for use with monkeys such as the CSST [69]. Together this battery of tasks offers the advantage that (1) it can be administered and performed by aged human and nonhuman primates alike; (2) the tasks are carefully controlled and allow analyses of performance patterns that can differentiate among subjects, both human and monkey, with different neuropathologies; and (3) there exists an accumulated wealth of information on structure-function relationships from human and animal studies assessing and carefully characterizing the effects of specific brain damage using these tasks.

In our cohort, animals range in age from 5 to 31 years of age. Based on an extensive survival study at Yerkes Regional Primate Research Center, which suggests a 1:3 ratio between monkey and human years of age, we have characterized young monkeys as 5 to 10 years of age, middle-aged monkeys as 13 to 19 years of age, early-aged monkeys as 20 to 24 years of age, and advanced-aged monkeys as >25 years of age.

A.   DEFINITION OF COGNITIVE IMPAIRMENT

Within this group of animals, we developed a cognitive impairment index (CII) as a measure of cognitive function in aging. This measure provides a convenient index for ranking and comparing individual animals. The CII was derived based on the principal components analysis [4], which indicated that overall impairments were predicted by a weighted average of each subject's scores on the DNMS, the DNMS-2 minute delay, and DRST-spatial (see test descriptions below). To simplify this, the scores on each of the three tasks for each individual were converted to a z-score relative to the mean performance of young adults (the baseline reference group). The CII was then computed as a simple average of the three standardized scores, with positive numbers indicating increasing impairments in z-units from the mean of the baseline reference group of young adult monkeys.

With this index, we established a cutoff for mild impairment as a CII that is 1.0 to 2.0 standard deviations above the mean for young adult monkeys. Thus, monkeys with a CII 1.0 to 2.0 SD above the mean of the young animals are considered to be mildly impaired, whereas monkeys with CIIs of 2.0 SDs or more above the mean of the young are considered severely impaired. Monkeys with CIIs below 1.0 are considered in the nonimpaired range. Based on these criteria for levels of impairment, we determine that animals in the normal range of performance and in the mild impairment range are equivalent to what has been termed "successful aging" in the human literature. Similarly, animals that fall into the severely impaired range are equivalent to "unsuccessful aging," as observed in human clinical studies.

Within our cohort of animals, based on the CII measurement, 4.55% of animals in the 13- to 19-year-old age group were mildly impaired and 22.7% were severely impaired. In the 20- to 24-year-old age range, 20.69% of the animals were mildly impaired and 20.69% of the animals were severely impaired. Finally, 19.35% of the animals in the 25- to 31-year-old age range were mildly impaired while 32.3% were severely impaired (Table 2.1). Overall, the percent of animals in the mild impairment range remained relatively stable through middle age and advanced age but the percent of animals in the severely impaired range (unsuccessful aging) increased by almost 15% from middle age and advanced age. As expected, the overall number of animals demonstrating significant cognitive impairment increased with age but there were still a considerable number of animals with mild or no cognitive impairment (Figure 2.1).

While the CII is an important measure of cognitive function, we thought it was important to also look at animals' performance on individual tests of memory and executive function. Using the same criterion as with the CII for level of impairment (mild impairment = 1.0–2.0 SD from the mean of the young on each test; and severe impairment equal to or greater than 2.0 SD from the mean of the young on each test), we determined the percent of animals that fall within the normal, mildly impaired, and severely impaired range on each individual test in our study. The results are outlined in the subsections below.

B.   DELAYED NONMATCHING TO SAMPLE (DNMS)

1.   Overview of DNMS

The DNMS task is a benchmark recognition memory task that assesses the subject's ability to identify a novel stimulus from a familiar stimulus following a specific

TABLE 2.1
Cognitive Impairment Index

13–19 Year Olds	CII (n = 22)
0–1.0 SD from Mean	16 (72.7%)
1.0–2.0 SD from Mean	1 (4.55%)
2.0+ SD from Mean	5 (22.7%)

20–24 Year Olds	CII (n = 29)
0–1.0 SD from Mean	17 (58.6%)
1.0–2.0 SD from Mean	6 (20.69%)
2.0+ SD from Mean	6 (20.69%)

25–31 Year Olds	CII (n = 31)
0–1.0 SD from Mean	15 (48.4%)
1.0–2.0 SD from Mean	6 (19.35%)
2.0+ SD from Mean	10 (32.3%)

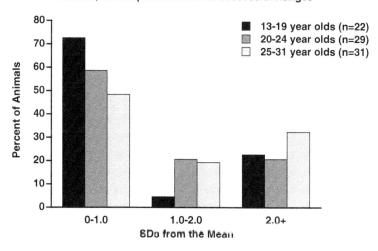

Cognitive Impairment Index: Percent of Animals in the Normal, Mild Impairment and Unsuccessful Ranges

FIGURE 2.1 Cognitive impairment index: percent of animals in the normal, mild impairment, and unsuccessful ranges.

delay interval. Although originally developed for assessment of memory in animals, it also has been used with human subjects. Various forms of this task have been used to assess memory function in monkeys following specific lesions of the forebrain, including transection of the fornix [70–72], limited or combined lesions of the hippocampus and amygdala [71–75], or medial dorsal thalamus [76].

This task is administered in three phases. First, in the acquisition phase, the animal must learn the rule of the task to reach criterion. After criterion is reached, a delay component is added where the animal must remember the stimulus over an increasing delay. Finally, in surgical animal models, there is the postoperative re-learning phase of the DNMS where the animal must reestablish a level of learning criterion after a surgical procedure. Depending on the experimental paradigm, deficits on the acquisition or post-operative re-learning phase of the DNMS task have been reported following damage to the hippocampus [71, 74, 77, 78], and to a greater extent in monkeys with combined damage to the amygdala and hippocampus [73, 74]. More recently, impairments have been found following damage to extrahippocampal regions, including rhinal cortex, entorhinal cortex, perirhinal cortex, and adjacent parahippocampal cortices [79–84], regions that are critical components of temporal lobe neuronal circuitry linking the hippocampus and amygdala with the rest of the forebrain. In humans, the DNMS task also has been shown to be sensitive to selected temporal lobe damage [85] and to a variety amnestic disorders [86], as well as to Alzheimer's disease and normal aging [67].

In aged monkeys, results from studies in several laboratories have shown an impairment in the acquisition and delay phases of the DNMS task [4, 10, 33, 36, 37, 39, 40]. The findings appear to be quite consistent across these studies and show that, as a group, aged monkeys are mildly impaired on the acquisition and delay conditions of the DNMS task. Another consistent finding is variability in the performance of aged animals. Whereas some aged monkeys evidence impairment, others perform the task as proficiently as young adults [36, 37, 39].

2.   Successful vs. Unsuccessful Aging in Performance on DNMS

This pattern of variability in performance on the DNMS task by aged animals is confirmed in the data from our cohort (see Table 2.2). On the acquisition phase, none of the animals in the 13- to 19-year-old age group fell within the mild impairment range (1.0–2.0 SD from the mean) while 21.7% of the animals in this group were in the severe impairment range (greater than 2.0 SD from the mean of the young). Whereas in the 20- to 24-year-old age range, 13.8% and 27.6% of the animals were 1.0–2.0 SD and greater than 2.0 SD, respectively, from the mean of the young. Finally, in the 25- to 31-year-old age range, 9.68% of the animals were mildly impaired and 35.48% were severely impaired. A similar pattern of impairments was observed in the delay components of the DNMS (Table 2.2). It has been suggested that the degree of impairment on the DNMS may be related to the extent of limbic system dysfunction [37, 39]. Consistent with this notion is the suggestion that the nature of the deficit on DNMS in impaired aged monkeys is due to a disproportionate sensitivity to proactive interference [14, 15]. It is of interest that, when aged monkeys were tested on a version of the DNMS task that contains an extensive degree of interference (i.e., using the same pair of objects throughout the task), their performance declined precipitously to a level comparable to that of their performance on

TABLE 2.2
Delayed Nonmatching to Sample

13–19 Year Olds	Errors (n = 23)	2 min Delays (n = 23)	10 min Delays (n = 19)
0–1.0 SD from Mean	18 (78.3%)	19 (82.6%)	13 (68.4%)
1.0–2.0 SD from Mean	0 (0%)	0 (0%)	1 (5.26%)
2.0+ SD from Mean	5 (21.7%)	4 (17.39%)	5 (26.32%)
20–24 Year Olds	**Errors (n = 29)**	**2 min Delays (n = 29)**	**10 min Delays (n = 27)**
0–1.0 SD from Mean	17 (58.6%)	22 (75.9%)	16 (59.3%)
1.0–2.0 SD from Mean	4 (13.8%)	2 (6.90%)	3 (11.1%)
2.0+ SD from Mean	8 (27.6%)	5 (17.24%)	8 (29.6%)
25–31 Year Olds	**Errors (n = 31)**	**2 min Delays (n = 30)**	**10 min Delays (n = 15)**
0–1.0 SD from Mean	17 (54.8%)	24 (80.0%)	10 (66.7%)
1.0–2.0 SD from Mean	3 (9.68%)	3 (10%)	1 (6.67%)
2.0+ SD from Mean	11 (35.48%)	3 (10%)	4 (26.67%)

the delayed response task [87]. Whether this simply reflects an increase in task difficulty or a shift in the underlying locus of neuronal circuitry is unclear.

C.   DELAYED RECOGNITION SPAN TASK (DRST)

1.   Overview of DRST

This task is a short-term memory test that was designed to investigate recognition memory in monkeys following bilateral removal of the hippocampus [88]. It requires the subject to identify, trial-by-trial, a new stimulus among an increasing array of serially presented, familiar stimuli. The task is administered using different classes of stimulus material, spatial vs. nonspatial (color, pattern, objects), to characterize possible material-specific recognition memory impairments. An expanded form of this task has been used in the same manner to assess recognition in a variety of neurological patient populations including those of Alzheimer's disease [67, 89], Huntington's disease or Korsakoff's disease [68], and Parkinson's disease [90]. In normal aged human subjects, recognition span memory is impaired in several stimulus classes, including spatial position and visual patterns [68, 91].

2.   Successful vs. Unsuccessful Aging in Performance on DRST

In our study, this task is administered using two different classes of stimulus material: spatial location or object shape. This allows us to characterize any recognition memory deficits that may occur as a general impairment or one that is material specific.

a.   Delayed Recognition Span Test: Spatial

Unlike the pattern of number of animals considered impaired with increasing age on learning the DNMS basic task, few animals were impaired (1.0–2.0 or greater than 2 Standard Deviations from the mean of the young monkeys) on DRST task. In fact, none of the animals in the 13- to 19-year-old range were impaired, and only 6.89% of animals in the 20- to 24-year-old age range fell within the mild impairment range. None of the animals in this age range were classified as severely impaired. Similarly, 6.45 % and 3.22% of animals in the 25- to 31-year-old range were mildly and severely impaired, respectively, on the spatial DRST (see Table 2.3).

b.   Delayed Recognition Span Test: Object

An almost identical pattern was observed on the object DRST. The performance of a very small number of animals was in the mild and severe impairment ranges (see Table 2.3).

D.   CONCEPTUAL SET SHIFTING TASK

1.   Overview of Conceptual Set-Shifting

Executive function is one of the first cognitive abilities to be compromised in aging and age-related disease [5, 6, 67] and is considered a primary function of the prefrontal cortices [47, 92–94]. As summarized above, we developed a task suitable

---

TABLE 2.3
Delayed Recognition Span Test

13–19 Year Olds	Object (n = 20)	Spatial (n = 23)
0–1.0 SD from Mean	18 (90.0%)	23 (100%)
1.0–2.0 SD from Mean	1 (5.0%)	0 (0%)
2.0+ SD from Mean	1 (5.0%)	0 (0%)
20–24 Year Olds	**Object (n = 26)**	**Spatial (n = 29)**
0–1.0 SD from Mean	21 (80.77%)	27 (93.10%)
1.0–2.0 SD from Mean	5 (19.23%)	2 (6.89%)
2.0+ SD from Mean	0 (0%)	0 (0%)
25–31 Year Olds	**Object (n = 16)**	**Spatial (n = 31)**
0–1.0 SD from Mean	13 (81.3%)	28 (90.32%)
1.0–2.0 SD from Mean	3 (18.75%)	2 (6.45%)
2.0+ SD from Mean	0 (0%)	1 (3.22%)

for testing monkeys based on the principles of the standard frontal lobe set-shifting task used in humans, the Wisconsin Card Sorting Test (WCST) [53, 54]. Our test, the Conceptual Set Shifting Task (CSST), uses a subset of the same stimuli as the WCST to assess abstraction, establishment, maintenance, and shifting of sets and perseveration in a manner that parallels that used in human clinical studies.

2. Successful vs. Unsuccessful Aging in Performance on CSST

Of the 128 animals in our group, 66 were tested on the CSST. Performance on the CSST appears to be affected early in aging and may become the most compromised with advanced age. In contrast to tests of memory where the performance of a few subjects reached the severe impairment range, a large number of animals were in the mild and severe impairment range on the CSST. In fact, on various measures of performance on the CSST, 12 middle-aged animals were mildly impaired and between 25 and 41% were severely impaired. In contrast, in the aged animals, 0 to 32% of the animals were mildly impaired and 0 to 36% were severely impaired (Table 2.4). These findings would suggest that executive system functions may be among the most sensitive domains affected with advancing age.

E. SUMMARY OF BEHAVIORAL FINDINGS

Based on the performance of these 128 monkeys on two tests of recognition memory, one test of executive function and a composite score of cognitive function, we have

TABLE 2.4
Conceptual Set-Shifting Task

13–19 Year Olds	Int Lrn (n = 16)	Shift (n = 17)	PE (n = 17)
0–1.0 SD from Mean	10 (62.5%)	8 (47.1%)	9 (53.0%)
1.0–2.0 SD from Mean	2 (12.5%)	2 (11.7%)	2 (11.7%)
2.0+ SD from Mean	4 (25.0%)	7 (41.2%)	6 (35.3%)

20–24 Year Olds	Int Lrn (n = 19)	Shift (n = 19)	PE (n = 19)
0–1.0 SD from Mean	14 (73.7%)	10 (52.6%)	10 (52.6%)
1.0–2.0 SD from Mean	2 (10.6%)	6 (31.6%)	2 (10.5%)
2.0+ SD from Mean	3 (15.8%)	3 (15.8%)	7 (36.8%)

25–31 Year Olds	Int Lrn (n = 10)	Shift (n = 10)	PE (n = 10)
0–1.0 SD from Mean	6 (60%)	8 (80.0%)	9 (90.0%)
1.0–2.0 SD from Mean	0 (0%)	2 (20%)	0 (0%)
2.0+ SD from Mean	4 (40%)	0 (0%)	1 (10%)

demonstrated a pattern of variable levels of performance on these tasks. While overall as groups, the 20- to 24- and 25- to 31-year-olds are impaired on these tests, there is considerable variability in performance. Many animals show no impairment and few show mild to severe impairments on tests of memory. On a test of executive function, more animals demonstrate mild and severe impairments, but still more than 50% show no impairment. This pattern of variability in performance is similar to what is observed in human clinical studies. In human studies, those individuals demonstrating no impairment (equivalent to scores below 1.0 SD in our study) might be considered among the more pristine among those successfully aging. While those demonstrating mild impairments (1.0 to 2.0 SD above the mean of the young in our study) might be considered to be more typically those who are successfully aging, but evidence some degree of cognitive decline associated with typical aging, and finally those demonstrating significant cognitive impairment (greater than 2.0 SD from the mean of the young in our study) are deemed as "unsuccessful aging" and may reflect the human classification of "mild cognitive impairment," keeping in mind that monkeys do not develop the pathological or behavioral profile of Alzheimer's disease [95].

V.   NEUROBIOLOGICAL BASIS FOR COGNITIVE DECLINE

Several possibilities have been advanced to account for mild or marked age-related cognitive decline, ranging from widespread cortical neuronal loss and neurotransmitter depletion, to amyloid deposition and to the development of neuritic plaques. While likely contributing to cognitive dysfunction, we believe that these factors are unlikely primary candidates to account for age-related cognitive decline. With few exceptions, neurons in the cerebral cortex do not undergo marked loss [95] and the presence and the extent of neuritic plaques or amyloid burden are quite variable and are not correlated with cognitive decline [96]. Rather, we have accumulated evidence over the past several years that lead us to the view that alteration and loss of white matter may be the principal neurobiological change that underlies age-related cognitive decline [3]. In electron microscopic (EM) studies of the effects of aging in the cerebral cortex [97, 98], corpus callosum [98], and optic nerve [99] of monkeys, myelin sheaths have been found to show marked age-related changes, including the accumulation of dense cytoplasm and the formation of fluid-filled balloons. In addition, the formation of sheaths with redundant myelin and thick sheaths occur with continued formation of myelin with age [100]. Of particular interest, the frequency of these alterations in myelin with age correlates significantly with the cognitive decline exhibited by monkeys. In support of this, using diffusion tensor magnetic resonance imaging (DT-MRI), we have recently reported significant age-related loss of fractional anisotropy (FA) in forebrain white matter of the frontal lobe. Reduced FA is regarded as a marker of white matter abnormalities and, like the EM measures, correlates with cognitive decline [101]. Further, unpublished data from our group on conduction across the corpus callosum indicates that, with age, there is a significant alteration in the profile of conduction parameters. This result could be explained if the myelin dystrophy observed in the corpus callosum [98] disrupts conduction in a fraction of the nerve fibers and suggests that alterations in myelin integrity and consequent disruption of conduction may alter the signal strength and hence the information transfer that is critical for neuronal circuits to operate properly. Finally, using designed-based stereology and MRI in separate studies, our group has demonstrated nerve fiber loss with age from the optic nerves [99], a 40% loss of nerve fibers in the anterior commissure of aged rhesus monkeys, and a significant loss of white matter volume on with MRI, with an accompanying increase in ventricular size (Wisco, Killiany, and Rosene, unpublished observations). These observations lend further support to the notion that there is likely to be a global loss of myelinated nerve fibers with age. Extensive multidisciplinary investigations into the precise mechanisms of these age-related changes in white matter and their relationship to cognitive decline are the focus of our current studies with the continued use of our nonhuman primate model of normal aging.

ACKNOWLEDGMENTS

The authors wish to acknowledge support from NIH grants PO1-AG0001 (DLR), R37-AG17609 (MBM), and R55-AG12610.

REFERENCES

1. Albert, M.S., Neuropsychological and neurophysiological changes in healthy adult humans across the age range, *Neurobiol. Aging*, 14, 623, 1993.
2. Perls, T.T., The different paths to 100, *Am. J. Clin. Nutr.*, 83, 484S, 2006.
3. Peters, A. and Rosene, D.L., In aging, is it gray or white, *J. Comp. Neurol.*, 462, 139, 2003.
4. Herndon, J.G. et al., Patterns of cognitive decline in aged rhesus monkeys, *Behav. Brain Res.*, 87, 25, 1997.
5. Moore, T.L. et al., Impairment in abstraction and set shifting in aged rhesus monkeys, *Neurobiol. Aging*, 24, 125, 2003.
6. Moore, T.L. et al., Executive system dysfunction occurs as early as middle-age in the rhesus monkey, *Neurobiol. Aging*, in press, 2006.
7. Lasarge, C.L. et al., Deficits across multiple cognitive domains in a subset of aged Fischer 344 rats. *Neurobiol. Aging*, June 22, 2006.
8. Tapp, P.D. et al., Frontal lobe volume, function, and beta-amyloid pathology in a canine model of aging, *J. Neurosci.*, 24, 8205, 2004.
9. Tapp, P.D. et al., Concept abstraction in the aging dog: development of a protocol using successive discrimination and size concept tasks, *Behav. Brain Res.*, 153, 199, 2004.
10. Bachevalier, J., Behavioral changes in aged rhesus monkeys, *Neurobiol. Aging*, 14, 619, 1993.
11. Moss, M.B. et al., Recognition span in aged monkeys, *Neurobiol. Aging*, 18, 13, 1997.
12. Arnsten A.F.T. and Jentsch J.D., The alpha-1 adrenergic agonist, cirazoline, impairs spatial working memory performance in aged monkeys, *Pharmacol. Biochem. Behavior*, 58, 55, 1997.

13. Arnsten, A.F.T., et al., Dopamine D1 receptor mechanisms in the cognitive perform-ance of young adult and aged monkeys, *Psychopharmacology*, 116, 143, 1994.
14. Bartus, J.M., Fleming, D., and. Johnson, H.R., Aging in the rhesus monkey: debili-tating effects on short-term memory, *J. Gerontol.*, 34, 209, 1978.
15. Bartus, R.T. and Dean, R.L., Recent memory in aged non-human primates: hyper-sensitivity to visual interference during retention, *Expl. Aging Res.*, 5, 385, 1979.
16. Bartus, R.T., Dean, R.L., and Fleming, D.L., Aging in the rhesus monkey: effects on visual discrimination learning and reversal learning, *J. Gerontol.*, 34, 209, 1979.
17. Baxter, M.G. and Gallagher, M., Neurobiological substrates of behavioral decline: models and data analytic strategies for individual differences in aging, *Neurobiol. Aging*, 17, 491, 1996.
18. Poon, L.W., Differences in human memory with aging: nature, causes and clinical implications, in *Handbook of the Psychology of Aging*, Birren J.E. and Shaie K.W., Eds., Van Nostrand Reinhold, New York, 1985, 427.
19. Light, L., Memory and aging: four hypotheses in search of data, *Annu. Rev. Psychol.*, 42, 333, 1991.
20. Albert, M.S., Age-related changes in cognitive function, in *Clinical Neurology of Aging*, Albert, M.A. and Knoefel J.E., Eds., Oxford University Press, New York, 1994, 314.
21. Powell, D.H., *Profiles in Cognitive Aging*, Harvard University Press, Cambridge, MA, 1994.
22. Schonfield, D. and Robertson, B.A., Memory storage and aging, *Canad. J. Psych.*, 20, 228, 1966.
23. Harwood, E. and Naylor, G.F.K., Recall and recognition in elderly and young subjects, *Austr. J. Psych.*, 21, 251, 1969.
24. Howell, S.C., Familiarity and complexity in perceptual recognition, *J. Gerontol.*, 27, 364, 1972.
25. Erber, J.T., Age differences in recognition memory, *J. Gerontol.*, 29, 177, 1974.
26. Rabinowitz, J., Priming in episodic memory, *J. Gerontol.*, 41, 204, 1986.
27. Talland, G.A., Age and the immediate memory span, *Gerontologist*, 7, 4, 1967.
28. Schonfield, D., Age and remembering, Proc. Sem., Duke University Council on Aging and Human Development, Durham, NC, 1969.
29. Park, D. et al., Forgetting of pictures over a long retention interval in old and young adults, *Psychol. Aging*, 3, 94, 1988.
30. Kubo, N. et al., Behavioral compensations in a positional learning and memory task by aged monkeys, *Behav. Processes*, 56, 15, 2001.
31. Marriott, J.G. and Abelson, J.S., Age differences in short-term memory of test-sophisticated rhesus monkeys, *Age*, 3, 7, 1980.
32. Medin, D.L. and Davis, R.T., in *Behavior of Non-Human Primates*, Shrier, A.M. and Stollmitz, F., Eds., Academic Press, New York, 1974, 1.
33. Rapp, P.R. and Amaral, D.G., Evidence for a task-dependent memory dysfunction in the aged monkey, *J. Neurosci.*, 9, 3568, 1989.
34. Calhoun, M.E. et al., Reduction in hippocampal cholinergic innervation is unrelated to recognition memory impairment in aged rhesus monkeys, *J. Comp. Neurol.*, 475, 238, 2004.
35. Killiany, R.J. et al., Recognition memory function in early senescent rhesus monkeys, *Psychobiology*, 28, 45, 2000.
36. Presty, S.K. et al., Age differences in recognition memory of the rhesus monkey (*Macaca mulatta*), *Neurobiol. Aging*, 8, 435, 1987.

37. Moss, M.B., Rosene, D.L., and Peters, A., Effects of aging on visual recognition memory in the rhesus monkey, *Neurobiol. Aging*, 9, 495, 1988.

38. Bachevalier, J.L. et al., Aged monkeys exhibit behavioral deficits indicative of widespread cerebral dysfunction, *Neurobiol. Aging*, 12, 99, 1991.

39. Rapp, P.R. and Amaral, D.G., Recognition memory deficits in a subpopulation of aged monkeys resemble the effects of medial temporal lobe damage, *Neurobiol. Aging*, 12, 481, 1991.

40. Arnsten, A.F.T. and Goldman-Rakic, P.S., Analysis of α-2 adrenergic agonist effects on the delayed nonmatch-to-sample performance of aged rhesus monkeys, *Neurobiol. Aging*, 11, 583, 1990.

41. Stuss, D.T., Interference effects on memory function in posteukotomy patients: an attentional perspective, in *Frontal Lobe Function and Dysfunction*, Levin, H.S., Eisenberg, H.M., and Benton, A.L., Eds., Oxford University Press, Oxford, 1991, 157.

42. Shimamura, A.P., Janowsky, J.S., and Squire, L.R., What is the role of frontal lobe damage in memory disorders? in *Frontal Lobe Function and Dysfunction*, Levin, H.S., Eisenberg, H.M. and Benton, A.L., Eds., Oxford University Press, Oxford, 1991, 173.

43. Moore, T.L. et al., Lesions of dorsal prefrontal cortex produce an executive function deficit in the rhesus monkey, *Soc. Neurosci. Abst.*, 27, Prog. #533.6, 2001.

44. Jacobsen, C.F., An experimental analysis of the frontal association areas in primates, *Arch. Neurol. Psychiat.*, 33, 558, 1935.

45. Mishkin, M., Effects of small frontal lesions on delayed alternation in monkeys, *J. Neurophysiol.*, 20, 615, 1957.

46. Butter, C.M., Mishkin, M., and Mirsky, A.F., Emotional responses toward humans in monkeys with selective frontal lesions, *Physiol. Behav.*, 3, 213, 1968.

47. Goldman, P.S. and Rosvold, H.E., Localization of function within the dorsolateral prefrontal cortex of the rhesus monkey, *Exp. Neurol.*, 27, 291, 1970.

48. Gross, C.G., Comparison of the effects of partial and total lateral frontal lesions on test performance by monkeys, *J. Comp. Physiol. Psychol.*, 56, 41, 1963.

49. Iversen, S.D., Interference and inferotemporal memory deficits, *Brain Res.*, 19, 277, 1970.

50. Battig, K., Rosvold, H.E., and Mishkin, M., Comparison of the effects of frontal and caudate lesions on delayed response and alternation in monkeys, *J. Comp. Physiol. Psych.*, 53, 400, 1960.

51. Goldman, P.S. et al., Analysis of the delayed-alternation deficit produced by dorsolateral prefrontal lesions in the rhesus monkey, *J. Comp. Physiol. Psychol.*, 77, 212, 1971.

52. Pohl, W.G., Dissociation of spatial discrimination deficits following frontal and parietal lesions in monkey, *J. Comp. Physiol. Psychol.*, 82, 227, 1973.

53. Berg, E.A., A simple objective test for measuring flexibility in thinking, *J. General Psychol.*, 39, 15, 1948.

54. Grant, D.A. and Berg, E.A., A behavioral analysis of degree of reinforcement and ease of shifting to new responses in a Weigl-type card sorting problem, *J. Exp. Psychol.*, 34, 404, 1948.

55. Dias, R., Robbins, T.W., and Roberts, A.C., Primate analogue of the Wisconsin Card Sorting Test: effects of excitotoxic lesions of the prefrontal cortex in the marmoset, *Behav. Neurosci.*, 110, 872, 1996.

56. Moore, T.L. et al., Impairment of executive function induced by hypertension in the rhesus monkey (*Macaca mulatta*), *Behav. Neurosci.*, 116, 387, 2002.

57. Royall, D.R., Executive cognitive impairment: a novel perspective on dementia. *Neuroepidemiology*, 19, 293, 2000.
58. Tierney M.C., Cognitive tests that best discriminate between presymptomatic AD and those who remain nondemented, *Neurology*, 57, 163, 2001.
59. Daigneault S., Braun C.M., and Whitaker H.A. Early effects of normal aging on perseverative and non-perseverative prefrontal measures, *Develop. Neuropsych.*, 8, 99, 1992.
60. Talland, G.A., Effects of aging on the formation of sequential and spatial concepts, *Percept. Mot. Skills*, 13, 210, 1961.
61. Albert, M.S., Duffy, F.H., and Naeser, M.A., Nonlinear changes in cognition and their neurophysiological correlates, *Canad. J. Psych.* 41, 141, 1987.
62. Lezak, M., *Neuropsychological Assessment*, 2nd ed., Oxford University Press, New York, 1983.
63. Albert, M.S., Wolfe, J., and Lafleche, G., Differences in abstraction ability with age. *Psych. and Aging*, 5, 94, 1990.
64. Bromley, D., Effects of age on intellectual output, *J. Gerontol.*, 12, 318, 1957.
65. Mack, J.L. and Carlson, N.J., Conceptual deficits and aging: the category test, *Percept. Motor Skills*, 46, 123, 1978.
66. Hess, T.M. and Slaughter, S.L., Aging effects on prototype abstraction and concept identification, *J. Gerontol.*, 41, 214, 1986.
67. Albert, M.S. and Moss, M.B., The assessment of memory disorders in patients with Alzheimer's disease, in *Neuropsychology of Memory*, Squire, L. and Butters, N., Eds., Guilford Press, New York, 1984.
68. Moss, M.B., Rosene, D.L., and Peters, A., The effects of aging on visual recognition memory in the rhesus monkey, *Primate Report*, 14, 133, 1986.
69. Moore, T.L. et al., A non-human primate test of abstraction and set shifting: an automated adaptation of the Wisconsin card sorting test, *J. Neurosci. Meth.*, 146. 165, 2005.
70. Gaffan, D., Recognition impaired and association intact in the memory of monkeys after transection of the fornix, *J. Comp. Physiol. Psychol.*, 86, 1100, 1974.
71. Mahut, H., Zola-Morgan, S., and Moss, M.B., Hippocampal resections impair associative learning and recognition memory in the monkey, *J. Neurosci.*, 2, 1214, 1982.
72. Saunders, R.C., Murray, E.A., and Mishkin, M., Further evidence that amygdala and hippocampus contribute equally to recognition memory, *Neuropsychologia*, 22, 758, 1984.
73. Mishkin, M., Memory in monkeys severely impaired by combined but not by separate removal of amygdala and hippocampus, *Nature*, 273, 297, 1978.
74. Zola-Morgan, S. and Squire, L.R., Medial temporal lesions in monkeys impair memory on a variety of tasks sensitive to human amnesia, *Behav. Neurosci.*, 99, 22, 1985.
75. Alverez, P., Zola-Morgan, S., and Squire, L.R., Damage limited to the hippocampal region produces long-lasting memory impairment in monkeys, *J. Neurosci.*, 15, 3796, 1995.
76. Aggleton, J.P. and Mishkin, M., Visual recognition impairment following medial thalamic lesions in monkeys, *Neuropsychologia*, 21, 189, 1983.
77. Zola-Morgan, S. and Squire, L.R., Memory impairment in monkeys following lesions limited to the hippocampus, *Behav. Neurosci.*, 100, 155, 1986.
78. Beason-Held, L.L. et al., Hippocampal formation lesions produce memory impairment in the rhesus monkey, *Hippocampus*, 9, 562, 1999.

79. Murray, E.A. and Mishkin, M., Visual recognition in monkeys following rhinal cortical ablations combined with either amygdalectomy or hippocampectomy, *J. Neurosci.* 6, 1991, 1986.

80. Gaffan, D. and Murray, E.A., Monkeys (Macaca fascicularis) with rhinal cortex ablations succeed in object discrimination learning despite 24-hr intertrial intervals and fail at matching to sample despite double sample presentations, *Behav. Neurosci.*, 106, 30, 1992.

81. Meunier M. et al., Effects on visual recognition of combined and separate ablations of the entorhinal and perirhinal cortex in rhesus monkeys, *J. Neurosci.*, 13, 5418, 1993.

82. Eacott, M.J., Gaffan, D., and Murray, E.A., Preserved recognition memory for small sets, and impaired stimulus identification for large sets, following rhinal cortex ablations in monkeys, *Eur. J. Neurosci.* 6, 1466, 1994.

83. Zola-Morgan, S., Squire, L.R., and Amaral, D.G., Lesions of the hippocampal formation but not lesions of the fornix or the mammillary nuclei produce long-lasting memory impairments in monkeys, *J. Neurosci.*, 9, 898, 1989.

84. Zola-Morgan, S. et al., Lesions of perirhinal and parahippocampal cortex that spare the amygdala and hippocampal formation produce severe memory impairment, *J. Neurosci.* 9, 4355, 1989.

85. Comparet, P., Darriet, D., and Jaffard, R., Demonstration of dissociation between frontal and temporal lesions in man on two versions of delayed non-matching recognition tests used in monkeys, *CR Acad. Sci.*, 314, 515, 1992.

86. Squire L.R., Zola-Morgan S., and Chen, K.S., Human amnesia and animal models of amnesia: performance of amnesic patients on tests designed for the monkey, *Behav. Neurosci.*, 102, 210, 1988.

87. Rapp, P.R., Neuropsychological analysis of learning and memory in the aged non-human primate, *Neurobiol. Aging*, 14, 627, 1993.

88. Rehbein, L. Long-Term Effects of early Hippocampectomy in the Monkey, unpublished doctoral thesis, Northwestern University, Boston, 1985.

89. Salmon, D.P. et al., Recognition memory span in mild and moderately demented patients with Alzheimer's disease, *J. Clin. Exp. Neuropsych.*, 4, 429, 1989.

90. Lange, K.W. et al., L-dopa withdrawal in Parkinson's disease selectively impairs cognitive performance in tests sensitive to frontal lobe function, *Psychopharmacology*, 107, 394, 1992.

91. Inouye, S.K. et al., Cognitive performance in a high-functioning community-dwelling elderly population, *J. Gerontol.*, 48, 146, 1993.

92. Milner, B., Disorders of memory after brain lesions in man. Preface: material-specific and generalized memory disorder, *Neuropsychologia*, 6, 175, 1968.

93. Milner, B., Aspects of human frontal lobe, in *Function Epilepsy and the Functional Anatomy of the Frontal Lobe*, Jasper H.H., Riggio S., and Goldman-Rakic P.S., Eds., Raven Press, New York, 1995.

94. Mishkin, M., Perseveration of central sets after frontal lesions in monkeys, in *The Frontal Granular Cortex and Behavior*, Warren, J.M. and Akert, K. Eds., McGraw-Hill, New York, 1964, 219–241.

95. Peters A., et al., Are neurons lost from the primate cerebral cortex during normal aging? *Cereb. Cortex*, 8, 295, 1998.

96. Sloan, J.A. et al., Lack of correlation between plaque burden and cognition in the aged monkey, *Acta Neuropath.*, 94, 471, 1997.

97. Peters, A., Moss, M.B., and Sethares, C., Effects of aging on myelinated nerve fibers in monkey primary visual cortex, *J. Comp. Neurol.*, 419, 364, 2000.

98. Peters A. and Sethares C., Aging and the myelinated fibers in prefrontal cortex and corpus callosum of the monkey, *J. Comp. Neurol.*, 442, 277, 2002.

99. Sandell, J.H. and Peters, A., Effects of age on nerve fibers in the rhesus monkey optic nerve, *J. Comp. Neurol.*, 429, 541, 2001.

100. Peters, A., Sethares C., and Killiany R.J., Effects of age on the thickness of myelin sheaths in monkey primary visual cortex, *J. Comp. Neurol.*, 435, 241, 2001.

101. Makris, N. et al., Cortical thinning of the attention and executive function networks in adults with Attention-Deficit/Hyperactivity Disorder, *Cerebral Cortex*, in press, 2006.

3 Neuropsychology of Cognitive Aging in Rodents

Joshua S. Rodefer and Mark G. Baxter

CONTENTS

I.   OVERVIEW

Advancing chronological age is associated with impairments in cognition in rodents, as it is in other species. The behavioral assessment of cognitive function in rodent models of aging provides a basis for understanding biological factors that contribute to these impairments. Advantages of rodent models of cognitive aging include their relatively brief lifespan relative to primates, the large range of behavioral tasks that have been developed for testing cognitive abilities in rodents, the anatomical homology of many brain structures between rodents and primates, the ability to carry out genetic manipulation in rodents (especially in mice), and the absence of many age-related neurodegenerative conditions observed in humans that complicate the study of phenomena associated with "normal" aging (as opposed to pathology).

Our goals in this chapter are twofold. First, we discuss some measurement and methodological issues surrounding the assessment of cognitive abilities in aged rodents. Some of these issues become especially critical when, as is commonly done in this work, one attempts to draw conclusions about the relationship between cognitive aging and neurobiological changes in the aged brain. Second, we provide a relatively brief and selective review of effects of cognitive aging on some of the major behavioral domains that can be readily assessed in rodents, as well as some neurobiological substrates that have been proposed to underlie some of these impairments.

II.   MEASUREMENT AND METHODOLOGICAL ISSUES

A.   MEASUREMENT AND RELIABILITY

With regard to the study of individual differences in cognitive performance in aging rodents, consideration of measurement issues is paramount. For example, in the absence of information about test-retest reliability of behavioral assessments, the use of behavioral scores as a basis for correlation with neurobiological measures is problematic. This is not a trivial problem, with many paradigms complicated by practice and carryover effects between assessments. Indeed, spatial learning in the water maze is one of the most problematic tasks in this regard because learning of new problems in the water maze occurs much more rapidly than initial acquisition. Initial acquisition curves are most commonly used as a basis for correlation with neurobiological parameters and it is not really possible to retest each rodent in the water maze as if they were encountering the problem for the first time. Of course, this also speaks to a neuropsychological issue as well as a measurement issue; initial acquisition of the water maze taps into a number of capacities other than spatial learning, including inhibition of prepotent responding (learning to swim away from the wall of the tank) and possibly attentional and cue-selection processes (learning which cues are stably related to the platform location).

Some solutions to this problem include examining correlations of performance across behavioral tasks that presumably depend on the same neurobiological substrate (e.g., the hippocampus). One of the first studies to employ this approach found that subgroups of rats identified as "impaired" and "unimpaired" based on their acquisition of spatial learning in the water maze honored those subgroup distinctions when tested on the Barnes circular platform task and in recovery from gustatory neophobia, both tasks that depend on the integrity of the hippocampus [1], but did not differ in simple reaction time tested in a separate assessment, despite this task revealing differences between young and aged rats overall. More recently, test-retest reliability of the water maze was demonstrated more directly by training rats in a standard protocol and retesting them several weeks later in a rapid-acquisition protocol in a new maze in a different physical room. Subgroups of "impaired" and "unimpaired" rats identified during initial training also differed in retention performance in a probe trial conducted 30 minutes after the rapid training protocol [2]. Performance in the water maze also correlated with acquisition of a reference memory problem in the radial arm maze, but not with working memory errors measured in the same paradigm [3], again confirming the reliability of the assessment in the water maze.

These considerations are important because reliability of behavioral scores constrains the magnitude of correlations with neurobiological measures. If the coefficient of correlation for two different assessments of a particular cognitive ability is 0.7 and the test-retest reliability of a neurobiological measure is 0.9, then the largest correlation that can be observed between these measures is 0.63, although the "true" population correlation between the measures may be 1.0 [4]. Thus, the use of behavioral scores that have poor reliability for correlational analysis makes the determination of correlations with neurobiological markers problematic. Even if the assessment itself is reliable, it is important to ascertain that the measure is reliably indicating the cognitive ability of interest (e.g., spatial learning). Swim times to the platform in the water maze may be very reliable across different assessments but may also include a component of motor ability, which may also be reliable from a testing standpoint but is not an indicator of the cognitive process of interest.

The relative merits of subdividing aged rats into "impaired" and "unimpaired" subgroups have been commented on previously [5]. In the context of measurement reliability, a binary classification may be more reliable than the absolute value of an individual behavioral score. Conversely, this approach discards a considerable amount of information provided by the absolute score value. It may be the case that a subgrouping approach may be more appropriate if there are concerns about the reliability of absolute scores, although it still would be important to confirm that subgroup classifications are reliable across assessments in some way.

B.   BEHAVIORAL TESTING ISSUES

Issues of behavioral control and specificity of age-related behavioral impairments are also critical to this area of research. We have already alluded to these concerns in the context of measurement issues. This relates not just to the reliability of a behavioral measure in the context of test-retest reliability, but also in terms of its relationship to the latent cognitive variable of interest. It is fairly obvious (but worth restating) that we cannot measure attention, memory, etc., directly, but rather must infer the integrity of these cognitive domains from performance on behavioral tasks. In a sense, this is the converse of the issue addressed in the section above; it is important to know that tasks that presumably measure the same cognitive ability provide performance measures that correlate with one another, but it is equally important to know that these measures are assessing the cognitive process of interest rather than a general age-related decline in behavioral performance or some other factor, such as sensorimotor ability. Indeed, it has been argued in studies of human cognitive aging that practically all the age-related variance in performance on cognitive tasks can be accounted for by a deficit in perceptual speed [6]. In this view, it would be pointless to discuss how age-related impairments in episodic memory retrieval, for example, are related to particular biological changes, because the age-related differences in performance on episodic retrieval owe to a core deficit in perceptual speed rather than a specific impairment in memory per se.

Nevertheless, dissociations in performance in cognitive aging have already been identified in aging rodents. One of the first studies to address this issue found that deficits in spatial learning in aging rats were independent of deficits in motor performance, indicating that spatial learning deficits could not be easily explained by noncognitive impairments [7]. As already discussed, age-related changes in reaction time were independent of age-related changes in spatial learning and recovery from gustatory neophobia [1, 8]. Similarly, age-related impairments on a putatively prefrontal cortex-dependent attentional set-shifting task were independent of age-related impairments in spatial learning in the water maze [9]. Taken together, these findings argue against a unitary decline in behavioral performance in aged rats that might explain apparent cognitive impairments by a single factor.

Of course, this does not mean that the behavioral scores themselves are pure measures of the cognitive processes that are of interest. Rats that are poor swimmers may perform poorly in the water maze for reasons that have nothing to do with disruption in spatial learning. It may be possible to use measures of performance in the water maze that are less contaminated by possible motor impairments, for example, bias of search during interpolated probe trials [10, 11]. It is better, however, to show that swimming ability per se either does not differ between young and aged rats or, if it does, that swimming ability is independent of performance on measures of cognitive performance. In this vein, visually cued water maze tasks are commonly included as behavioral controls and given after the conclusion of standard, hidden-platform testing in the water maze. The argument is that if rats perform normally when swimming to a visible platform (requiring no learning about its location), then any deficit in locating a hidden platform, which must be done based on the relationships between distal spatial cues, is not due to some impairment in swimming ability or motivation to escape from the water. Similarly, tests of object recognition memory may show that performance is intact at very brief delays but not at longer ones, indicating that the motivation to explore a novel object is intact, even if memory for whether objects are novel or not is impaired [12]. If in a particular experiment aged rats are impaired, for example, in both spatial and visually cued tasks, this does not necessarily mean that their impairment in the spatial task is due exclusively to some nonmnemonic factor, but it makes it very challenging to absolutely exclude this possibility directly. Indeed, blind young rats can perform very well in the standard hidden-platform water maze task [13]. Nonetheless, the inclusion of such behavioral controls is essential if age-related changes in a particular behavioral measure of performance are to be attributed with relative confidence to a deficit in the cognitive process the task purports to measure, rather than some less specific perform-ance deficit.

C.   NEUROPSYCHOLOGICAL SPECIFICITY

We already have alluded to the issue of how behavioral tasks are associated with the integrity of particular neural systems. For example, spatial learning in the water maze is heavily identified with the hippocampal system. The question of whether a particular behavioral task is a reliable measure of a cognitive latent variable of interest (e.g., spatial learning) is not quite the same as whether that task is reliably associated with changes in the integrity of function within a particular brain region. That is to say, a particular subpopulation of aged rats could reliably demonstrate impairments on several different tests of spatial learning, but this does not necessarily mean that these impairments owe to neurobiological changes in hippocampal func-tion specifically. For example, impaired performance in the water maze has been associated with damage to the frontal cortex, parietal cortex, and temporal cortex [14–17], although some of these deficits are not always found [18, 19].

Of course, this problem is not unique to the water maze. Many different manip-ulations can affect multiple-choice serial reaction time performance, a test of atten-tion [20], although the presence of many measures of performance and parametric manipulations of task difficulty in that task allow the dissociation of many different causes of overall impairment in performance. These problems also are not unique to the study of aging. Indeed, they are not dissimilar to core issues in the use of neuropsychological assessment to localize brain damage in humans before the advent of neuroimaging techniques. Sensitivity and specificity are two qualities that are important in behavioral tasks used for neuropsychological assessment. Sensitivity denotes the reliability with which a behavioral deficit is observed after damage to a specific brain region; specificity denotes the extent to which the particular deficit is restricted to a specific locus of brain region. By these criteria, one might say that spatial learning in the water maze is extremely sensitive to hippocampal damage because it is unusual to find instances in which hippocampal damage is documented but spatial learning is normal, but it also is relatively unspecific because impairments in spatial learning in the water maze can be seen in animals that have damage to brain regions other than the hippocampus.

D.   NEUROBIOLOGICAL CORRELATIONS

Just because performance in a behavioral task correlates with a particular neuro-chemical measure does not imply that changes in that neurochemical marker are responsible for the impairment in performance of the behavioral task. It is again fairly obvious to state that correlation does not imply causation and that observing associations between changes in biological markers and age-related impairments in cognition — some of which we will review in subsequent sections — does not imply that changes in the marker necessarily cause the cognitive impairment. There are, however, some experimental approaches that can be brought to bear on this problem. One is to use an intervention to modify the neurobiological parameter of interest to see if this moderates the cognitive impairment. For example, if low levels of a growth factor are associated with impairment in a particular aspect of memory, that growth factor may be replaced in aged, memory-impaired animals to see if memory is restored. The logic of this approach may not be entirely secure — if aspirin relieves a headache, it does not mean that the headache was caused by an aspirin deficiency — but it does provide data more supportive of causality. It also may be possible to model some neurobiological changes in a young animal to determine if these reproduce the pattern of cognitive impairment in aging. One example of this approach is the study of the role of basal forebrain cholinergic neurons in age-related impairments in spatial learning. Although correlations are observed between cholinergic markers and age-related impairments in spatial learning and memory, removal of hippocampal cholinergic input in young rats did not impair spatial learning in a water maze protocol sensitive to the effects of normal aging [21], nor did it cause aged, unimpaired rats to develop spatial learning impairment [22]. These types of approaches, as well as others, can be used to complement correlational studies done in aged rodents.

III.   NEUROPSYCHOLOGY OF AGED RODENTS

A.   SPATIAL LEARNING

Although a comprehensive review of studies examining spatial learning in aged animals is beyond the scope of this chapter, we will attempt to summarize recent reports in a number of areas relating to spatial cognition in aged subjects.

1.   Age-Related Impairments in Spatial Learning

As has already been noted, spatial learning in the water maze is commonly used to assess hippocampal-dependent cognitive function in aged rodents. This is probably because the water maze does not require food or water restriction, which may place differential physiological stress on aged rodents, and because learning in the water maze proceeds rapidly and efficiently. However, it has been noted that aged rats may have exacerbated responses to the stress of submersion in water [23, 24], which may need to be considered in these experiments. These impairments are also seen in other spatial tasks, including the Barnes circular maze [25], which uses escape from bright light in an open field as a motivator, as well as the more standard radial arm maze [26]. Aged mice are also impaired in spatial tasks in the water maze, although measures of performance different than those used in rats may be maximally sensitive to these impairments [27]. In general, spatial learning impairments appear to emerge gradually as chronological age increases. Even 11-month-old Fischer-344 rats are impaired relative to 4-month-old Fischer-344 rats on a demanding measure of spatial memory, the number of platform crossings on probe trials [28].

2.   Behavioral Strategies

Barnes and co-workers [29] were the first to report that aged rats were less likely than young rats to use place strategies to solve a simple spatial discrimination in a

T-maze in which egocentric (body-turn) and visual cue-guided strategies were also able to support accurate discrimination behavior. Subsequent reports indicated that aged rats used different behavioral strategies in the Morris and T-water mazes, and detection of age-related spatial learning deficits depended on the task used and the strategies employed [30]. In particular, these authors noted that the acquisition of spatial tasks using egocentric strategies was unimpaired in aged rats. Complementary observations were reported by Nicolle et al. [31] in aged mice using a cue-competition paradigm in the water maze. In this task, mice learn to swim to a visible platform in a fixed location. Probe trials are given in which the visible platform is moved to a different location in the maze: mice either swim toward the visible platform in its new location (a cue strategy) or swim toward its previous location first (a place strategy). The prevalence of a cue strategy increased with age, with 23-month-old mice using a cue strategy exclusively. Aged rats were impaired on a number of behavioral assessments in the radial arm water maze, and committed both reference and working memory errors compared to young rats across all days of testing, thus suggesting that aged-rats may have employed nonspatial strategies in learning new platform locations [32].

3.   Structural and Anatomical Analyses

Despite overwhelming behavioral and electrophysiological data on hippocampal dysfunction in aging, a clear understanding of the anatomical and structural basis for these cognitive declines is lacking. Cell sizes and numbers do not differ in the subdivisions of entorhinal cortex between young and aged rats despite behavioral differences in the water maze, suggesting that parameters other than neuronal size and number may be relevant for understanding age-related cognitive declines [33]. In a more recent study, this group examined hippocampal cell genesis in its relation to spatial learning and again found that behavioral deficits did not appear to correlate with adult hippocampal neurogenesis [34] (see also Chapter 6). These studies are consistent with reports that total neuron number in the entorhinal, perirhinal, and postrhinal cortices is largely preserved during normal aging. Moreover, individual variability in hippocampal-dependent learning in aged rats does not correlate with neuron number in any area examined [35]. Thus, age-related cognitive decline can occur in the absence of significant neuronal death in any major area of the hippocampal system. In contrast, a significant age-related relationship between deficit in spatial learning and the loss of p75-positive neurons in the basal, but not rostral, forebrain has been reported. Although there was no learning impairment at 6 months of age, fully one-half the rats were impaired at 12 months and 71% displayed deficits at age 26 months [36]. Another study examined basal forebrain cholinergic neurons in young and aged, male and female Fischer 344 rats that had been trained on the Morris water maze [37]. Young rats' performance was superior to aged rats' performance, but young male rats were better at finding the precise platform location compared to young females. When examining structural differences, young male and female rats had larger basal forebrain cholinergic neurons compared to the aged groups, but this was largely a function of a difference between aged and young male rats. In no case, however, was there a correlation between neuron size and spatial memory performance. Examination of postsynaptic densities in hippocampal excitatory synapses in aged spatial learning-impaired and unimpaired rats found a significant decrease in postsynaptic density area in aged-impaired compared to aged-unimpaired rats, suggesting that hippocampal synapses might become less efficient in aged-impaired animals, which might manifest as behavioral deficits in cognitive tasks [38].

4.   Signal Transduction

Brightwell and colleagues [39] investigated the effectiveness of signal transduction in aged rats with impaired spatial performance. Individual proteins from the CREB family can function as either enhancers (e.g., CREB1) or repressors (e.g., CREB2) and influence the short-term to long-term memory transitions. Aged animals that were impaired in the Morris water maze were found to have lower levels of CREB1 in the hippocampus compared to both younger animals and aged non-impaired animals, suggesting dysregulation of CREB1 levels may lead to some aspects of spatial learning deficits in aged subjects. Aged rats with impaired spatial memory, compared to young rats, demonstrated increased protein kinase C (PKC)-gamma immunoreactivity in the CA1 region of the hippocampus, but not in the dentate gyrus [40]. Furthermore, this increased PKC-gamma activity in CA1 was significantly correlated with spatial memory deficits. These data are consistent with a report that demonstrated a significant relationship between choice accuracy and PKC-gamma immunogenicity in the hippocampal CA1 region, but not amygdala, of aged animals [41].

5.   NMDA Receptors

Adams et al. [42] investigated the association between levels of the NR1 subunit of N-methyl-D-aspartate (NMDA) receptors and performance in the Morris water maze task. Although neither global nor region-specific differences in hippocampal NR1 levels were observed, there was a selective association between individual behavioral performance and NR1 immunofluorescence levels in the CA3 region, suggesting that NMDA abundance in the CA3 region is critical for spatial learning over the lifespan. More recently, Clayton and colleagues [43] used antisense oligonucleotides to knock down the NR2B subunit expression in the hippocampus, suggesting a key role for reduced NR2B expression in aged-related cognitive deficits in older animals. Another way to examine NMDA subunit involvement in learning and memory is by pharmacological manipulation. Suldinac is a nonsteroidal anti-inflammatory drug (NSAID) that is a nonselective cyclooxygenase (COX) inhibitor. Chronic administration of suldinac, but not its non-COX active metabolite, ameliorated age-related decreases in the NR1 and NR2B NMDA receptor subunits and prevented similar age-related increases in the pro-inflammatory cytokine interleukin-1beta (IL-1beta) in the hippocampus. Moreover, suldinac reversed age-related deficits in radial arm maze deficits [44]. In a fashion consistent with these data, others have reported that chronic aspirin (a NSAID) treatment improves spatial learning in both adult and aged rats [45].

6. Hormones and Stress

Although much research suggests that ovarian hormone levels are important in cognition, the effect of manipulating hormone levels in aged animals has been less well explored. Foster and colleagues [46] reported that estradiol did not enhance acquisition of cue and spatial discrimination in the Morris water maze, but the researchers noted a dose by age interaction such that a high dose of estradiol did produce higher retention scores in aged animals. Markham et al. [47] also noted an age and hormone interaction. Ovarian hormone replacement early in life can be detrimental to cognitive performance, whereas ovarian hormone replacement when rats are at least 14 to 16 months old has a beneficial effect on spatial learning. These studies contrast with recent work by Bimonte-Nelson and colleagues [48], who reported that a lack of ovarian hormones over a longer period (e.g., greater than 1.5 months) improved spatial memory in aged female rats. These seemingly contradictory data might be explained not by levels of estradiol, but by lower levels of progesterone being related to the ovarectomized-induced enhancement of spatial learning. This idea was supported by a subsequent study that demonstrated that progesterone supplementation reversed the cognitive enhancement produced in aged ovarectomized rats [49]. Recently, Ziegler and Gallagher [50] attempted to elucidate whether estrogen is critical to spatial learning in middle-aged females that generally have declining ovarian hormone cyclicity. Estradiol was administered in a phasic pattern to simulate normal cyclic behavior, yet estradiol did not have any effect in either young or middle-aged rats, nor on any behavioral measure. The lack of significant effects where others have previously observed cognitive effects of estradiol might be explained by methodological or training differences across laboratories.

Bimonte-Nelson and colleagues [51] also reported on the importance of hormone-related cognitive enhancements in aged male rats by demonstrating that testosterone, which is aromatized to estrogen, improved working memory. In contrast, administration of dihydrotestosterone, which is not aromatized to estrogen, did not attenuate age-related deficits in working memory. Thus, hormone therapy in aged males and females may have beneficial effects on some aspects of cognition when the age of the subjects is taken into consideration.

Bizon et al. [52] examined the function of the hypothalamic-pituitary-adrenal (HPA) axis in young and aged animals. Plasma corticosterone levels in cognitively impaired aged animals were slower to return to baseline following restraint stress compared to both younger rats and cognitively unimpaired aged rats. Analysis of neurobiological data revealed that glucocorticoid receptor mRNA was reduced in the hippocampus and medial prefrontal cortex in aged cognitively impaired rats compared to either young or aged unimpaired groups. Moreover, the decreased mRNA levels in these regions were significantly correlated with impaired performance in the water maze task. In a subsequent study to evaluate the role of neurogenesis in aged animals, Bizon and colleagues demonstrated that nonimpaired aged rats did not demonstrate enhanced hippocampal neurogenesis compared to cognitively impaired aged rats. Thus, aged rats that maintain cognitive function do so while still enduring the same significant reductions in hippocampal neurogenesis that are characteristic of cognitively impaired aged subjects [53]. This contrasts somewhat with a previous study that reported spatial memory performance of aged rats was predictive of hippocampal neurogenesis ([54]; see also Chapter 6).

In a creative study, Gatewood and co-workers [55] examined the effect of motherhood on age-related deficits in a food-reinforced spatial learning task by comparing age-matched nulliparous, primiparous, and multiparous females (0, 1, and 2 pregnancies and lactations, respectively) at ages from 6 to 24 months. Primiparous and multiparous females demonstrated significantly accelerated acquisition and showed decreased memory decline up to 24 months of age when compared to the nulliparous subjects. Furthermore, amyloid precursor protein, a marker of neurodegeneration, was decreased in the CA1 and dentate gyrus regions of the hippocampus in multiparous females compared to nulliparous and primiparous females. Moreover, the level of amyloid precursor protein was inversely related to spatial learning performance, suggesting that natural reproductive related hormone levels and postpartum experiences may decrease vulnerability for age-related cognitive decline in females. The role of maternal behaviors was indirectly assessed by Lehmann and colleagues [56], who examined the effects of maternal separation and handling on long-term cognitive outcome. Rats that had been handled extensively early in life were observed to have superior spatial cognition, a decreased stress response, and no decrease in hippocampal neuronal counts when compared to those rats that were either not handled or underwent early maternal separation [56].

7.   Plasticity and Cognition

Aging has been documented to be related to specific impairments in learning and memory, many of which are associated with selective damage to the amygdala and hippocampal regions that are important in long-term potentiation (LTP) and long-term depression (LTD) [for review, see 57]. Almaguer and colleagues [58] compared aged rats that were cognitively impaired to both young rats and aged, nonimpaired rats and noted that stimulation of the perforant path produced reduced LTP in the aged impaired rats, whereas aged rats that were nonimpaired were comparable to young animals. Barnes et al. [59] demonstrated that aged, spatially impaired rats had a higher threshold for LTP induction compared to middle-aged and younger controls, suggesting that the fewer perforant path synaptic contacts in aged, spatially impaired rats require greater depolarization and convergence before any modifications of synaptic strength can be produced. Schulz and co-workers [60] attempted to find behavioral and neurobiological correlates with aged rats that were divided into superior and inferior learners and then examined in a battery of behavioral assessments. In aged superior rats, levels of LTP in CA1 correlated with hippocampal mediated tasks (e.g., spatial preference learning and water maze escape). Unfortunately, there were no significant correlations observed in the aged inferior learning group, which may suggest an effect of overall impairment or other yet unknown factors. Subsequently, Schulz and colleagues [61] probed striatal parameters for associations with age-related cognitive decline. Superior and inferior learners were again compared and individual differences in the different behaviors of the aged rats were accounted for by variability in some striatal parameters for both superior (e.g., LTP) and inferior (e.g., NR2 subunit expression) rats [61].

Rosenzweig et al. [62] attempted to examine the flexibility of hippocampal spatial mapping in an elegant methodology by monitoring rats that were attending to a spatial reference that was in conflict with another frame of reference. When adult and aged rats attempted to find an unmarked goal, aged rats were impaired in their ability to find the unmarked goal and in their ability to realign the hippocampal map based on the changing contextual information. Wilson and colleagues [63] observed spatial performance of young and aged rats in the Morris water maze and then examined firing patterns of hippocampal place cells when animals were in familiar and novel environments, in an attempt to better understand how spatial representations distinguish familiar and altered environments. One consistent pattern to emerge from the data was that the (in)ability of the hippocampus to encode subtle differences in contextual environmental information may represent a major component of memory deficits [63]. Subsequently, Wilson and colleagues [64] expanded on this model and better characterized the ability of the hippocampal place cells to form new representation but also noted the delay in some spatial representations being anchored to external cues and landmarks. Taken in sum with previous work by Wilson's colleagues and others [62], these descriptions and observation help converge seemingly divergent data into a more comprehensive model of hippocampal function and aging.

8.   Treatment: Diet and Exercise

Research has demonstrated that vegetables and fruit that are high in antioxidant activity can have beneficial cognitive effects (see Chapter 15). Andres-Lacueva and colleagues [65] reported that aged rats fed a diet rich in blueberries had better water maze performance than those on a control diet, and behavioral performance was associated with brain levels of several blueberry-derived anthocyanins isolated in cortical tissue. This work is in agreement with the previous report by Casadesus et al. [66], who assessed changes in hippocampal plasticity parameters (e.g., neurogenesis; extracellular kinase activation; levels of insulin growth factor-1, IGF-1) in aged animals that were supplemented with a blueberry-rich diet. Parameters of hippocampal plasticity were enhanced in supplemented animals and cell proliferation, extraceullular receptor kinase activation, and IGF-1 levels all correlated with improved spatial task performance, suggesting that hippocampal plasticity may contribute to enhanced learning and memory measures observed in aged animals on a blueberry-rich diet. Many have also explored the role of exercise-induced cognitive enhancement. Albeck and colleagues [67] found that aged rats that exercised for 7 weeks performed significantly better in the water maze than controls, an improvement that reflected cognitive improvement because the groups did not differ in swim speed.

9.   Treatment: Drug

Compounds having activity at the nicotinic acetylcholine (nACh) receptor have been identified as having potential therapeutic benefits in aged populations. SIB-1553A is a novel nACh ligand that has subtype selectivity for alpha2-beta4 subunits. Administration of SIB-1553A was reported to be effective in enhancing T- and water-maze performance in aged rats [68]. Manipulations of other cholinergic receptor subtypes have also been found to have a positive effect on some types of learning in aged animals. Lazaris and colleagues [69] examined the effects of bilateral injections of methoctramine into the dorsolateral striatum of cognitively impaired aged female rats. The selective muscarinic M2 cholinergic antagonist improved procedural working memory, but was without effect on spatial memory. In contrast, a recent study by Rowe and colleagues [70] reported that the selective M2 antagonist, BIBN-99, significantly improved spatial learning and memory in aged animals during testing and the enhanced performance was observed to persist for up to 24 days post drug administration.

The noradrenergic system has also been suggested to play an important role in enhanced learning in aged animals. Chopin and colleagues [71] demonstrated that the selective alpha(2) antagonist dexefaroxan attenuated age-related memory deficits in 24-month-old rats, as well as reversing cognitive impairments induced by nucleus basalis magnocellular lesions. Recently, Ramos et al. [72] examined the effects of the beta-1 adrenergic antagonists in aged animals and found that the mixed beta-1/beta-2 antagonist propanolol had no effect on spatial memory but that the selective beta-1 ligand betaxolol produced dose-dependent enhancement of spatial cognition in aged subjects. Thus, the use of more selective beta-adrenergic compounds warrants further investigation.

The use of monoamine oxidase inhibitors has also been investigated. Kiray and colleagues [73] examined the effects of deprenyl, an irreversible monoamine oxidase B inhibitor, on spatial memory in aged rats. Initially, the effects of deprenyl were examined in combination with estradiol on aged female rat cognition and a synergistic effect between deprenyl and estradiol was observed. Subsequently, the actions of deprenyl were examined in aged male rats. Spatial learning in males, like females, was enhanced by deprenyl administration [74]. Other examination of antidepressant treatment has revealed that chronic treatment with the tricyclic antidepressant amitriptyline from middle age on prevents normal age-related deficits in water maze learning. Administration of amitriptyline also decreases plasma corticosterone levels, suggesting altered anxiety and stress-related behaviors [75].

The identification of effective cognitive enhancing compounds continues to be an unmet need. Hernandez and colleagues [76] examined the effects of two acetylcholinesterase inhibitors, galantamine and donepezil, on spatial learning. Both galantamine and donepezil dose-dependently enhanced cognitive performance while modestly increasing choline acetyltransferase activity in the basal forebrain and hippocampus. In a similar fashion, Aura and Riekkinen [77] demonstrated that the acetylcholinesterase inhibitor tetrahydroaninoacridine and the NMDA allosteric modulator D-cycloserine both enhanced spatial navigation. However, if aged rats were pretrained on the task, then any drug-enhanced effect on behavior was eliminated. Moreover, pretraining did not reverse age-related deficits; thus, compounds with apparent cognitive-enhancing capabilities may function by enhancing procedural aspects of learning in aged animals. Thus, while a number of compounds have been suggested to have demonstrated effectiveness in reversing age-related deficits, procedural and methodological issues are important considerations.

Administration of the 5-HT(6) receptor antagonist SB-271046 improved acquisition and consolidation in a water maze task in aged rats. Treatment with SB-271046 improved swim strategy, escape latencies, and task recall, suggesting that the drug may enhance cognitive processes as well as ameliorate age-related cognitive deficits observed in older animals [78]. In addition, Froestl et al. [79] examined the effects of the novel GABA(B) receptor antagonist SGS742. Chronic administration of SGS742 was reported to upregulate GABA(B) receptors in the frontal cortex of rats and produce cognitive enhancing effects in aged rats in both radial and water maze tasks.

B. FEAR CONDITIONING

Although the spatial water maze has been frequently used as a common measure of hippocampus-dependent learning, other animal paradigms have attempted to contribute to and expand our understanding of the role of the hippocampus in learning and memory. Fear conditioning is a hippocampally mediated form of associative learning that requires an animal to associate a conditioned stimulus (CS) and a fear-producing unconditioned shock stimulus (US). For delay conditioning, the foot shock immediately follows the tone, whereas in trace conditioning, the tone and shock are often separated by a short interval (15 to 20 seconds) and then the retention of this learning is tested a discrete time late (e.g., 24 hours).

1. Age-Related Impairment in Fear Conditioning

Blank and colleagues [80] first reported data suggesting that the trace fear conditioning procedure was sensitive to the effects of aging. By examining behavioral freezing in mice, they demonstrated that aged mice were impaired when compared to their younger controls. McEchron et al. [81] continued in this vein when they examined the effects of trace fear conditioning in aged rats. Both freezing and heart rate were sensitive measures for detecting age-related changes in trace fear conditioning. Although aged animals were not impaired at short durations of delay, they were significantly impaired in the 20-second long trace fear conditioning when compared to their younger control subjects. These data are in agreement with the recent work of Villarreal et al. [82], who demonstrated that aged rats were impaired in trace, but not delay, fear conditioning. The differences between these two tasks is the imposed delay between the tone and shock. These data, when taken in sum, suggest that aged animals are not impaired in the sensory-motor abilities to perform the task, but rather display a deficit that is characteristic of compromised hippocampal functioning and processing.

2. Neurobiological Associations

Gale and colleagues [83] examined the neurobiological role of the basolateral amygdala in maintaining stable memories of fear. Animals that had received lesions of the basolateral amygdala after fear conditioning displayed robust freezing deficits compared to sham controls. Moreover, these deficits were observed independent to the training-to-lesion interval. Indeed, rats with lesions showed robust deficits during both recent (1 day) and distant (16 months) memory tests. Thus it would appear that the basolateral amygdale might be important for encoding and storage function of emotionally and/or fear-related conditioning. The role of amount of contextual information within an environment on emotional memory was reported by Doyere and colleagues [84]; and in an interesting finding they reported that performance task deficits in aged animals were restricted to particular procedures that employed poor cues within the environment. When aged rats were tested in a more cue-rich environment, task performance improved, suggesting that aged animals may be able to employ different or enhanced learning strategies under different environmental conditions.

Monti et al. [85] took a different approach when exploring conditioned fear in aged rats. They examined whether changes in the functional state of proteins that were known to be involved with hippocampal learning could be associated with age-related decline in hippocampal-mediated behaviors in aged rats. These authors found that aged-related impairments in freezing were causally associated with a dysregulation in CREB activation, and specifically to the increased phosphorylation in aged rats after learning.

A similar approach was investigated by Kasckow and colleagues [86]. Noting that aging in rodents was accompanied by age-related changes in the immune system, they sought to identify relevant changes in the hypothalamic-pituitary-adrenal (HPA) axis. Despite finding decreased ACTH and corticosterone release following dexamethasone administration in aged-animals, testing revealed no significant associations between HPA-related data and the decreased freezing times observed in aged animals relative to middle- or younger-aged animals. The authors noted that any decrease in pituitary-related functions might be overcome by an associated increase in adrenal-related activity in aged animals.

A neuroimmune approach of age-related cognitive decline was investigated by Barrientos et al. [87]. They reported that peripheral injection of *Escherichia coli* produced both anterograde and retrograde amnesia in 24-month-old rats, but not in younger animals. Indeed, aging alone did not produce significant impairments in freezing time, nor in water maze acquisition time, but the immune challenge did produce decreased accuracy in swimming following a longer delay, suggesting a deficit in long-term memory consolidation. Moreover, immune challenge produced marked increased levels of the pro-inflammatory cytokine, interleukin 1-beta (IL-1-beta) in the hippocampus that is associated with aged-related memory impairments. Combined with the immune challenge observations, these data suggest that aged animals may be vulnerable to cognitive impairments produced by immune challenge, and that the behavioral effects of the immune challenge were observed for an extended duration following challenge.

3.   Modulating Changes in Fear Conditioning

Attempts to identify effective pharmacological agents to combat cognitive decline in aged populations is a continuing goal. Gould and Feiro [88] explored context and cued fear conditioning to see if galantamine, an acetylcholinesterase (AChE) inhibitor and nicotinic acetylcholine receptor allosteric modulator, would prove effective in reducing impairments. Aged C57BL/6 mice were not impaired in the acquisition of auditory cued or contextual fear conditioning, and were not impaired in the retention of contextual fear conditioned memories. However, mice were significantly impaired in the retention of auditory fear cued conditioned memories. Moreover, galantamine significantly improved the age-related deficits in the retention of cued fear conditioning. Feiro and Gould [89] also examined the interactive effects of nicotinic and muscarinic receptor antagonists. Administration of the muscarinic receptor antagonist scopolamine uniformly disrupted contextual fear conditioning across all ages, and younger animals were more sensitive to the disruptive effect of scopolamine in auditory cued fear conditioning than were aged rats. In contrast, the nicotinic receptor antagonist mecamylamine had no effect on contextual or auditory-cued conditioned fear in young or old animals. Examination of combined drug administration of subthreshold doses disrupted fear conditioning in younger animals, but not in aged animals, suggesting that cholinergic involvement in conditioned fear is differentially affected by age.

The involvement of nicotinic receptors in fear conditioning was further examined by Caldarone and colleagues [90], who investigated mice lacking the beta-2 subunit of the nicotinic receptor. The absence of the beta-2 subunit in young animals had no effect on contextual or tone-conditioned fear, but aged knockout males were impaired in freezing to both context and tone-conditioned fears compared to wildtype controls. These findings are consistent with previous reports that nicotinic acetylcholine receptors that lack the beta-2 subunit are not critical for normal performance in a fear conditioning task, but are likely involved in the maintenance and preservation of neuronal functioning during the aging process.

Another pathway that may have a role in age-related cognitive decline is that of oxidative stress. Quinn and colleagues [91] examined the effects of a diet high in the antioxidant alpha-lipoic acid in Tg2576 mice, a transgenic model of the cerebral amyloidosis associated with Alzheimer's disease. Aged mice that received the antioxidant-enhanced diet for 6 months demonstrated improved performance in context fear conditioning and in Morris water maze performance compared to the normal-diet controls. Although beta-amyloid levels remained unchanged, these data suggest that chronic dietary manipulation can improve some aspects of learning and memory in aged populations.

In a similar fashion, chronic administration of nonsteroidal anti-inflammatory drugs (NSAIDs) has been reported to have neuroprotective effects in aging. Administration of the nonselective cyclooxygenase (COX) inhibitor sulindac for 2 months produced significant improvement in Fischer-344 rats in contextual fear conditioning [44]. Interestingly, administration of the COX inhibitor also decreased the age-related decline of N-methyl-D-aspartate receptor subunits (NR1, NR2B) that are typically associated with age-related memory decreases. In addition, COX inhibitor administration also prevented the age-related increases in the proinflammatory cytokine, interleukin 1-beta (IL-1-beta) in the hippocampus, supporting the inflammation hypothesis of aging and suggesting therapeutic value of NSAID administration in aged populations.

Increased levels of IL-1-beta are implicated in impaired cognitive performance and in the decline of synaptic plasticity in the hippocampus. However, IL-1-beta is an inactive precursor that is cleaved into its active and mature form by caspase-1. Thus, one way to target this system might be to interfere with the production of the active form of IL-1-beta. Gemma and colleagues [92] used a selective caspase-1 inhibitor to reduce levels of IL-1-beta for one month. Aged control rats had impaired memory for the training context compared to younger animals, but chronic inhibition of caspase-1 activity attenuated this age-related memory impairment. When examined, hippocampal levels of IL-1-beta in aged animals approached levels of younger control subjects.

C.   CLASSICAL CONDITIONING

The effects of age on conditioned responses using an eyeblink conditioning paradigm have not been examined in great depth. Weiss and Thompson [93] reported that middle-aged and older rats (18 and 30 months old) were significantly impaired in the ability to form conditioned responses when compared to younger rats (3 and 12 months of age). The lack of deficits in evoking a blink response supported the notion of a deficit in associative conditioning. Subsequent work explored strain differences in aged rat performance, building upon the observation that while aged Fischer-344 rats demonstrate significant impairment in forming conditioned responses, even younger Fischer-344 animals perform submaximally. Examination of the F1 generation of a hybrid cross (Fischer-344 × Brown Norway) revealed that hybrid rats aged 9 to 24 months learned conditioned responses quickly. Aged (36-month-old) F1 hybrid subjects were significantly impaired across all training days, but performed at a significantly greater level than aged Fischer-344 rats [94]. These data suggest that strain differences can be significant, and that the relatively poor performance of younger Fischer rats may be indicative of neurobiological deficits that impair ability in conditioned eyeblink paradigms. Vogel and colleagues [95] examined the development of age-related cognitive impairments in C57BL/6 mice. Measures with a more cerebellar component (e.g., eyeblink-conditioning, rotorod) were shown to be sensitive to age-related changes earlier than other tasks. Specifically, animals 9 to 18 months old demonstrated deficits in conditioned responses compared to younger 4-month-old animals. In a similar fashion, 4-month-old animals performed significantly better than 12- to 18-month-old animals in the latency to fall during the rotorod procedure. In contrast, aged mice were not impaired by the hippocampally dependent Morris water maze task when compared to younger animals.

D.   ATTENTION AND EXECUTIVE FUNCTION

The effects of aging on performance in attention-related tasks have been somewhat limited by the number of rodent models that assess frontal cognition. Muir et al. [96] demonstrated age-related changes in attentional functioning in 7- vs. 13- to 14-month-old rats in the 5-choice serial reaction time task by manipulating the attentional loading of the task. Subsequently, as animals aged, the difference between younger (10 to 11 months old) and aged (23 to 24 months old) performance became greater, such that significant differences in performance could be observed in baseline measures without any manipulations of the attentional load of the task. This was similar to results reported by Grottick and Higgins [97], who found that aged (24 months old) rats were impaired in 5-CSRTT performance compared to younger (12 months old) subjects. Increasing the difficulty of the task impaired the performance of younger rats, producing comparable performance to older rats. Likewise, decreasing the task difficulty for older subjects produced performance comparable to younger animals.

There have been a few recent studies of executive function in aged rodents. Barense and colleagues [9] examined cognitive decline in aged Long-Evans rats in an attentional set-shifting task. Older rats (27 to 28 months old) were significantly impaired in performance compared to younger (4 months old) subjects across all tasks measured, which included reversal learning and attentional shifts. However, significant impairment was only observed in extradimensional shift (EDS) learning, which required rats to change the dimension of the compound stimulus they were using to solve the discrimination — for example, rats using odor to solve the discriminations had to start using digging medium instead. In addition, impaired performance on EDS was uncorrelated with performance in the Morris water maze, suggesting that age-related declines in frontal- and hippocampal-mediated functions are dissociable. More recently, similar age-related impairments in frontal function have been found in Sprague-Dawley rats. Rodefer and Nguyen [98] demonstrated that older rats demonstrated consistent impairment in discrimination learning but, in a fashion similar to Barense and colleagues, only found significant impairment in EDS learning. Impaired reversal learning in aged rats has also been reported in an automated olfactory discrimination paradigm [99]; perhaps the increased difficulty of discrimination learning in this setting reveals impairments that are not reliable when reversal learning is tested in the set-shifting task.

IV. SUMMARY

Impairments in multiple behavioral domains are observed in aged rodents and a wide variety of neurobiological parameters have been investigated in conjunction with these impairments. These paradigms also provide a setting in which to test possible pharmacological and environmental manipulations that may be able to ameliorate age-related cognitive decline. Careful behavioral design and the use of multiple measures of performance [100] will enhance the ability of experiments in aged rodents to tell us about the biological substrates of cognitive impairment in human brain aging, and will increase the applicability of these models for preclinical development and testing of agents that may be effective cognitive enhancers.

ACKNOWLEDGMENTS

Preparation of this chapter was supported in part by the Wellcome Trust (MGB).

REFERENCES

1. Gallagher, M. and Burwell, R.D., Relationship of age-related decline across several behavioral domains, *Neurobiol. Aging*, 10, 691, 1989.
2. Colombo, P.J., Wetsel, W.C., and Gallagher, M., Spatial memory is related to hippocampal subcellular concentrations of calcium-dependent protein kinase C isoforms in young and aged rats, *Proc. Natl. Acad. Sci. U.S.A.*, 94, 14195, 1997.
3. Colombo, P.J. and Gallagher, M., Individual differences in spatial memory and striatal ChAT activity among young and aged rats, *Neurobiol. Learn. Mem.*, 70, 314, 1998.
4. Nunnally, J.C. and Bernstein, I.H., *Psychometric Theory*, 3rd ed., McGraw-Hill, New York, 1994.
5. Baxter, M.G. and Gallagher, M., Neurobiological substrates of behavioral decline: models and data analytic strategies for individual differences in aging, *Neurobiol. Aging*, 17, 491, 1996.
6. Salthouse, T.A., Speed of behavior and its implications for cognition, in *Handbook of the Psychology of Aging*, 2nd ed., Birren, J.E. and Schaie, K.W., Eds., Van Nostrand Reinhold, New York, 1985, 400.
7. Gage, F.H., Dunnett, S.B., and Björklund, A., Spatial learning and motor deficits in aged rats, *Neurobiol. Aging*, 5, 43, 1984.
8. Burwell, R.D. and Gallagher, M., A longitudinal study of reaction time performance in Long-Evans rats, *Neurobiol. Aging*, 14, 57, 1993.
9. Barense, M.D., Fox, M.T., and Baxter, M.G., Aged rats are impaired on an attentional set-shifting task sensitive to medial frontal cortex damage in young rats, *Learn. Mem.*, 9, 191, 2002.
10. Markowska, A.L. et al., Variable-interval probe test as a tool for repeated measurements of spatial memory in the water maze, *Behav. Neurosci.*, 107, 627, 1993.
11. Gallagher, M., Burwell, R., and Burchinal, M., Severity of spatial learning impairment in aging: development of a learning index for performance in the Morris water maze, *Behav. Neurosci.*, 107, 618, 1993.
12. Bussey, T.J., Muir, J.L., and Aggleton, J.P., Functionally dissociating aspects of event memory: the effects of combined perirhinal and postrhinal cortex lesions on object and place memory in the rat, *J. Neurosci.*, 19, 495, 1999.
13. Lindner, M.D. et al., Blind rats are not profoundly impaired in the reference memory Morris water maze and cannot be clearly discriminated from rats with cognitive deficits in the cued platform task, *Cog. Brain Res.*, 5, 329, 1997.
14. Nagahara, A.H., Otto, T., and Gallagher, M., Entorhinal/perirhinal lesions impair performance on two versions of place learning in the Morris water maze, *Behav. Neurosci.*, 109, 3, 1995.
15. Liu, P. and Bilkey, D.K., Perirhinal cortex contributions to performance in the Morris water maze, *Behav. Neurosci.*, 112, 304, 1998.
16. DiMattia, B.D. and Kesner, R.P., Spatial cognitive maps: differential role of parietal cortex and hippocampal formation, *Behav. Neurosci.*, 102, 471, 1988.
17. Kolb, B., Sutherland, R.J., and Whishaw, I.Q., A comparison of the contributions of the frontal and parietal association cortex to spatial localization in rats, *Behav. Neurosci.*, 97, 13, 1983.
18. Burwell, R.D. et al., Corticohippocampal contributions to spatial and contextual learning, *J. Neurosci.*, 24, 3826, 2004.
19. de Bruin, J. P.C. et al., A behavioural analysis of rats with damage to the medial prefrontal cortex using the Morris water maze: evidence for behavioural flexibility, but not for impaired spatial navigation, *Brain Res.*, 652, 323, 1994.

20. Robbins, T.W., The 5-choice serial reaction time task: behavioural pharmacology and functional neurochemistry, *Psychopharmacology*, 163, 362, 2002.

21. Baxter, M.G. et al., Selective immunotoxic lesions of basal forebrain cholinergic cells: effects on learning and memory in rats, *Behav. Neurosci.*, 109, 714, 1995.

22. Baxter, M.G. and Gallagher, M., Intact spatial learning in both young and aged rats following selective removal of hippocampal cholinergic input, *Behav. Neurosci.*, 110, 460, 1996.

23. Mabry, T.R., Gold, P.E., and McCarty, R., Age-related changes in plasma catecholamine responses to acute swim stress, *Neurobiol. Learn. Mem.*, 63, 260, 1995.

24. Mabry, T.R. et al., Age and stress history effects on spatial performance in a swim task in Fischer-344 rats, *Neurobiol. Learn. Mem.*, 66, 1, 1996.

25. Barnes, C.A., Memory deficits associated with senescence: a neurophysiological and behavioral study in the rat, *J. Comp. Physiol. Psychol.*, 93, 74, 1979.

26. Chrobak, J.J. et al., Within-subject decline in delayed-non-match-to-sample radial arm maze performance in aging Sprague-Dawley rats, *Behav. Neurosci.*, 109, 241, 1995.

27. Frick, K.M. et al., Reference memory, anxiety and estrous cyclicity in C57BL/6NIA mice are affected by age and sex, *Neuroscience*, 95, 293, 2000.

28. Frick, K.M. et al., Age-related spatial reference and working memory deficits assessed in the water maze, *Neurobiol. Aging*, 16, 149, 1995.

29. Barnes, C.A., Nadel, L., and Honig, W.K., Spatial memory deficit in senescent rats, *Can. J. Psych.*, 34, 29, 1980.

30. Begega, A. et al., Effects of ageing on allocentric and egocentric spatial strategies in the Wistar rat, *Behav. Processes*, 53, 75, 2001.

31. Nicolle, M.M., Prescott, S., and Bizon, J.L., Emergence of a cue strategy preference on the water maze task in aged C57B6 x SJL F1 hybrid mice, *Learn. Mem.*, 10, 520, 2003.

32. Shukitt-Hale, B. et al., Effect of age on the radial arm water maze-a test of spatial learning and memory, *Neurobiol. Aging*, 25, 223, 2004.

33. Merrill, D.A., Chiba, A.A., and Tuszynski, M.H., Conservation of neuronal number and size in the entorhinal cortex of behaviorally characterized aged rats, *J. Comp. Neurol.*, 438, 445, 2001.

34. Merrill, D.A. et al., Hippocampal cell genesis does not correlate with spatial learning ability in aged rats, *J. Comp. Neurol.*, 459, 201, 2003.

35. Rapp, P.R. et al., Neuron number in the parahippocampal region is preserved in aged rats with spatial learning deficits, *Cereb. Cortex*, 12, 1171, 2002.

36. Greferath, U. et al., Impaired spatial learning in aged rats is associated with loss of p75-positive neurons in the basal forebrain, *Neuroscience*, 100, 363, 2000.

37. Veng, L.M., Granholm, A.C., and Rose, G.M., Age-related sex differences in spatial learning and basal forebrain cholinergic neurons in F344 rats, *Physiol. Behav.*, 80, 27, 2003.

38. Nicholson, D.A. et al., Reduction in size of perforated postsynaptic densities in hippocampal axospinous synapses and age related spatial learning impairments, *J. Neurosci.*, 24, 7648, 2004.

39. Brightwell, J.J., Gallagher, M., and Colombo, P.J., Hippocampal CREB1 but not CREB2 is decreased in aged rats with spatial memory impairments, *Neurobiol. Learn. Mem.*, 81, 19, 2004.

40. Colombo, P.J. and Gallagher, M., Individual differences in spatial memory among aged rats are related to hippocampal PKCgamma immunoreactivity, *Hippocampus*, 12, 285, 2002.

41. Rossi, M.A., Mash, D.C., and deToledo-Morrell, L., Spatial memory in aged rats is related to PKCgamma-dependent G-protein coupling of the M1 receptor, *Neurobiol. Aging*, 26, 53, 2005.
42. Adams, M.M. et al., Hippocampal dependent learning ability correlates with N-methyl-D-aspartate (NMDA) receptor levels in CA3 neurons of young and aged rats, *J. Comp. Neurol.*, 432, 230, 2001.
43. Clayton, D.A. et al., A hippocampal NR2B deficit can mimic age-related changes in long-term potentiation and spatial learning in the Fischer 344 rat, *J. Neurosci.*, 22, 3628, 2002.
44. Mesches, M.H. et al., Sulindac improves memory and increases NMDA receptor subunits in aged Fischer 344 rats, *Neurobiol. Aging*, 25, 315, 2004.
45. Smith, J.W. et al., Chronic aspirin ingestion improves spatial learning in adult and aged rats, *Pharmacol. Biochem. Behav.*, 71, 233, 2002.
46. Foster, T.C. et al., Interaction of age and chronic estradiol replacement on memory and markers of brain aging, *Neurobiol. Aging*, 24, 839, 2003.
47. Markham, J.A., Pych, J.C., and Juraska, J.M., Ovarian hormone replacement to aged ovariectomized female rats benefits acquisition of the morris water maze, *Horm. Behav.*, 42, 284, 2002.
48. Bimonte-Nelson, H.A. et al., Ovarian hormones and cognition in the aged female rat. I. Long-term, but not short-term, ovariectomy enhances spatial performance, *Behav. Neurosci.*, 117, 1395, 2003.
49. Bimonte-Nelson, H.A. et al., Ovarian hormones and cognition in the aged female rat. II. progesterone supplementation reverses the cognitive enhancing effects of ovariectomy, *Behav. Neurosci.*, 118, 707, 2004.
50. Ziegler, D.R. and Gallagher, M., Spatial memory in middle-aged female rats: assessment of estrogen replacement after ovariectomy, *Brain Res.*, 1052, 163, 2005.
51. Bimonte-Nelson, H.A. et al., Testosterone, but not nonaromatizable dihydrotestosterone, improves working memory and alters nerve growth factor levels in aged male rats, *Exp. Neurol.*, 181, 301, 2003.
52. Bizon, J.L. et al., Hypothalamic-pituitary-adrenal axis function and corticosterone receptor expression in behaviourally characterized young and aged Long-Evans rats, *Eur. J. Neurosci.*, 14, 1739, 2001.
53. Bizon, J.L., Lee, H.J., and Gallagher, M., Neurogenesis in a rat model of age-related cognitive decline, *Aging Cell*, 3, 227, 2004.
54. Drapeau, E. et al., Spatial memory performances of aged rats in the water maze predict levels of hippocampal neurogenesis, *Proc. Natl. Acad. Sci. U.S.A.*, 100, 14385, 2003.
55. Gatewood, J.D. et al., Motherhood mitigates aging-related decrements in learning and memory and positively affects brain aging in the rat, *Brain Res. Bull.*, 66, 91, 2005.
56. Lehmann, J. et al., Comparison of maternal separation and early handling in terms of their neurobehavioral effects in aged rats, *Neurobiol. Aging*, 23, 457, 2002.
57. Rosenzweig, E.S. and Barnes, C.A., Impact of aging on hippocampal function: plasticity, network dynamics, and cognition, *Prog. Neurobiol.*, 69, 143, 2003.
58. Almaguer, W. et al., Aging impairs amygdala-hippocampus interactions involved in hippocampal LTP, *Neurobiol. Aging*, 23, 319, 2002.
59. Barnes, C.A., Rao, G., and Houston, F.P., LTP induction threshold change in old rats at the perforant path-granule cell synapse, *Neurobiol. Aging*, 21, 613, 2000.
60. Schulz, D. et al., Water maze performance, exploratory activity, inhibitory avoidance and hippocampal plasticity in aged superior and inferior learners, *Eur. J. Neurosci.*, 16, 2175, 2002.

61. Schulz, D. et al., Behavioural parameters in aged rats are related to LTP and gene expression of ChAT and NMDA-NR2 subunits in the striatum, *Eur. J. Neurosci.*, 19, 1373, 2004.
62. Rosenzweig, E.S. et al., Hippocampal map realignment and spatial learning, *Nat. Neurosci.*, 6, 609, 2003.
63. Wilson, I.A. et al., Place cell rigidity correlates with impaired spatial learning in aged rats, *Neurobiol. Aging*, 24, 297, 2003.
64. Wilson, I.A. et al., Cognitive aging and the hippocampus: how old rats represent new environments, *J. Neurosci.*, 24, 3870, 2004.
65. Andres-Lacueva, C. et al., Anthocyanins in aged blueberry-fed rats are found centrally and may enhance memory, *Nutr. Neurosci.*, 8, 111, 2005.
66. Casadesus, G. et al., Modulation of hippocampal plasticity and cognitive behavior by short-term blueberry supplementation in aged rats, *Nutr. Neurosci.*, 7, 309, 2004.
67. Albeck, D.S. et al., Mild forced treadmill exercise enhances spatial learning in the aged rat, *Behav. Brain Res.*, 168, 345, 2006.
68. Bontempi, B. et al., SIB-1553A, (±)-4-[[2-(1-methyl-2-pyrrolidinyl)ethyl]thio]phenol hydrochloride, a subtype-selective ligand for nicotinic acetylcholine receptors with putative cognitive-enhancing properties: effects on working and reference memory performance in aged rodents and nonhuman primates, *J. Pharm. Exp. Ther.*, 299, 297, 2001.
69. Lazaris, A. et al., Intrastriatal infusions of methoctramine improve memory in cognitively impaired aged rats, *Neurobiol. Aging*, 24, 379, 2003.
70. Rowe, W.B. et al., Long-term effects of BIBN-99, a selective muscarinic M2 receptor antagonist, on improving spatial memory performance in aged cognitively impaired rats, *Behav. Brain Res.*, 145, 171, 2003.
71. Chopin, P., Colpaert, F.C., and Marien, M., Effects of acute and subchronic administration of dexefaroxan, an alpha(2)-adrenoceptor antagonist, on memory performance in young adult and aged rodents, *J. Pharmacol. Exp. Ther.*, 301, 187, 2002.
72. Ramos, B.P. et al., The beta-1 adrenergic antagonist, betaxolol, improves working memory performance in rats and monkeys, *Biol. Psychiatry*, 58, 894, 2005.
73. Kiray, M. et al., Positive effects of deprenyl and estradiol on spatial memory and oxidant stress in aged female rat brains, *Neurosci. Lett.*, 354, 225, 2004.
74. Kiray, M. et al., Deprenyl and the relationship between its effects on spatial memory, oxidant stress and hippocampal neurons in aged male rats, *Physiol. Res.*, 55, 205, 2005.
75. Yau, J.L., Hibberd, C., Noble, J., and Seckl, J.R., The effect of chronic fluoxetine treatment on brain corticosteroid receptor mRNA expression and spatial memory in young and aged rats, *Brain Res. Mol. Brain Res.*, 106, 117, 2002.
76. Hernandez, C.M. et al., Comparison of galantamine and donepezil for effects on nerve growth factor, cholinergic markers, and memory performance in aged rats, *J. Pharmacol. Exp. Ther.*, 316, 679, 2006.
77. Aura, J. and Riekkinen, P., Jr., Pre-training blocks the improving effect of tetrahydroaminoacridine and D-cycloserine on spatial navigation performance in aged rats, *Eur. J. Pharmacol.*, 390, 313, 2000.
78. Foley, A.G. et al., The 5-HT(6) receptor antagonist SB-271046 reverses scopolamine-disrupted consolidation of a passive avoidance task and ameliorates spatial task deficits in aged rats, *Neuropsychopharmacology*, 29, 93, 2004.
79. Froestl, W. et al., SGS742: the first GABA(B) receptor antagonist in clinical trials, *Biochem. Pharmacol.*, 68, 1479, 2004.

80. Blank, T. et al., Small-conductance, Ca2+-activated K+ channel SK3 generates age-related memory and LTP deficits, *Nat. Neurosci.*, 6, 911, 2003.

81. McEchron, M.D., Cheng, A.Y., and Gilmartin, M.R., Trace fear conditioning is reduced in the aging rat, *Neurobiol. Learn. Mem.*, 82, 71, 2004.

82. Villarreal, J.S., Dykes, J.R., and Barea-Rodriguez, E.J., Fischer 344 rats display age-related memory deficits in trace fear conditioning, *Behav. Neurosci.*, 118, 1166, 2004.

83. Gale, G.D. et al., Role of the basolateral amygdala in the storage of fear memories across the adult lifetime of rats, *J. Neurosci.*, 24, 3810, 2004.

84. Doyere, V. et al., Age-related modifications of contextual information processing in rats: role of emotional reactivity, arousal and testing procedure, *Behav. Brain Res.*, 114, 153, 2000.

85. Monti, B., Berteotti, C., and Contestabile, A., Dysregulation of memory-related proteins in the hippocampus of aged rats and their relation with cognitive impairment, *Hippocampus*, 15, 1041, 2005.

86. Kasckow, J.W. et al., Stability of neuroendocrine and behavioral responsiveness in aging Fischer 344/Brown-Norway hybrid rats, *Endocrinology*, 146, 3105, 2005.

87. Barrientos, R.M. et al., Peripheral infection and aging interact to impair hippocampal memory consolidation, *Neurobiol. Aging*, 27, 723, 2006.

88. Gould, T.J. and Feiro, O.R., Age-related deficits in the retention of memories for cued fear conditioning are reversed by galantamine treatment, *Behav. Brain Res.*, 165, 160, 2005.

89. Feiro, O. and Gould, T.J., The interactive effects of nicotinic and muscarinic cholinergic receptor inhibition on fear conditioning in young and aged C57BL/6 mice, *Pharmacol. Biochem. Behav.*, 80, 251, 2005.

90. Caldarone, B.J., Duman, C.H., and Picciotto, M.R., Fear conditioning and latent inhibition in mice lacking the high affinity subclass of nicotinic acetylcholine receptors in the brain, *Neuropharmacology*, 39, 2779, 2000.

91. Quinn, J.F. et al., Chronic dietary alpha-lipoic acid reduces deficits in hippocampal memory of aged Tg2576 mice, *Neurobiol. Aging*, 28(2), 213–225, 2007.

92. Gemma, C. et al., Improvement of memory for context by inhibition of caspase-1 in aged rats, *Eur. J. Neurosci.*, 22, 1751, 2005.

93. Weiss, C. and Thompson, R.F., The effects of age on eyeblink conditioning in the freely moving Fischer-344 rat, *Neurobiol. Aging*, 12, 249, 1991.

94. Weiss, C. and Thompson, R. F., Delayed acquisition of eyeblink conditioning in aged F1 hybrid (Fischer-344 x Brown Norway) rats, *Neurobiol. Aging*, 13, 319, 1992.

95. Vogel, R.W. et al., Age-related impairment in the 250-millisecond delay eyeblink classical conditioning procedure in C57BL/6 mice, *Learn. Mem.*, 9, 321, 2002.

96. Muir, J.L., Fischer, W., and Björklund, A., Decline in visual attention and spatial memory in aged rats, *Neurobiol. Aging*, 20, 605, 1999.

97. Grottick, A.J. and Higgins, G.A., Assessing a vigilance decrement in aged rats: effects of pre-feeding, task manipulation, and psychostimulants, *Psychopharmacology (Berl)*, 164, 33, 2002.

98. Rodefer, J.S. and Nguyen, T.N., Naltrexone reverses age-induced cognitive deficits in rats, *Neurobiol. Aging*, in press, 2007.

99. Schoenbaum, G. et al., Teaching old rats new tricks: age-related impairments in olfactory reversal learning, *Neurobiol. Aging*, 23, 555, 2002.

100. Olton, D.S., Age-related behavioral impairments: benefits of multiple measures of performance, *Neurobiol. Aging*, 14, 637, 1993.

Section II

Quantifying Aging-Related Changes in the Brain

4 Design-Based Stereology in Brain Aging Research

Christoph Schmitz and Patrick R. Hof

CONTENTS

I.   INTRODUCTION

In recent years, the application of design-based stereologic methods to the analysis of the central nervous system has contributed considerably to our understanding of the functional and pathological morphology of the aging brain. Design-based stereology has become the method of choice in quantitative histological analysis. Its advantages over other quantitative techniques in respect to rigor, accuracy, and consistency of results have been documented extensively in the scientific literature.

Originally, design-based stereology was described as a set of methods that provide a three-dimensional interpretation of structures based on observations made on two-dimensional sections [1]. However, in the current use of design-based stereology, many methods make use of three-dimensional sections. The term "design-based" indicates that the methods and the sampling schemes that define the newer methods in stereology are "designed," that is, defined *a priori*, in such a manner that one need not take into consideration the size, shape, spatial orientation, and spatial distribution of the cells to be investigated [2]. Eliminating the need for information about the geometry of the cells under investigation results in more robust data because potential sources of systematic errors in the calculations are eliminated [2–4].

Design-based stereology can be divided into analyses of the global and local characteristics of tissues, the most important of which are volume, number, connectivity, spatial distribution, and length of linear biological structures. These characteristics can be expressed as absolute values (e.g., the volume of the granule cell layer in the human hippocampus, the number of granule cells in the human hippocampal granule cell layer, etc.) or as relative values (e.g., the volume fraction of the human hippocampus occupied by the granule cell layer, the density of granule cells within the human hippocampal granule cell layer, etc.). Both global and local characteristics can be analyzed by a variety of stereologic methods.

This chapter is divided into three parts. The first part provides an overview of recent progress in brain aging research on humans, non-human primates, and rodents with design-based stereology and reviews the main outcome of such investigations. The second part of the chapter provides an introduction into the use of design-based stereologic methods that most neuroscientists interested in their use would need to analyze volumes of brain regions, numbers of cells (neurons, glial cells) within these brain regions, mean volumes (nuclear, perikaryal) of these cells, length densities of linear biological structures such as vessels and nerve fibers, and the cytoarchitecture of brain regions (i.e., the spatial distribution of cells within a region of interest). The chapter closes with a short outlook on the future of design-based stereology in brain aging research.

II.   RECENT PROGRESS IN BRAIN AGING RESEARCH
WITH DESIGN-BASED STEREOLOGY

The application of design-based stereologic methods to the analysis of the central nervous system has considerably contributed to our understanding of the functional and pathological morphology of the aging brain. The main outcome of such investigations revealed first that there is no substantial global neuron or synapse loss in the aging brain, as previously thought [1, 5]. Rather, certain brain regions show a regionally specific loss of neurons and synapses during aging, and various types of neurons change their gene expression profiles during aging ("functional loss"). Second, the patterns of age-related neuron loss in nonhuman primates and rodents are not entirely comparable to those seen in the human brain, which should be considered when using animal models of brain aging. Third, neuron and synapse loss observed in pathological conditions such as Alzheimer's disease seem to be the result of the disease process but not a consequence of normal aging. It should also be noted that design-based stereologic studies in brain aging research are always performed on postmortem autopsy tissue. Accordingly, all findings discussed in the following represent results from cross-sectional studies rather than longitudinal studies.

A. DESIGN-BASED STEREOLOGIC ANALYSES OF THE AGING HUMAN BRAIN

Pakkenberg and Gundersen [6] performed the most comprehensive investigation of age-related alterations in the total number of neurons in the human cerebral cortex. Analyzing 94 brains covering the age range from 20 to 90 years, they found an average total number of 23 billion neocortical neurons in male brains (and 19 billion in female brains). Only approximately 10% of all neocortical neurons were lost over the lifespan in both sexes. In a follow-up study, total numbers of glial cells in the neocortex were compared between six aged individuals (age range 81 to 98 years) and six young individuals (age range 18 to 35 years) [7]). No differences between the groups were found (36 billion vs. 39 billion glial cells).

These reports of only minor alterations in global neuron and glial cell numbers are in contrast with reports of regional neuron loss in the aging human cerebral cortex. Kordower and colleagues [8] found on average an approximately 40% loss of layer II entorhinal cortex neurons and an approximately 25% loss of perikaryal volume of these neurons in the brains of individuals with mild cognitive impairment (but no Alzheimer's disease), compared with individuals with no cognitive impairment. Both loss and atrophy of layer II entorhinal cortex neurons significantly correlated with performance on clinical tests of declarative memory. Age-related loss of layer II entorhinal cortex neurons in neurologically normal subjects was recently confirmed in an independent sample [9], whereas earlier studies found no age-related loss of these cells in cognitively normal individuals [10, 11].

According to West [12], the human hippocampus also shows a regionally specific pattern of age-related neuron loss across the age range of 13 to 85 years, with substantial loss of neurons in the subiculum (52%) and the hilus of the dentate gyrus (31%) but no significant changes in the remaining hippocampal subdivisions. This specific loss of neurons in the hippocampus and the entorhinal cortex may qualify as a morphological correlate of senescent decline in memory in that they can be expected to compromise the functional integrity of brain regions known to be intimately involved in memory processing.

Concerning synapse loss in the aging human cerebral cortex, Scheff and colleagues [13] found that the synaptic volume density in lamina III and V of the superior-middle frontal cortex did not correlate with age in a sample of 37 cognitively normal individuals ranging in age from 20 to 89 years. Corresponding data for the hippocampus have not been published. On the other hand, there seems to occur a 30 to 40% reduction in the total length of myelinated fibers within the white matter of the human brain, with a particular decline of myelinated fibers with the smallest diameter [14, 15].

The human locus coeruleus does not show age-related loss of neurons [16, 17], and in the cerebellum, substantial loss of Purkinje and granule cells during aging was only observed in the anterior lobe (approximately 40% [18]). In the substantia nigra, conflicting data have been reported, of either no age-related loss of melanin-containing neurons [19] or an approximately 40% loss of these neurons during aging [20, 21]. Nevertheless, the well-established decrease in dopaminergic nigrostriatal function with age seems to be related to phenotypic age-related changes (functional loss) rather than to frank neuronal degeneration. This is supported by reports of dramatic age-related loss of neurons immunoreactive for tyrosine hydroxylase (on average, approximately 45% [19]), the dopamine transporter (on average, approximately 75% [20]), guanosine triphosphate cyclohydrolase I (a critical enzyme in catecholamine function, on average approximately 80% [22]), and nuclear receptor-related factor 1 (associated with the induction of dopaminergic phenotypes in developing and mature midbrain neurons, on average approximately 45% [22]). A similar situation was reported for the human basal forebrain, with a dramatic age-related loss of approximately 60% of neurons expressing the calcium-binding protein calbindin [23], without concomitant loss of neurons immunoreactive for choline acetyltransferase [23, 24], low-affinity nerve growth factor receptor (p75[NTR]) [23]), or vesicular acetylcholine transporter [24].

B.   DESIGN-BASED STEREOLOGIC ANALYSES OF THE BRAIN OF NONHUMAN PRIMATES AND RODENTS

The patterns of age-related neuron loss (including functional loss) in the brain of nonhuman primates and rodents are not identical to that in the human brain and conflicting data have been reported. For example, similar to humans, mice do not show age-related reductions in global cortical neuron number [25]; however, unlike in humans, preserved numbers of entorhinal cortex neurons have been reported in old rhesus monkeys (considered the best, commonly available model of aging in humans) and in old rats [26–28]. Rhesus monkeys showed no age-related alterations in numbers of Nissl-stained neurons, neurofilament protein-containing layer IVB cells, or Meynert cells in the primary visual cortex (area V1) [29, 30]. On the other hand, an age-related loss of about 30% of neurons in cortical area 8A was reported in rhesus monkeys, with no concomitant neuron loss in area 46 [31].

Basal forebrain cholinergic neurons projecting to area 8A were also reduced by approximately 50% during aging in rhesus monkeys, whereas corresponding neurons projecting to area 46 were not [31]. Smith and colleagues [32] reported an approximately 45% loss of cholinergic neurons in the intermediate division of the Ch4 region of the basal forebrain in old rhesus monkeys that was reversible by growth factor gene therapy. Also, Wu et al. [33] found, similar to humans, an age-related loss of approximately 50% of neurons immunoreactive for calbindin without concomitant loss of neurons immunoreactive for choline acetyltransferase or high- and low-affinity neurotrophin receptors in the common marmoset (*Callithrix jacchus*). No age-related alterations in the number of basal forebrain cholinergic neurons were found in the mouse brain [25], whereas a 30% decrease in both cholinergic and total neuron number was detected in the horizontal limb/nucleus basalis of aged rats [34].

Similar to humans, rhesus monkeys, tree shrews, rats, and mice showed no age-related loss of neurons in the hippocampal dentate gyrus and in the CA1-CA3 fields [35–40]. However, unlike in humans, neither rhesus monkeys nor rodents displayed age-related loss of neurons in the subiculum, the hilus of the dentate gyrus, and the parahippocampal region [37, 41]. No age-related loss of synapses was found in the supragranular layer of the dentate gyrus of rhesus monkeys [42] and in the CA1 stratum radiatum in rats [43], whereas aging mice showed an average 20% loss of synaptophysin-immunoreactive presynaptic boutons in the molecular layer of the dentate gyrus [44]. Aging rats showed a significant 15% decline in neurons immunoreactive for the 67-kDa isoform of glutamic acid decarboxylase in area CA1 but not in dentate gyrus or area CA3 [45], and a conserved number of glucocorticoid receptor-immunoreactive neurons in area CA1/2 [46]. Aged female mice displayed an average 20% increase in the numbers of astrocytes and microglial cells in the dentate gyrus and area CA1 [47], whereas male mice did not [48].

Conflicting data also exist concerning age-related alterations in the substantia nigra of nonhuman primates. The total number of neurons in the substantia nigra was found to be either conserved [49] or reduced [50] in old rhesus monkeys, and conserved in old squirrel monkeys [51]. On the other hand, as in humans, all studies performed thus far on monkeys found an age-related reduction in the number of tyrosine hydroxylase-immunoreactive neurons in the substantia nigra [51, 52]. The finding of an age-related increase in neuromelanin-containing neurons in the substantia nigra of both squirrel monkeys [51] and rhesus monkeys [49], however, does not match the situation reported in elderly humans [19–21].

In the cerebellum, conserved numbers of Purkinje and granule cells were found in lobule IV, VII, and X of the vermis of aged rats [53]. In contrast, an age-related decline of approximately 25% in the total number of cerebellar Purkinje cells was reported in mice, without concomitant loss of cerebellar granule cells [38]. Neurons in the fifth cervical and fourth lumbar dorsal root ganglion were found to be preserved but showed an approximately 15% reduction in their mean cross-sectional area [54].

Recently, the nature and effects of brain microvascular pathology in aging and Alzheimer's disease have become a main focus of interest in brain aging research [55, 56]. In this regard, a study by Villena and co-workers [57] should be mentioned, which appears thus far to be the only design-based stereologic study performed on capillary networks in normal aging. The authors investigated the dorsal lateral geniculate nucleus of aging rats and found an increase in mean values of capillary profile density, capillary volume fraction, length and surface area per unit volume, and capillary average diameter between 3 and 18 months of age, and a significant decrease in mean capillary volume fraction (−18.75%) and mean capillary average diameter (−5.5%) between 18 and 24 months.

C.   DESIGN-BASED STEREOLOGIC ANALYSES OF THE BRAIN IN ALZHEIMER'S DISEASE

In Alzheimer's disease (AD) research, three main questions have been addressed with design-based stereologic methods: (1) Is the pattern of neuron loss in AD similar to the pattern of neuron loss in normal aging? (2) Which of the neuropathological hallmarks of AD (formation of plaques, neurofibrillary tangles, and neuron loss) correlates best with the cognitive status of the patients? (3) What are the interactions between the neuropathological hallmarks of AD? Several design-based stereologic studies focusing on the hippocampus in AD showed (unlike in normal aging) substantial neuron loss in area CA1 [11, 58–60]. This selective neuron loss was preceded by plaque formation in preclinical AD, a period during which there are abundant amyloid deposits in the brain but no evidence of cognitive decline [58]. The number of Nissl stained neurons plus the number of extracellular tangles in severe cases of AD was only approximately 70% of the number of Nissl stained neurons in unaffected controls in area CA1 of the hippocampus, indicating that a substantial number of CA1 neurons died in AD without the formation of NFT [59]. This situation was different from the situation in cortex area 9 (outlined below) [61]. Furthermore, evidence was found that dementia in extreme aging depended more on the damage of hippocampal subdivisions commonly less affected in AD than on severe NFT formation and neuron loss in area CA1 and entorhinal cortex [62].

In the entorhinal cortex of AD patients with severe cognitive impairment a dramatic loss of approximately 90% of layer II neurons (and approximately 70% of layer IV neurons, respectively) was found [10]. Entorhinal neuron loss positively correlated with the Clinical Dementia Rating score of the individuals, as well as with the formation of neurofibrillary tangles (NFT) and neuritic plaques, but was not related to diffuse plaques or total plaques [10]. The latter result was in contrast to a study by Bussière and colleagues [63], who estimated the total volume occupied by amyloid deposits in the entorhinal cortex and subiculum as an effective predictor of dementia severity. In a detailed follow-up study, however, Giannakopoulos et al. [64] demonstrated that NFT counts in the entorhinal cortex and prefrontal cortex area 9 and neuron numbers in the CA1 field of the hippocampus were the best predictors of the Mini-Mental State Examination score of the patients. The authors could also show that high total NFT counts, but not amyloid volume, were strongly associated with a lower number of unaffected neurons in the CA1 field of the hippocampus, entorhinal cortex, and prefrontal cortex area 9, indicating that the formation of plaques is not the primary cause of neuron loss in AD. Furthermore, Bussière et al. [61] demonstrated that in prefrontal cortex area 9, a substantial number of pyramidal cells persisted either unaffected or in a transitional stage of NFT formation in severe cases of AD. These results suggested that certain affected neurons might respond positively to therapeutic strategies aimed at protecting the cells that are prone to neurofibrillary degeneration in AD.

Design-based stereologic investigations into alterations of capillary networks in AD were only reported in a study by Bouras and colleagues [65]. The authors measured total capillary lengths and numbers, as well as mean length-weighted diameters, total NFT and neuron numbers, and amyloid volume in entorhinal cortex and area CA1 of the hippocampus in 19 very old individuals with variable degrees of cognitive decline. This study found that the total capillary length and capillary segment numbers in hippocampus and entorhinal cortex did not predict the cognitive status of the cases. However, the mean capillary diameter in these regions was correlated to clinical dementia rating scores, independently of other pathologic lesions such as NFT. This suggests that changes in some capillary morphometric parameters are independent predictors of AD-related neuron loss and cognitive decline.

Various transgenic animal models of AD have been investigated with design-based stereologic methods. However, age-related hippocampal neuron loss was found only in mice overexpressing both human mutated APP751 (carrying the Swedish and London mutations KM670/671NL and V717I) and human mutated presenilin-1 (PS-1 M146L) [66], and in mice carrying knocked-in mutations in PS-1 (M233T and L235P) and overexpressing human mutated APP (KM670/671NL and V717I) [67]. Similar to the situation in the human brain, both animal models showed no correlation between the amount of neuron loss and the formation of plaques. On the other hand, neither model developed NFT, indicating other factors than plaque and NFT formation in neuron loss in AD. The mice overexpressing both human mutated APP751 and human mutated PS-1 also showed a complex pattern of age-related reductions in the numbers of synaptophysin-immunoreactive presynaptic boutons in various subregions of the hippocampus [44]. For a comprehensive overview of investigations into synapse and neuron loss in transgenic mouse models of AD, see [68].

III. DESIGN-BASED STEREOLOGIC METHODS FOR BRAIN AGING RESEARCH

A. How to Obtain Rigorous Results in Brain Aging Research with Design-Based Stereology

Design-based stereologic methods have been developed to make valid statements about a brain region of interest (ROI), or a population of cells or linear biological structures within the ROI. Many studies state that the presented results are unbiased (i.e., without systematic error) because they are based on the use of design-based stereology. However, the use of design based stereology does not guarantee unbiasedness of the corresponding estimates per se [69]. Rather, a number of prerequisites must be met to eliminate (or at least minimize) bias in design-based stereologic analyses. First, one needs access to the entire ROI. In design-based stereology, this is achieved by systematic-random sampling of sections from exhaustive section series encompassing the entire ROI [70, 71]. Second, the entire ROI (or objects to be counted within it) must be recognizable by an appropriate (i.e., sensitive and specific) stain or marker. Third, all parts of the ROI must have the same chance to contribute to the sampling. This is achieved by selecting microscopic fields on the sampled sections in a systematic-random manner (see next subsection). Finally, the estimates must be independent of the size, shape, spatial orientation, and spatial distribution of the objects within the ROI. This is achieved by the three-dimensional design of almost all probes described in the next subsection. This, however, requires the use of thick (i.e., 3D) sections instead of thin (2D) sections [72–78].

Prior to preparing such 3D sections, which can be as thick as 500 μm when investigating the human brain [79], there are a number of issues to be considered. First, different fixation and embedding protocols can result in very different tissue shrinkage [72, 80–82]. Thus, estimates of the volume of brain regions or cells (but also length estimates, investigations on neuron density, and analyses of the spatial distribution of cells) will depend on the protocols used, and comparisons among groups should be restricted to materials processed under identical conditions. In contrast, estimates of total numbers of cells performed with design-based stereology are not affected by tissue shrinkage during fixation and embedding. Second, methacrylate and paraffin embedding may cause inhomogeneous compression of tissue sections along the z-axis during cutting of the tissue, which can result in differences in particle densities along this axis [74, 78, 83]. Third, the estimates must be affected neither by loss of structures at the upper or the lower surface of the sections when hit by the knife during cutting the tissue, nor by incomplete staining of the tissue. The latter problem may occur particularly in the middle of the section thickness when analyzing sections processed with immunohistochemistry. In this case, incomplete antibody penetration can be minimized by free-floating staining procedures. Fourth, irrespective of the embedding medium and the cutting and staining procedures, one has to consider shrinkage of the sections along the z-axis [72, 75, 84]. This shrinkage may be surprisingly high [77] and may vary from one part of a section to another. Measurements of the section thickness (preferably for each investigated microscopic field) with the z-axis position encoder of a computer-controlled, semiautomated stereology system (described in the next subsection) can give reasonably accurate readings of the formal section thickness. However, this depends on adequate staining of the entire section thickness, the use of an oil objective for the measurements, Köhler illumination, and an appropriately opened condenser. Correction for actual section thickness is crucial, particularly for estimates of the volume of brain regions, investigations of total numbers of neurons, and analyses of the spatial distribution of cells.

B.   DEFINING THE BORDERS OF A BRAIN REGION

Design-based stereologic investigations usually begin with the identification of the boundaries of the ROI on a systematic-random series of sections (Figure 4.1a). Estimates of the volume of the selected ROI or the number of cells within this ROI depend on the delineation criteria, which may or may not be easily identifiable. For example, the boundaries between the white matter and the granule and pyramidal cell layers in the mouse hippocampus can easily be identified on Nissl-stained sections, but in many cases, the delineation may be more difficult. For example, the cerebellar Purkinje cell layer is of particular interest in aging research because Purkinje cells are known to be lost during aging in both rodents and primates [38, 85]. On the other hand, it is virtually impossible to delineate exactly the Purkinje cell layer. To circumvent this problem, a first step can be only a rough delineation of the ROI at low magnification, including the entire ROI in the traced area (i.e., the entire cerebellum). Then, at a higher magnification, the traced area can be scanned systematically and investigated only within those microscopic fields that belong to the ROI (e.g., only those microscopic fields showing the boundary between the molecular layer and the granule cell layer in the cerebellum, where the Purkinje cell layer is situated).

The most challenging issue is to identify reliably cortical areas in the human brain. Cortical areas are delineated by the pial surface, the cortex-white matter transition, and their borders with neighboring areas. Defining the pial surface and the cortex-white matter border is usually not a problem on histological sections. However, the crucial step in identifying a cortical area is the localization of its borders with neighboring areas. In this respect, a cortical area is defined as a cortical tissue volume characterized by a homogeneous microstructural organization (i.e., by its cytoarchitecture). Thus, a regional border must be established at locations where the cytoarchitecture of the cortex changes considerably. All classical anatomical maps of the primate cerebral cortex (including human) are based on this axiom, but they suffer from several limitations. In particular, these maps do not reflect intersubject variability in the size of cortical areas and the location of their borders [86], although several cytoarchitectural studies have indicated the existence of a considerable degree of intersubject variability [87–90]. In addition, these "classical" cortical maps are usually two-dimensional, highly schematic drawings, which do not provide the information necessary for correlations with recently developed functional imaging techniques in the living human brain. Finally, there are striking differences between the maps of different authors in terms of the number, localization, extent, and contour of cortical areas (see [91]).

Macroscopic landmarks such as sulcal and gyral patterns of the cortical surface are rarely useful to identify reliably borders of cortical areas because cytoarchitectural borders among areas do not coincide consistently with sulcal fundi or other macroscopic landmarks [89, 92].

Consequently, the definition of borders of cortical areas in the human brain should be performed in each individual brain using a standardized, reproducible, and statistically testable observer-independent method. One possibility to achieve this is using the so-called "grey level index" (GLI) method, extensively reviewed in [93–95]. Another option is to elucidate regional characteristics and boundaries of cortical areas with a chemoarchitectural approach, that is, making use of differences in the regional distribution of certain subsets of neurons [61, 90, 96–103].

In summary, there are many possibilities for the identification of boundaries of the ROI in design-based stereologic studies. Accordingly, each design-based stereologic study should provide a description of the methods selected to identify these boundaries, and a discussion of the extent to which the obtained results depend on the delineation criteria.

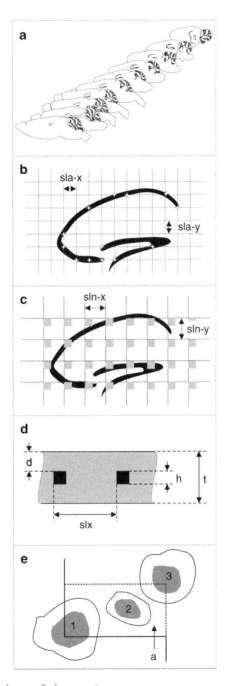

FIGURE 4.1 (see caption on facing page)

C. Estimating the Volume of a Brain Region

Estimates of the volume of a ROI can be performed with Cavalieri's principle [104] from the profile areas of the cut sections of the ROI (Figure 4.2). An initial random cut through the ROI is required, with subsequent cuts at regular intervals. Provided the sections through the ROI are systematic-random, (i.e., taken at consistent intervals with an equal probability of being sampled), Cavalieri's principle yields an unbiased estimate of the volume of the ROI by multiplying the sum of the profile areas of the ROI on all sections by the distance between them.

The profile areas of the sections through the ROI can be measured by tracing the boundaries of the ROI on video images displayed on a computer, and letting the software calculate the profile area, or by using point counting on a randomly placed rectangular lattice of known side lengths on the surface of a section and counting the intersections of the lattice with the ROI (Figure 4.1b). Provided the position of the lattice on the ROI is random (i.e., all parts of the region have an equal probability of being hit by the lattice), this method gives an unbiased estimate of the profile area of this region by multiplying the sum of the counted intersections (or points) with the uniform area, determined by the side lengths of the lattice, represented by each intersection (or point) [71].

Estimates of the volume of an ROI with Cavalieri's principle can be biased when investigating thick sections under the microscope [71, 105]. This potential bias can be nearly eliminated if the ROI is cut into an exhaustive series of sections of uniform thickness, a systematic-random series of these sections with a random start is selected

FIGURE 4.1 Estimating the volume of a brain region and the total number of neurons within it with design-based stereology. The procedure is shown for the pyramidal and granule cell layers of the rat hippocampus as practical illustrations: (a) a systematic random series of sections through the entire region of interest is selected, with a different random start for each brain (e.g., every sixth section: sections no. 3, 9, …); (b) the projection areas (i.e., the cross-sectional areas) of the hippocampus cell layers are estimated by randomly placing a rectangular lattice with side lengths sla-x and sla-y on the surface of a section. Then the intersections of the lattice and the cell layers are counted (arrows). (c to e) The total number of neurons within the cell layers is determined by randomly placing a rectangular lattice with side lengths sln-x and sln-y on the surface of a section. This lattice determines the positions of unbiased virtual counting spaces (gray squares in c; black squares in d) with base area a (unbiased counting frame; shown in e) and height h at a depth d within a section with thickness t. Neurons are counted if they come into focus within h and if they are found within the unbiased counting frame (neuron 2 in e). Neurons are also counted if they hit the inclusion lines (dashed lines and neuron 3 in e) but not the exclusion lines (solid lines and neuron 1 in e) of an unbiased counting frame. Alternatively, one can define a unique, punctate identifier for each neuron (e.g., the midpoint of the nucleus or the nucleolus, the top of the nucleus, known as the characteristic point; [108]), and count all punctate identifiers positioned within the unbiased virtual counting spaces spread over the regions of interest.

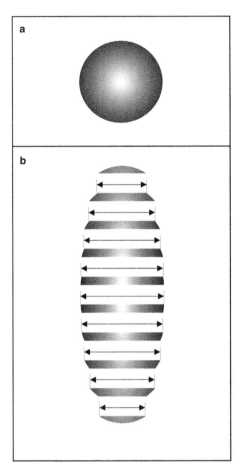

FIGURE 4.2 Estimating the volume of a brain region with Cavalieri's principle: (a) schematic drawing of a spherical brain region; (b) after cutting the brain region into an exhaustive series of sections of uniform thickness, the top profile area of each (or every nth) section is measured (arrows). To obtain an unbiased estimate of the volume of this brain region one has to multiply the sum of the profile areas of the brain region on all sections by the (uniform) section thickness. In the example shown here, the first section of this brain region (shown on top in b) is not considered for the analysis. This is due to the fact that it does not show a top profile area.

for analysis, and the analysis is performed using objectives with short depth of focus, under Köhler illumination, and open condenser. The variability of estimates of the volume of an ROI with Cavalieri's principle depends on the number of analyzed sections and, if point counting is used, the distance between the points [71, 106, 107].

D. DETERMINING THE NUMBER OF CELLS WITHIN A GIVEN TISSUE VOLUME

Estimating the number of cells by microscopic inspection of series of sections leads to the problem that cutting a given tissue volume into sections results in cutting the cells within this tissue and, therefore, the number of cell fragments in the sections differs from the number of cells within the tissue. In consequence, estimates of cell numbers based solely on counts of cell fragments in sections are biased (Figure 4.3). In design-based stereology, this problem is solved by counting a cell only if its "characteristic point" [108] is found within an "unbiased virtual counting space" [109, 110] (usually referred to as "optical disector" [3, 84, 111] or "counting box" [112]) placed within the section. This characteristic point can be the top of the nucleus, the top of the nucleolus, or any other (zero-dimensional) point that can be registered at only one position in space. The practical implementation of this procedure is shown in Figure 4.4. At each investigated microscopic field, an "unbiased counting frame" [113] is placed on the section. A cell is counted only if its characteristic point is both found within the unbiased counting frame (defining the base area of the unbiased virtual counting space) and comes into focus within a certain thickness of the section (defining the height of the unbiased virtual counting space). Cell counts carried out with unbiased virtual counting spaces are unbiased in that they are not influenced by the size, shape, spatial orientation, or spatial distribution of the cells under study.

There are two potential sources of bias in cell counts with unbiased virtual counting spaces. The first one may arise from loss of nucleoli or neurons at the upper or the lower surface of sections when hit by the knife during sectioning of the tissue ("lost caps"; [114]). Lost caps can be prevented using adequate histologic techniques [77]. Nevertheless, it is recommended to always place the upper surface of the unbiased virtual counting spaces a few micrometers below the upper surface of the sections, and the lower surface of the unbiased virtual counting spaces a few micrometers above the lower surface of the sections (i.e., introducing "guard zones"; see Figure 4.1d). This also helps to prevent potential bias in cell number estimates by uneven or wavy surfaces of the sections. The second potential source of bias is incomplete staining of the tissue, particularly in the middle of the section thickness. This problem may particularly arise when using immunohistochemical preparations (see, e.g., [115]). Therefore, it is always recommended first to carry out a small pilot study on the sections prior to design-based stereologic analysis, to figure out the thickness of the sections showing adequate staining. Then, the height of the unbiased virtual counting spaces (h in Figure 4.1d) is adjusted appropriately.

It should be mentioned that certain conditions such as design based stereologic applications in electron microscopy might prevent the use of thick sections and unbiased virtual counting spaces. In these situations, one can investigate two thin (2D) adjacent sections (the "disector"; [116]) which, however, prevents the use of characteristic points identifying the cells under study. Rather, a cell is then counted only if it is located within the unbiased counting frame and is not touching its exclusion lines (see Figure 4.1e), or if it is outside the counting frame and hits an inclusion line of the frame (see Figure 4.1e). Furthermore, the cell is counted only

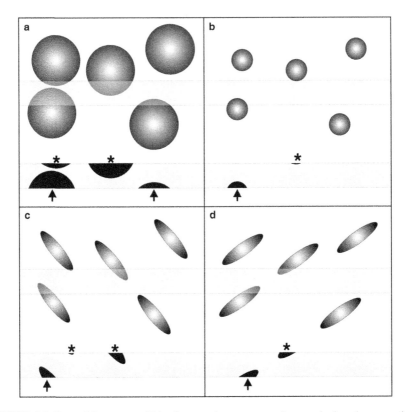

FIGURE 4.3 Potential sources of bias in counting neurons when analyzing tissue sections. Note that all examples shown here comprise the same number and density of neurons (gray elements). Also, when focusing on the midpoints of the neurons, the spatial distribution of these neurons is the same in all cases. The difference between (a) and (b) is the size of the neurons, whereas the difference between (c) and (d) is the spatial orientation of the neurons. A virtual section through the tissue is indicated by a gray bar at the bottom of each example. Neuron fragments at the upper surface of the section are indicated by asterisks, and neurons fragments at the lower surface of the section are indicated by arrows. One could count all neuron fragments, and the result would be 4 counted neuron fragments in (a), 2 in (b), 3 in (c), and 2 in (d). Alternatively, one could count only those neuron fragments found at the upper surface of the section, resulting in 2 in (a), 1 in (b), 2 in (c), and 1 in (d). One could also count only fragments at the lower surface of the section, yielding 2 in (a), and 1 each in (b), (c), and (d). Accordingly, estimates of neuron numbers within a given tissue volume based solely on counts of neuron fragments in the sections might not represent the true number of neurons within this tissue volume.

if it appears in the lower section but not in the upper section (or vice versa). When using the disector, one has to make sure that the distance in the z-direction between the sections is smaller than the smallest z-axis height of the cells under study, taking into account any kind of z-axis compression or shrinkage of the tissue as a result of histologic processing. Otherwise, cells could be positioned between the sections and would not be registered, introducing bias to the cell counts. From the practical use of the disector, it is generally valid that the distance between the sections should be one third of the smallest z-axis height of the cells under study, which can be established by a small pilot study.

E. DETERMINING THE TOTAL NUMBER OF NEURONS WITHIN A GIVEN BRAIN REGION

In design-based stereology it is not necessary to count all neurons to analyze the total number of neurons within a given ROI. Rather, one can select a proper sample of unbiased virtual counting spaces to be investigated and derive an estimated total number of neurons within the ROI from the number of neurons in the sample and the sampling probability. This is illustrated (for a single section) in Figure 4.1. Unbiased virtual counting spaces are placed in a systematic and random manner within a series of systematically and randomly sampled sections throughout the ROI (Figures 4.1a and c) and neurons are counted with unbiased virtual counting spaces (Figures 4.1d and e) or with the disector (as discussed above).

Estimated total numbers of neurons within a given ROI can be obtained in two ways. One possibility is to determine the mean neuron density within all investigated unbiased virtual counting spaces (N_V) and multiply this average neuron density by the global volume of the investigated ROI (V_{Ref}; estimated with Cavalieri's principle as explained above) ("$V_{Ref} \times N_V$" method; [117]). Alternatively, one can multiply the number of neurons counted within all unbiased virtual counting spaces with the reciprocal value of the sampling probability ("fractionator" method; [84]). The sampling probability depends on the following three fractions: (1) the "section sampling fraction" (i.e., the number of investigated sections compared to the total number of sections), (2) the "area sampling fraction" (i.e., the base area of the unbiased virtual counting spaces [a in Figure 4.1e] compared to the product of the side lengths of the rectangular lattice used for placing the unbiased counting frames within the sections [$sln\text{-}x \times sln\text{-}y$ in Figure 4.1c]), and (3) the "thickness sampling fraction" (i.e., the height of the unbiased virtual counting spaces [h in Figure 4.1d] compared to the average section thickness after histologic processing [t in Figure 4.1d]).

The advantage of the fractionator method over the $V_{Ref} \times N_V$ method is that it does not require estimates of the global volume of the ROI. Thus, estimating the total number of neurons within a given ROI with the fractionator method is (from an economical point of view) more efficient than doing the same with the $V_{Ref} \times N_V$ method. Interestingly, estimated total numbers of neurons obtained with the fractionator method are also more precise (i.e., from a statistical point of view more efficient) than corresponding estimates obtained with the $V_{Ref} \times N_V$ method [110].

The variability of estimated total numbers of neurons within a given brain region obtained with the fractionator method or the $V_{Ref} \times N_V$ method depends on the number of analyzed sections, the number of counted neurons, and the three-dimensional cytoarchitecture of the investigated brain region [109, 110, 118–120].

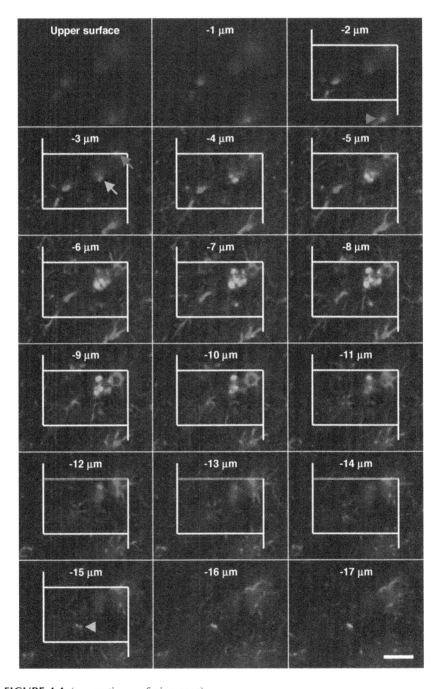

FIGURE 4.4 (see caption on facing page)

F.   ESTIMATING MEAN CELLULAR/NUCLEAR SIZE

For estimating mean cellular/perikaryal or nuclear volumes of neurons (so-called local volumes) with design-based stereology, several methods are available and are summarized in Figure 4.5. Among them, the "nucleator" method [121], the "rotator" method [122], and the "optical rotator" method [123] have been developed to obtain unbiased estimates of "number-weighted" mean local volumes (i.e., each neuron has the same probability of being selected for investigation). Alternatively, one can estimate "volume-weighted" mean local volumes with the "point sampled intercepts" method [124]. Here, the probability of a neuron being selected for investigation depends on its individual size.

An important question with regard to the application of these methods in brain aging research is the use of appropriate sections. This is based on the fact that the nucleator method, the rotator method, and the point sampled intercepts method require the use of "isotropic uniform random" sections [125] or "vertical" sections [126], that is, sections with a certain plane of section. It is generally possible to prepare such sections from a given brain region (for the corresponding protocols see [126–129]). In practice, however, investigations on isotropic uniform random or vertical sections are affected by the problem that the plane of section is unknown, resulting in potential loss of orientation within the sections. The optical rotator method can be used to measure local volumes of neurons within (thick) conventional coronal, sagittal, or horizontal sections, but requires that the sections show only a minimum shrinkage in the z-axis. This can generally be achieved by embedding tissue in methacrylate before sectioning (see, e.g., [75, 130, 131]) or in paraffin. In most applications in brain aging research, however, embedding in methacrylate is not possible because it makes immunohistochemistry impossible. Paraffin sections

FIGURE 4.4 (SEE COLOR INSERT FOLLOWING PAGE 204) The optical disector for investigating the number of cells within a given tissue volume. The procedure is shown for cells immunoreactive for GFAP (in red) and BrdU (in green) within the dentate gyrus of a 24-month-old mouse. The upper surface of a section is visualized with confocal microscopy, as well as the same microscopic field at 17 consecutive focal planes below the upper surface, with a distance of 1 μm between the focal planes. An unbiased counting frame is shown between -2 μm and -15 μm at each focal plane, with exclusion lines in white and inclusion lines in yellow. Thus, an unbiased virtual counting space with a height of 13 μm is generated within the tissue section. The top of the cells is used as sampling unit. The top of a BrdU-immunoreactive cell comes into focus at -2 μm (red arrowhead; with the cell visible until -17 μm). However, this cell is not counted because it is not found within the unbiased virtual counting space, and does not hit one of the inclusion lines of the unbiased counting frame. Another top of a BrdU-immunoreactive cell is detected at -3 μm (red arrow; with the cell also visible until -17 μm). This cell is counted because its top hits the inclusion line of the unbiased counting frame at -3 μm. Furthermore, at -3 μm, the top of a BrdU-immunoreactive cell also comes into focus (green arrowhead; with the cell visible until -13 μm). This cell is counted because its top lies within the unbiased virtual counting space at -3μm. Another BrdU-immunoreactive structure appears at -15 μm (green arrowhead); however, it is not recognized as a cell when going to deeper focal planes. (Scale bar = 20 μm.)

cannot be used in combination with immunofluorescent detection of antigens and might be affected by inhomogeneous compression of tissue sections along the z-axis during cutting of the tissue (as explained above). Frozen or vibratome sections, which are the most appropriate kinds of sections in brain aging research, however, can show considerable shrinkage in the z-axis [75, 77]), preventing the use of the optical rotator in most applications.

A general solution for this problem does not exist. One possibility is to test (in a pilot study) the hypothesis that estimates of local volumes obtained on isotropic uniform random or vertical sections with the nucleator method, the rotator method or the point sampled intercepts method do not differ from corresponding estimates obtained on conventional coronal, sagittal, or horizontal sections [129]. Another possibility might be to prevent shrinkage in section thickness by omitting dehydration of sections and coverslipping them with glycerol, even when immuno-histochemical detection of antigens was visualized with 3,3'-diaminobenzidine [132].

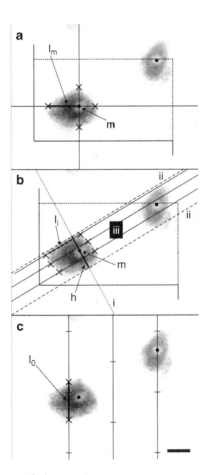

FIGURE 4.5 (see caption on facing page)

The variability of estimated local volumes obtained with the methods described here depends mainly on the number of investigated neurons. Detailed investigations into this issue, however, have not been published.

G. ESTIMATING TOTAL LENGTHS AND LENGTH DENSITIES OF CAPILLARIES AND FIBERS

Only a few studies in brain aging research have addressed alterations in total lengths and length densities of capillaries and fibers with design-based stereologic methods (e.g., [55, 65]). This might be due to the fact that in the past, corresponding estimates

FIGURE 4.5 The nucleator, rotator, and point sampled intercepts methods for estimating the mean cellular or nuclear volume of cells. The procedures are shown for NeuN-immunoreactive cells in layer V of an adult mouse neocortex as an example. (a) When using the nucleator method, a certain point within each cell needs to be determined as sampling unit. For obtaining unbiased estimates, the position of this point must be either uniformly random within the cell or must be the midpoint of the cell [121]. For practical use, it is convenient to select the midpoint of the nucleolus as the sampling unit. Note that for both cells shown in (a), the midpoint of the nucleolus is found within the selected focal plane, either within an unbiased counting frame (cell on the right) or hitting the inclusion (dotted) lines but not the exclusion (solid) lines of the unbiased counting frame (cell on the left). Accordingly, both cells would be considered for analysis. The distance from the midpoint of the nucleolus to the cellular or nuclear boundary (l) is measured in four mutually orthogonal directions (which can also be done in three or more directions, thus influencing the precision of the estimates). Then the average of the third powers of these measurements serves as basis for obtaining an unbiased estimate of the cellular or nuclear volume (for details, see [121]). (m = midpoint of the nucleolus; l_m, = distance between the midpoint of the nucleolus and the nuclear boundary.) (b) Obtaining unbiased estimates with the rotator method also depends on the selection of a point with either uniformly random position within the cell or the midpoint of the cell [122]. First, an axis is created along the shortest aspect of the sampled cell on the section through the midpoint of the nucleolus ("i" in Figure 4.5b). Then the top and the bottom positions of the cellular or nuclear profile are marked with respect to the defined axis ("ii"; light dashed lines in Figure 4.5b) to measure the height of the cellular or nuclear profile ("h"; thick solid line in Figure 4.5b). Next, three parallel test lines are generated perpendicular to the defined axis ("iii"; light solid lines in Figure 4.5b). The position of the test lines on the defined axis must be uniformly random (i.e., the position of the first test line in an interval of h/3 is randomly chosen, with the distance between the lines being h/3). Then the lengths of the intercepts of the test lines between the defined axis and the cellular or nuclear boundary (l_i; thick dashed line) are measured. These measurements serve as the basis for obtaining an unbiased estimate of the cellular or nuclear volume (for details, see [122]). (m = midpoint of the nucleolus; l_i – length of the intercept of a test line between a defined axis and the nuclear boundary.) (c) When using the point sampled intercepts method, all cellular or nuclear profiles found in a given focal plane are considered for analysis. A test system of parallel lines is randomly placed on the section. Then the length of the intercept of the test line between the cellular or nuclear boundaries (l_0) is measured for each sampled cell or nucleus. These measurements serve as the basis for obtaining an unbiased estimate of the cellular or nuclear volume (for details, see [124]). (l_0 – length of a test line between the nuclear boundaries.) (Scale bar = 5 μm.)

required the use of isotropic uniform random sections [133, 134]. As explained above, however, this results in potential loss of orientation within the sections.

Recently, a design-based stereologic method, the "space balls," has been introduced to obtain unbiased estimates of total lengths and length densities of capillaries and fibers on (thick) conventional coronal, sagittal, or horizontal sections [135, 136]. First, microscopic fields are systematically and randomly sampled throughout the ROI (as shown in Figure 4.1c). Then, a sphere (a so-called "space ball") or a hemisphere is placed within the sections in each microscopic field, and the intersections between the sphere and the capillaries or fibers under study are counted (Figure 4.6). From these data, an average length density can be obtained [135, 136].

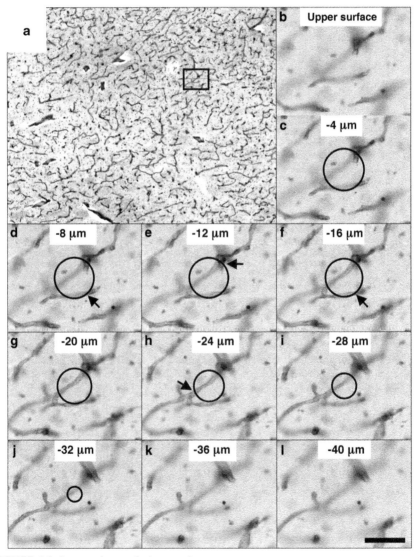

FIGURE 4.6 (see caption on facing page)

By combining this length density estimate with an estimate of the volume of the ROI (as explained above), an estimate of the total length of the capillaries or fibers under study within the ROI is obtained (see, e.g., [132]).

Note that estimates obtained with the space balls method are not unbiased in a strict sense. One source of bias is the ratio of the diameter of the space balls and the diameter of the capillaries or fibers under study. Another source of bias is the z-axis shrinkage of the tissue due to histologic processing (for details, see [134]). Unlike with three-dimensional reconstructions, it is not possible to correct for this shrinkage. Rather, length estimates obtained with the space balls method will be different if sections are cut in different planes and the capillaries or fibers under study have a preferential direction. Practical solutions to minimize this bias have been provided [134]. The variability of estimated total lengths and length densities of capillaries and fibers obtained with the space balls method depends mainly on the number of space balls applied.

For the sake of completeness, another possibility to quantify total lengths and length densities of capillaries and fibers with design-based stereology shall be mentioned — that is, the use of "isotropic virtual planes" [137]. In this case, the capillaries or fibers under study contained in thick (3D) sections are investigated with software-randomized isotropic virtual planes in volume probes in systematically sampled microscope fields. This, however, requires the analysis of virtual planes within thick sections, which can be tedious and cumbersome. Using the space balls method, the plane of analysis is always the focal plane of the microscopic fields.

FIGURE 4.6 The space balls method for estimating the total length of a linear biological structure within a given tissue. The procedure is shown for collagen IV-immunoreactive capillaries in the mediodorsal nucleus of the thalamus from a human brain. The postmortem brain was fixed by immersion in 10% formalin prior to histologic processing (for details, see [132]). The right hemisphere was embedded in gelatin, deeply frozen at –60°C, and cut into serial 600–700-μm-thick coronal sections. Approximately 4 cm × 4 cm small pieces containing the thalamus were cut out from these thick sections, frozen, and cut into 50-μm-thick coronal sections. To prevent shrinkage in section thickness, the sections were not dehydrated but mounted on gelatin-coated slides and coverslipped with 80% glycerol in TRIS-buffered saline. Panel (a) provides a low-power overview of capillaries in the mediodorsal nucleus. The square indicates the region at which the high-power photomicrographs (b–l) were taken. These show the upper surface of the section as well as the same microscopic field at 10 consecutive focal planes below the upper surface, with a distance of 4 μm between the focal planes. Between –4 μm and –32 μm, the intersections of a hemisphere (a [semi-]"space ball") and the focal plane at the investigated focal depth are shown as circles. This (semi-)space ball was centered at a depth of –4 μm and had a radius of 30 μm. At –8 μm, –12 μm, –16 μm, and –24 μm, intersections between the hemisphere and the capillaries in focus at the point of intersection were found (arrows). From the total number of intersections and the size of the hemisphere, the capillary length density of the investigated microscopic field can be calculated [135]. By placing (semi-)space balls in a systematic-random manner throughout the entire mediodorsal nucleus, an estimate of the average capillary length density within this region is obtained. Finally, by combining length density with an estimate of the volume of the region (as shown in Figure 4.2), one can obtain an unbiased estimate of the total capillary length in the structure. [Scale bar = 150 μm (a); 30 μm (high-power photomicrographs).]

H.   QUANTITATIVE ANALYSIS OF THE THREE-DIMENSIONAL CYTOARCHITECTURE OF A GIVEN BRAIN REGION

An attractive way to quantitatively study the three-dimensional cytoarchitecture of a given ROI with design-based stereology is to perform "nearest neighbor" analyses [138]. This method is based on the "nearest-neighbor distance distribution function" analysis founded in theoretical statistics [139]. In brief, this method consists of the following steps, which are shown in Figure 4.7. First, a systematic random series of thick sections is generated from the brain region of interest. When investigating

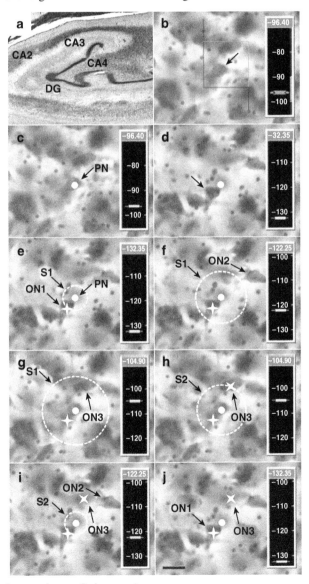

FIGURE 4.7 (see caption on facing page)

the rodent brain, a section thickness between 100 and 150 μm is appropriate; whereas for the human brain, a section thickness up to 750 μm can be used. Second, the sections are stained by a method that guarantees staining throughout the section thickness (e.g., gallocyanin; Figure 4.7a). Third, the volume of the ROI is estimated using Cavalieri's principle, and the total number of neurons within this ROI using

FIGURE 4.7 Analysis of the nearest-neighbor distance distribution function for neurons in a given brain region. The procedure is shown for the hippocampal hilus ("CA4") in a human brain. The brain was mounted with celloidin and cut into a complete series of 200-μm-thick frontal sections, which were stained with gallocyanin (for details, see [79]). (a) Overview of the hippocampal cell layers in the human brain (DG = dentate gyrus). (b) A microscopic field was systematically, randomly sampled within area CA4 at high magnification with a 20× oil objective (NA = 0.8) (for systematic-random sampling of microscopic fields, see Figure 4.1c). An unbiased virtual counting space with height of 10 μm (h in Figure 4.1d) was placed at a depth (d in Figure 4.1d) of 90 μm below the upper surface of the section. At a depth of 96.4 μm below the upper surface of the section, a neuron was sampled with the unbiased virtual counting space (arrow). (c) By mouse-clicking on the nucleolus of this neuron, it becomes categorized as a parent neuron (PN) and is marked (white dot). (d) At a depth of 132.35 μm in the same microscopic field (i.e., 35.95 μm below the focal plane of the PN), a second neuron is found (arrow). This neuron may be the nearest neighbor to the selected PN. (e) By mouse-clicking on the nucleolus of this offspring neuron (thereafter offspring neuron 1; ON1), it is marked by a white star. Then a sphere centered on the nucleolus of the PN is calculated and displayed, with the 3D distance between the nucleolus of the PN and the nucleolus of ON1 as the sphere's radius. From this sphere (thereafter sphere 1; S1), the intersection of the focal plane at the investigated focal depth and the sphere is shown as a circle. (f) At a depth of 122.25 μm in the same microscopic field (i.e., 25.85 μm below the focal plane of the PN), another neuron is found (ON2). However, ON2 is lying outside the circle representing the plane intersection of S1 at this focal depth. Accordingly, the distance between the nucleolus of ON2 and the PN is larger than the distance between the nucleolus of ON1 and the PN. Therefore, ON2 is not the nearest neighbor of the selected PN. (g) At a depth of 104.9 μm in the same microscopic field (i.e., 8.5 μm below the focal plane of the PN), another neuron appears (ON3). ON3 is lying within the circle representing the plane intersection of S1 at this focal depth. Accordingly, the distance between the nucleolus of ON3 and the PN is smaller than the distance between the nucleolus of ON1 and the PN. Therefore, ON1 is not the nearest neighbor of the selected PN, as initially thought. (h) ON3 is also marked by a white star. Another sphere (S2) is now centered on the nucleolus of the PN, with the distance between the nucleolus of the PN and the nucleolus of ON3 as the sphere's radius. From S2, the intersection of the sphere and the focal plane at the investigated focal depth is shown as a circle. S1 is no longer considered by the software, its radius being larger than the radius of S2. (i) Going back to a depth of 122.25 μm in the same microscopic field (i.e., to the focal plane at which ON2 was found), it can be seen that ON2 is lying outside the circle representing the plane section of S2 at this focal depth, and thus is not the nearest neighbor of the selected PN. (j) Back at a depth of 132.35 μm in the same microscopic field (i.e., where ON1 was found), no intersections of S2 and the focal plane at the investigated focal depth exist anymore, due to the fact that the radius of S2 is smaller than 35.95 μm (i.e., the distance between the investigated focal depth and the focal plane of PN). Accordingly, ON1 is not the nearest neighbor of the selected PN. As no other neuron is detected within S2, ON3 is the nearest neighbor of the selected PN, and the radius of S2 is its nearest-neighbor distance. [Scale bar = 1 mm (a); 25 μm (b to j).]

the fractionator method. Fourth, for a systematic-random set of approximately 1000 neurons, the nearest neighbor is identified in 3D (Figures 4.7b to j) and the nearest-neighbor distance of each of these neurons is measured. Fifth, the cumulative relative frequency distribution is calculated from these approximately 1000 nearest-neighbor distances, yielding the nearest-neighbor distance distribution function. Finally, graphical comparisons are performed between this nearest-neighbor distance distribution function and corresponding distribution functions obtained from computer simulations, modeling virtual ROIs with the same quantitative characteristics (i.e., volume, total number of neurons) as the investigated ROI (for details, see [138]). The results obtained with the nearest-neighbor method facilitate the determination of whether neurons within a given ROI exhibit spatial randomness, a clustered distribution, or a more dispersed distribution. The variability of nearest-neighbor analyses depends mainly on the number of investigated neurons.

For the sake of completeness another approach to study the spatial distribution of neurons also shall be mentioned, that is, "Voronoi tessellation" [140–142]. This method focuses on the region of space that any cell within an ROI occupies, the region of space that is closer to that cell than to any other. The results of the Voronoi tessellation method provide information concerning spatial distribution as follows: if the size of the Voronoi spaces (i.e., the regions of space that are closer to a given cell than to any other) do not vary much, the cells are regularly distributed. However, if the size of the Voronoi spaces varies considerably, cellular clusters are present. Unfortunately, algorithms to apply three-dimensional tessellations to histologic specimens are not available.

I.   EQUIPMENT REQUIRED FOR DESIGN-BASED STEREOLOGIC ANALYSES IN BRAIN AGING RESEARCH

The recent developments in design-based stereology have become possible only with the introduction of computer-interfaced microscopes and imaging instrumentation. Furthermore, the availability of semiautomated, computer-based stereology systems has substantially reduced both the observer's effort and potential errors associated with the use of design-based stereology. Moreover, these systems facilitate the combination of computer-based anatomical mapping and stereologic estimates (for illustrative examples, see [61, 143]. Currently, the following semiautomated, computer-based stereology systems are available: CAST (Visiopharm; Hørsholm, Denmark); Digital Stereology (Kinetic Imaging; Bromborough, U.K.); Stereologer (Systems Planning and Analysis; Alexandria, Virginia); Stereology Toolkit Plug-in for NOVA PRIME (Bioquant Image Analysis Corporation; Nashville, Tennessee); and StereoInvestigator (MBF Bioscience; Williston, Vermont). These systems integrate three-axes motor-driven specimen stages with a computer in order to acquire data from 3D structures, and implement (to various degrees) the stereologic probes described above.

The motorized stage is used to map brain regions and objects that are larger than a single microscopic field; to access specific locations throughout the entire ROI, regardless of optical magnification; and to perform systematic-random sampling. Furthermore, the microscope is usually equipped with a z-axis position encoder that measures accurately the actual focal position of the microscope stage. This is particularly important when performing 3D probes like the optical disector, the optical rotator, space balls, and nearest-neighbor analysis. The tissue specimen is usually viewed on a computer monitor via a high-resolution analog CCD video camera or a digital camera with more than ten frames per second. This allows focusing through the tissue in real-time. In addition, as stereologic applications have extended to confocal microscopy [144], electron microscopy [145], computed tomography [146], and magnetic resonance imaging [147], some commercial stereology systems provide image file readers that accept three-dimensional confocal and MRI image sets, as well as the file formats generated by a variety of electron microscopes and flatbed scanners. Once these image files are read, they can be analyzed by the system's analysis procedures.

It should be mentioned that some design-based stereologic analyses can still be performed with simple microscopes and with minimal or even without computer assistance (see, e.g., [148]). However, the advantages provided by design-based stereology are best obtained when it is integrated into computer-based microscopy systems that optimize data collection, storage, and analysis.

J. ADDITIONAL SOURCES OF INFORMATION

This chapter can only provide an introduction to design-based stereology, without claiming completeness in describing all design-based stereologic methods available and all of their applications in brain aging research. For more details, the reader may consult a variety of reviews [2–5, 70, 73, 83, 110, 136, 144, 149, 150–161] as well as several comprehensive books on stereology [162–170]. Of special interest might also be the Stereology Literature Database of the Enterprise Biology Software Project (Medina, WA), which currently lists more than 1100 papers reporting stereologic investigations of the brain.

IV. The Future of Design-Based Stereology in Brain Aging Research

In recent years, substantial progress has been made in brain aging research by the use of design-based stereologic methods. Based on the data reviewed here, several comments can be made with respect to the future of design-based stereology in brain aging research. First, more regions in the brain of humans, nonhuman primates, and rodents should be investigated for the presence of absolute neuron loss (Nissl stained neurons or neurons immunoreactive for NeuN) and functional loss (alterations in gene expression profiles of neurons). This is particularly the case for the striatum and the thalamus (to evaluate to which extent age-related cortical neuron loss is based on target loss) and for cytoarchitectonically defined cortical areas in the brain of humans and nonhuman primates. This should be accompanied by advanced integration of anatomical mapping with stereologic analyses. Second, better distinctions should be made between functional loss and absolute neuron loss. Third, analyses of selective functional loss and absolute neuron loss in different brain regions should be performed on the same brains rather than on different samples, in order to achieve more reliability in patterns of regionally specific neuron loss in brain aging.

Last but not least, brain aging research will greatly benefit from further integration of design-based stereology with confocal microscopy and electron microscopy. The optical resolution of confocal microscopy and electron microscopy, as well as the ability to collect registered series of focal planes, is ideally suited for the three-dimensional sampling of design-based stereology. The first attempts to integrate the collection of confocal and electron microscopic images with the implementation of design-based stereology have been undertaken [144, 145, 171]. Furthermore, computer-based microscopy systems integrating confocal illumination have been made commercially available. As with light microscopy, it is expected that the field of design-based stereologic analyses in brain aging research will considerably expand with the recognition that the integration of design-based stereology with confocal microscopy and electron microscopy is fundamental in revealing certain features of brain aging that would not have been detected otherwise.

ACKNOWLEDGMENTS

We would like to thank the Stanley Medical Research Institute and the US-National Alliance of Autism Research (to C.S. and P.R.H.), the Alzheimer Forschung Initiative e.V., the Internationale Stichting Alzheimer Onderzoek and the Hersenstichting (to C.S.), and NIH grants AG02219, AG05138, MH58911, and MH66392 (to P.R.H.).

REFERENCES

1. Haug, H., History of neuromorphometry, *J. Neurosci. Methods,* 18, 1, 1986.
2. West, M.J., Design-based stereological methods for counting neurons, *Prog. Brain Res.,* 135, 43, 2002.
3. West, M.J., New stereological methods for counting neurons, *Neurobiol. Aging,* 14, 275, 1993.
4. Gundersen, H.J.G. et al., The new stereological tools: disector, fractionator, nucleator and point sampled intercepts and their use in pathological research and diagnosis, *Acta Pathol. Microbiol. Immunol. Scand.,* 96, 857, 1988.
5. Hyman, B.T., Gomez-Isla, T., and Irizarry, M.C., Stereology: a practical primer for neuropathology, *J. Neuropathol. Exp. Neurol.,* 57, 305, 1998.
6. Pakkenberg, B. and Gundersen, H.J., Neocortical neuron number in humans: effect of sex and age, *J. Comp. Neurol.,* 384, 312, 1997.
7. Pakkenberg, B. et al., Aging and the human neocortex, *Exp. Gerontol.,* 38, 95, 2003.
8. Kordower, J.H. et al., Loss and atrophy of layer II entorhinal cortex neurons in elderly people with mild cognitive impairment, *Ann. Neurol.,* 49, 202, 2001.
9. Simic, G. et al., Hemispheric asymmetry, modular variability and age-related changes in the human entorhinal cortex, *Neuroscience,* 130, 911, 2005.
10. Gomez-Isla, T. et al., Profound loss of layer II entorhinal cortex neurons occurs in very mild Alzheimer's disease, *J. Neurosci.,* 16, 4491, 1996.
11. Price, J.L. et al., Neuron number in the entorhinal cortex and CA1 in preclinical Alzheimer disease, *Arch Neurol.,* 58, 1395, 2001.

12. West, M.J., Regionally specific loss of neurons in the aging human hippocampus, *Neurobiol. Aging,* 14, 287, 1993.
13. Scheff, S.W., Price, D.A., and Sparks, D.L., Quantitative assessment of possible age-related change in synaptic numbers in the human frontal cortex, *Neurobiol. Aging,* 22, 355, 2001.
14. Tang, Y. et al., Age-induced white matter changes in the human brain: a stereological investigation, *Neurobiol. Aging,* 18, 609, 1997.
15. Marner, L. et al., Marked loss of myelinated nerve fibers in the human brain with age, *J. Comp. Neurol.,* 462, 144, 2003.
16. Ohm, T.G., Busch, C., and Bohl, J., Unbiased estimation of neuronal numbers in the human nucleus coeruleus during aging, *Neurobiol. Aging,* 18, 393, 1997.
17. Mouton, P.R. et al., Absolute number and size of pigmented locus coeruleus neurons in young and aged individuals, *J. Chem. Neuroanat.,* 7, 185, 1994.
18. Andersen, B.B., Gundersen, H.J., and Pakkenberg, B., Aging of the human cerebellum: a stereological study, *J. Comp. Neurol.,* 466, 356, 2003.
19. Chu, Y. et al., Age-related decreases in Nurr1 immunoreactivity in the human substantia nigra, *J. Comp. Neurol.,* 450, 203, 2002.
20. Ma, S.Y. et al., Dopamine transporter-immunoreactive neurons decrease with age in the human substantia nigra, *J. Comp. Neurol.,* 409, 25, 1999.
21. Cabello, C.R. et al., Ageing of substantia nigra in humans: cell loss may be compensated by hypertrophy, *Neuropathol. Appl. Neurobiol.,* 28, 283, 2002.
22. Chen, E.Y. et al., Age-related decreases in GTP-cyclohydrolase-I immunoreactive neurons in the monkey and human substantia nigra, *J. Comp. Neurol.,* 426, 534, 2000.
23. Geula, C. et al., Loss of calbindin-D28k from aging human cholinergic basal forebrain: relation to neuronal loss, *J. Comp. Neurol.,* 455, 249, 2003.
24. Gilmor, M.L. et al., Preservation of nucleus basalis neurons containing choline acetyltransferase and the vesicular acetylcholine transporter in the elderly with mild cognitive impairment and early Alzheimer's disease, *J. Comp. Neurol.,* 411, 693, 1999.
25. Jucker, M. et al., Structural brain aging in inbred mice: potential for genetic linkage, *Exp. Gerontol.,* 35, 1383, 2000.
26. Merrill, D.A. et al., Conservation of neuron number and size in entorhinal cortex layers II, III, and V/VI of aged primates, *J. Comp. Neurol.,* 422, 396, 2000.
27. Gazzaley, A.H. et al., Preserved number of entorhinal cortex layer II neurons in aged macaque monkeys, *Neurobiol. Aging,* 18, 549, 1997.
28. Merrill, D.A., Chiba, A.A., and Tuszynski, M.H., Conservation of neuronal number and size in the entorhinal cortex of behaviorally characterized aged rats, *J. Comp. Neurol.,* 438, 445, 2001.
29. Hof, P.R. et al., Numbers of meynert and layer IVB cells in area V1: a stereologic analysis in young and aged macaque monkeys, *J. Comp. Neurol.,* 420, 113, 2000.
30. Kim, C.B., Pier, L.P., and Spear, P.D., Effects of aging on numbers and sizes of neurons in histochemically defined subregions of monkey striate cortex, *Anat. Rec.,* 247, 119, 1997.
31. Smith, D.E. et al., Memory impairment in aged primates is associated with local death of cortical neurons and atrophy of subcortical neurons, *J. Neurosci.,* 24, 4373, 2004.
32. Smith, D.E. et al., Age-associated neuronal atrophy occurs in the primate brain and is reversible by growth factor gene therapy, *Proc. Natl. Acad. Sci. U.S.A.,* 96, 10893, 1999.

33. Wu, C.K. et al., Selective age-related loss of calbindin-D28k from basal forebrain cholinergic neurons in the common marmoset (Callithrix jacchus), *Neuroscience,* 120, 249, 2003.

34. Smith, M.L. and Booze, R.M., Cholinergic and GABAergic neurons in the nucleus basalis region of young and aged rats, *Neuroscience,* 67, 679, 1995.

35. Rapp, P.R. and Gallagher, M., Preserved neuron number in the hippocampus of aged rats with spatial learning deficits, *Proc. Natl. Acad. Sci. U.S.A.,* 93, 9926, 1996.

36. Keuker, J.I. et al., Preservation of hippocampal neuron numbers and hippocampal subfield volumes in behaviorally characterized aged tree shrews, *J. Comp. Neurol.,* 468, 509, 2004.

37. Keuker, J.I., Luiten, P.G., and Fuchs, E., Preservation of hippocampal neuron numbers in aged rhesus monkeys, *Neurobiol. Aging,* 24, 157, 2003.

38. Rutten, B.P.F. et al., The aging brain: accumulation of DNA damage or neuron loss? *Neurobiol. Aging,* 28, 91, 2007.

39. Calhoun, M.E. et al., Hippocampal neuron and synaptophysin-positive bouton number in aging C57BL/6 mice, *Neurobiol. Aging,* 19, 599, 1998.

40. Rasmussen, T. et al., Memory impaired aged rats: no loss of principal hippocampal and subicular neurons, *Neurobiol. Aging,* 17, 143, 1996.

41. Rapp, P.R. et al., Neuron number in the parahippocampal region is preserved in aged rats with spatial learning deficits, *Cereb. Cortex,* 12, 1171, 2002.

42. Tigges, J., Herndon, J.G.. and Rosene, D.L., Preservation into old age of synaptic number and size in the supragranular layer of the dentate gyrus in rhesus monkeys, *Acta Anat.,* 157, 63, 1996.

43. Geinisman, Y. et al., Aging, spatial learning, and total synapse number in the rat CA1 stratum radiatum, *Neurobiol. Aging,* 25, 407, 2004.

44. Rutten, B.P. et al., Age-related loss of synaptophysin immunoreactive presynaptic boutons within the hippocampus of APP751SL, PS1M146L, and APP751SL/PS1M146L transgenic mice, *Am.. J. Pathol.,* 167, 161, 2005.

45. Shi, L. et al., Stereological quantification of GAD-67-immunoreactive neurons and boutons in the hippocampus of middle-aged and old Fischer 344 x Brown Norway rats, *J. Comp. Neurol.,* 478, 282, 2004.

46. Bhatnagar, M. et al., Neurochemical changes in the hippocampus of the brown Norway rat during aging, *Neurobiol. Aging,* 18, 319, 1997.

47. Mouton, P.R. et al., Age and gender effects on microglia and astrocyte numbers in brains of mice, *Brain Res.,* 956, 30, 2002.

48. Long, J.M. et al., Stereological analysis of astrocyte and microglia in aging mouse hippocampus, *Neurobiol. Aging,* 19, 497, 1998.

49. Pakkenberg, H. et al., A stereological study of substantia nigra in young and old rhesus monkeys, *Brain Res.,* 693, 201, 1995.

50. Siddiqi, Z., Kemper, T.L. and Killiany, R., Age-related neuronal loss from the substantia nigra-pars compacta and ventral tegmental area of the rhesus monkey, *J. Neuropathol. Exp. Neurol.,* 58, 959, 1999.

51. McCormack, A.L. et al., Aging of the nigrostriatal system in the squirrel monkey, *J. Comp. Neurol.,* 471, 387, 2004.

52. Emborg, M.E. et al., Age-related declines in nigral neuronal function correlate with motor impairments in rhesus monkeys, *J. Comp. Neurol.,* 401, 253, 1998.

53. Dlugos, C.A. and Pentney, R.J., Morphometric analyses of Purkinje and granule cells in aging F344 rats, *Neurobiol. Aging,* 15, 435, 1994.

54. Bergman, E. and Ulfhake, B., Loss of primary sensory neurons in the very old rat: neuron number estimates using the disector method and confocal optical sectioning, *J. Comp. Neurol.*, 396, 211, 1998.

55. Bailey, T.L. et al., The nature and effects of cortical microvascular pathology in aging and Alzheimer's disease, *Neurol. Res.*, 26, 573, 2004.

56. Zlokovic, B.V., Neurovascular mechanisms of Alzheimer's neurodegeneration, *Trends Neurosci.*, 28, 202, 2005.

57. Willem, A. et al., Stereological changes in the capillary network of the aging dorsal lateral geniculate nucleus, *Anat. Rec. A Discov. Mol. Cell. Evol. Biol.*, 274, 857, 2003.

58. West, M.J. et al., Hippocampal neurons in pre-clinical Alzheimer's disease, *Neurobiol. Aging*, 25, 1205, 2004.

59. Hof, P.R. et al., Stereologic evidence for persistence of viable neurons in layer II of the entorhinal cortex and the CA1 field in Alzheimer disease, *J. Neuropathol. Exp. Neurol.*, 62, 55, 2003.

60. West, M.J. et al., Differences in the pattern of hippocampal neuronal loss in normal ageing and Alzheimer's disease, *Lancet*, 344, 769, 1994.

61. Bussière, T. et al., Stereologic analysis of neurofibrillary tangle formation in prefrontal cortex area 9 in aging and Alzheimer's disease, *Neuroscience*, 117, 577, 2003.

62. von Gunten, A. et al., Stereologic analysis of hippocampal Alzheimer's disease pathology in the oldest-old: evidence for sparing of the entorhinal cortex and CA1 field, *Exp. Neurol.*, 193, 198, 2005.

63. Bussiere, T. et al., Stereologic assessment of the total cortical volume occupied by amyloid deposits and its relationship with cognitive status in aging and Alzheimer's disease, *Neuroscience*, 112, 75, 2002.

64. Giannakopoulos, P. et al., Tangle and neuron numbers, but not amyloid load, predict cognitive status in Alzheimer's disease, *Neurology*, 60, 1495, 2003.

65. Bouras, C. et al., Stereologic analysis of microvascular morphology in the elderly: Alzheimer's disease pathology and cognitive status, *J. Neuropathol. Exp. Neurol.*, 65, 235, 2006.

66. Schmitz, C. et al., Hippocampal neuron loss exceeds amyloid plaque load in a transgenic mouse model of Alzheimer's disease, *Am. J. Pathol.*, 164, 1495, 2004.

67. Casas, C. et al., Massive CA1/2 neuronal loss with intraneuronal and N-terminal truncated A42 accumulation in a novel Alzheimer transgenic model, *Am. J. Pathol.*, 165, 1289, 2004.

68. Brasnjevic, I. et al., Synapse and neuron loss in transgenic mouse models of Alzheimer's disease, in *Frontiers in Alzheimer's Disease Research*, Welsh, E.M., Ed., Nova Science Publishers, Hauppauge, 97, 2006.

69. Guillery, R.W. and Herrup, K., Quantification without pontification: choosing a method for counting objects in sectioned tissues, *J. Comp. Neurol.*, 386, 2, 1997.

70. Gundersen, H.J.G., Stereology of arbitrary particles, *J. Microsc.*, 143, 3, 1986.

71. Gundersen, H.J.G. and Jensen, E.B., The efficiency of systematic sampling and its prediction, *J. Microsc.*, 147, 229, 1987.

72. Dorph Petersen, K.A., Nyengaard, J.R., and Gundersen, H.J.G., Tissue shrinkage and unbiased stereological estimation of particle number and size, *J. Microsc.*, 204, 232, 2001.

73. Schmitz, C. and Hof, P.R., Design-based stereology in neuroscience, *Neuroscience*, 130, 813, 2005.

74. Hatton, W.J. and von Bartheld, C.S., Analysis of cell death in the trochlear nucleus of the chick embryo: calibration of the optical disector counting method reveals systematic bias, *J. Comp. Neurol.*, 409, 169, 1999.

75. Messina, A. et al., Requirements for obtaining unbiased estimates of neuronal numbers in frozen sections, *J. Neurosci. Methods*, 97, 133, 2000.

76. Perl, D.P. et al., Practical approaches to stereology in the setting of aging- and disease-related brain banks, *J. Chem. Neuroanat.*, 20, 7, 2000.

77. Schmitz, C. et al., Use of cryostat sections from snap-frozen nervous tissue for combining stereological estimates with histological, cellular, or molecular analyses on adjacent sections, *J. Chem. Neuroanat.*, 20, 21, 2000.

78. Gardella, D. et al., Differential tissue shrinkage and compression in the z-axis: implications for optical disector counting in vibratome-, plastic- and cryosections, *J. Neurosci. Methods*, 124, 45, 2003.

79. Heinsen, H., Arzberger, T., and Schmitz, C., Celloidin mounting (embedding without infiltration) — a new, simple and reliable method for producing serial sections of high thickness through complete human brains and its application to stereological and immunohistochemical investigations, *J. Chem. Neuroanat.*, 20, 49, 2000.

80. Bauchot, R., Les modifications du poids encephalique au cours de la fixation [Modifications of brain weight in the course of fixation], *J. Hirnforsch.* 9, 253, 1967.

81. Kretschmann, H.J., Tafesse, U., and Herrmann, A., Different volume changes of cerebral cortex and white matter during histological preparation, *Microsc. Acta*, 86, 13, 1982.

82. Quester, R. and Schroder, R., The shrinkage of the human brain stem during formalin fixation and embedding in paraffin, *J. Neurosci. Methods*, 75, 81, 1997.

83. Von Bartheld, C., Counting particles in tissue sections: choices of methods and importance of calibration to minimize biases, *Histol. Histopathol.*, 17, 639, 2002.

84. West, M.J., Slomianka, L., and Gundersen, H.J.G., Unbiased stereological estimation of the total number of neurons in the subdivisions of the rat hippocampus using the optical fractionator, *Anat. Rec.*, 231, 482, 1991.

85. Zanjani, H. et al., Cerebellar Purkinje cell loss in aging Hu-Bcl-2 transgenic mice, *J. Comp. Neurol.*, 475, 481, 2004.

86. Abbott, A., Neuroscience: a new atlas of the brain, *Nature*, 424, 249, 2003.

87. Filimonoff, I.N., Über die Variabilität der Großhirnrindenstruktur. Mitteilung II — Regio occipitalis beim erwachsenen Menschen, *J. Psychol. Neurol.*, 44, 2, 1932.

88. Zilles, K. et al., Quantitative analysis of sulci in the human cerebral cortex: development, regional heterogeneity, gender difference, asymmetry, intersubject variability and cortical architecture, *Human Brain Mapping*, 5, 218, 1997.

89. Amunts, K. et al., Brodmann's areas 17 and 18 brought into stereotaxic space — where and how variable? *Neuroimage*, 11, 66, 2000.

90. Sherwood, C.C. et al., Variability of Broca's area homologue in African great apes: implications for language evolution, *Anat. Rec.*, 271A, 276, 2003.

91. Braak, H., *Architectonics of the Human Telencephalic Cortex*, Springer, Berlin, 1980.

92. Geyer, S. et al., Two different areas within the primary motor cortex of man, *Nature*, 382, 805, 1996.

93. Schleicher, A. et al., Observer-independent method for microstructural parcellation of cerebral cortex: a quantitative approach to cytoarchitectonics, *Neuroimage*, 9, 165, 1999.

94. Schleicher, A. et al., A stereological approach to human cortical architecture: identification and delineation of cortical areas, *J. Chem. Neuroanat.*, 20, 31, 2000.

95. Schleicher, A. et al., Quantitative architectural analysis: a new approach to cortical mapping, *Anat. Embryol.*, 210, 373, 2005.

96. Hof, P.R. and Morrison, J.H., Neurofilament protein defines regional patterns of cortical organization in the macaque monkey visual system: a quantitative immunohistochemical analysis, *J. Comp. Neurol.*, 352, 161, 1995.

97. Hof, P.R., Mufson, E.J., and Morrison, J.H., Human orbitofrontal cortex: cytoarchitecture and quantitative immunohistochemical parcellation, *J. Comp. Neurol.*, 359, 48, 1995.

98. Nimchinsky, E.A. et al., Neurofilament and calcium-binding proteins in the human cingulate cortex, *J. Comp. Neurol.*, 384, 597, 1997.

99. Vogt, B.A. et al., Cytology of human caudomedial cingulate, retrosplenial, and caudal parahippocampal cortices, *J. Comp. Neurol.*, 438, 353, 2001.

100. Bussière, T. et al., Progressive degeneration of nonphosphorylated neurofilament protein-enriched pyramidal neurons predicts cognitive impairment in Alzheimer's disease: stereologic analysis of prefrontal cortex area 9, *J. Comp. Neurol.*, 463, 281, 2003.

101. Carmichael, S.T. and Price, J.L., Architectonic subdivision of the orbital and medial prefrontal cortex in the macaque monkey, *J. Comp. Neurol.*, 346, 366, 1994.

102. Dombrowski, S.M., Hilgetag, C.C., and Barbas, H., Quantitative architecture distinguishes prefrontal cortical systems in the rhesus monkey, *Cereb. Cortex*, 11, 975, 2001.

103. Ongur, D., Ferry, A.T., and Price, J.L., Architectonic subdivision of the human orbital and medial prefrontal cortex, *J. Comp. Neurol.*, 460, 425, 2003.

104. Cavalieri, B., *Geometria Indivisibilibus Continuorum*, Typis Clementis Ferronij, Bononiae, 1635 (reprinted as *Geometria Degli Indivisibili*, Unione Tipografico-Editrice Torinese, Torino, 1966).

105. Uylings, H.B., van Eden, C.G., and Hofman, M.A., Morphometry of size/volume variables and comparison of their bivariate relations in the nervous system under different conditions, *J. Neurosci. Methods*, 18, 19, 1986.

106. Glaser, E., Comments on the shortcomings of predicting the precision of Cavalieri volume estimates based upon assumed measurement functions, *J. Microsc.*, 218, 1, 2005.

107. Cruz-Orive, L.M., and García-Fiñana, M., A review of the article: comments on the shortcomings of predicting the precision of Cavalieri volume estimates based upon assumed measurement functions, by Edmund Glaser, *J. Microsc.*, 218, 6, 2005.

108. König, D. et al., Modelling and analysis of 3-D arrangements of particles by point processes with examples of application to biological data obtained by confocal scanning light microscopy, *J. Microsc.*, 161, 405, 1991.

109. Schmitz, C., Variation of fractionator estimates and its prediction, *Anat. Embryol.*, 198, 371, 1998.

110. Schmitz, C. and Hof, P.R., Recommendations for straightforward and rigorous methods of counting neurons based on a computer simulation approach, *J. Chem. Neuroanat.*, 20, 93, 2000.

111. West, M.J. and Slomianka, L., 2-D versus 3-D cell counting - a debate. What is an optical disector?, *Trends Neurosci.*, 24, 374, 2001.

112. Williams, R.W. and Rakic, P., Three-dimensional counting: an accurate and direct method to estimate numbers of cells in sectioned material, *J. Comp. Neurol.*, 278, 344, 1988.

113. Gundersen, H.J.G., Notes on the estimation of the numerical density of arbitrary particles: the edge effect, *J. Microsc.*, 111, 219, 1977.

114. Andersen, B.B. and Gundersen, H.J.G., Pronounced loss of cell nuclei and anisotropic deformation of thick sections, *J. Microsc.*, 196, 69, 1999.

115. Jinno, S. et al., Quantitative analysis of GABAergic neurons in the mouse hippocampus, with optical disector using confocal laser scanning microscopy, *Brain Res.*, 814, 55, 1998.

116. Sterio, D.C., The unbiased estimation of number and size of arbitrary particles using the disector, *J. Microsc.*, 134, 127, 1984.

117. West, M.J. and Gundersen, H.J.G., Unbiased stereological estimation of the number of neurons in the human hippocampus, *J. Comp. Neurol.*, 296, 1, 1990.

118. Cruz-Orive, L.M., Precision of the fractionator from Cavalieri designs, *J. Microsc.*, 213, 205, 2004.

119. Cruz-Orive, L.M. and Geiser, M., Estimation of particle number by stereology: an update, *J. Aerosol Med.*, 17, 197, 2004.

120. Slomianka, L. and West, M.J., Estimators of the precision of stereological estimates: an example based on the CA1 pyramidal cell layer of rats, *Neuroscience*, 136, 757, 2005.

121. Gundersen, H.J.G., The nucleator, *J. Microsc.*, 151, 3, 1988.

122. Vedel Jensen, E.B. and Gundersen, H.J.G., The rotator, *J. Microsc.*, 170, 35, 1993.

123. Tandrup, T., Gundersen, H.J.G., and Jensen, E.B., The optical rotator, *J. Microsc.*, 186, 108, 1997.

124. Gundersen, H.J.G. and Jensen, E.B., Stereological estimation of the volume-weighted mean volume of arbitrary particles observed on random sections, *J. Microsc.*, 138, 127, 1985.

125. Miles, R.E. and Davy, P.J., Precise and general conditions for the validity of a comprehensive set of stereological fundamental formulae, *J. Microsc.*, 107, 211, 1976.

126. Baddeley, A.J., Gundersen, H.J.G., and Cruz-Orive, L.M., Estimation of surface area from vertical sections, *J. Microsc.* 142, 259, 1986.

127. Mattfeldt, T., Mall, G., and Gharehbaghi, H., Estimation of surface area and length with the orientator, *J. Microsc.*, 159, 301, 1990.

128. Nyengaard, J.R. and Gundersen, H.J.G., The disector: a simple and direct method for generating isotropic, uniform random sections from small specimens, *J. Microsc.*, 165, 427, 1992.

129. Schmitz, C. et al., No difference between estimated mean nuclear volumes of various types of neurons in the mouse brain obtained on either isotropic uniform random sections or conventional frontal or sagittal sections, *J. Neurosci. Methods*, 88, 71, 1999.

130. Sousa, N., Paula-Barbosa, M.M., and Almeida, O.F., Ligand and subfield specificity of corticoid-induced neuronal loss in the rat hippocampal formation, *Neuroscience*, 89 1079, 1999.

131. Lukoyanov, N.V. et al., Synaptic reorganization in the hippocampal formation of alcohol-fed rats may compensate for functional deficits related to neuronal loss, *Alcohol*, 20, 139, 2000.

132. Kreczmanski, P.J. et al., Stereological studies of capillary length density in the frontal cortex of schizophrenics, *Acta Neuropathol.*, 109, 510, 2005.

133. Smith, C.S. and Guttman, L., Measurement of internal boundaries in three-dimensional structures by random sectioning, *Trans. AIME*, 197, 81, 1953.

134. Gundersen, H.J.G., Stereological estimation of tubular length, *J. Microsc.*, 207, 155, 2002.

135. Mouton, P.R. et al., Stereological length estimation using spherical probes, *J. Microsc.*, 206, 54, 2002.

136. Calhoun, M.E. and Mouton, P.R., Length measurement: new developments in neurostereology and 3D imagery, *J. Chem. Neuroanat.* 21, 61, 2001.

137. Larsen, J.O., Gundersen, H.J.G., and Nielsen, J., Global spatial sampling with isotropic virtual planes: estimators of length density and total length in thick, arbitrarily oriented sections, *J. Microsc.*, 191, 238, 1998.

138. Schmitz, C. et al., Altered spatial arrangement of layer V pyramidal cells in the mouse brain following prenatal low-dose X-irradiation. A stereological study using a novel three-dimensional analysis method to estimate the nearest neighbor distance distributions of cells in thick sections, *Cereb. Cortex*, 12, 954, 2002.

139. Diggle, P.J., *Statistical Analysis of Spatial Point Patterns*, Academic Press, New York, 1983.

140. Duyckaerts, C. and Godefroy, G., Voronoi tessellation to study the numerical density and the spatial distribution of neurones, *J. Chem. Neuroanat.*, 20, 83, 2000.

141. Duyckaerts, C., Godefroy, G., and Hauw, J.J., Evaluation of neuronal numerical density by Dirichlet tessellation, *J. Neurosci. Methods*, 51, 47, 1994.

142. Hof, P.R. et al., Loss and altered spatial distribution of oligodendrocytes in the superior frontal gyrus in schizophrenia, *Biol. Psychiatry*, 53, 1075, 2003.

143. Nimchinsky, E.A. et al., Spindle neurons of the human anterior cingulate cortex, *J. Comp. Neurol.*, 355, 27, 1995.

144. Peterson, D.A., Quantitative histology using confocal microscopy: implementation of unbiased stereology procedures, *Methods*, 18, 493, 1999.

145. Mayhew, T.M., How to count synapses unbiasedly and efficiently at the ultrastructural level: proposal for a standard sampling and counting protocol, *J. Neurocytol.*, 25, 793, 1996.

146. Pakkenberg, B. et al., Unbiased and efficient estimation of total ventricular volume of the brain obtained from CT-scans by a stereological method, *Neuroradiology*, 31, 413, 1989.

147. Roberts, N. et al., Unbiased estimation of human body composition by the Cavalieri method using magnetic resonance imaging, *J. Microsc.*, 171, 239, 1993.

148. Kaplan, S. et al., A simple technique for localizing consecutive fields for disector pairs in light microscopy: application to neuron counting in rabbit spinal cord following spinal cord injury, *J. Neurosci. Methods*, 145, 277, 2005.

149. Cruz-Orive, L.M. and Weibel, E.R., Recent stereological methods for cell biology: a brief survey, *Am. J. Physiol.*, 258, L148, 1990.

150. Oorschot, D.E., Peterson, D.A., and Jones, D.G., Neurite growth from, and neuronal survival within, cultured explants of the nervous system: a critical review of morphometric and stereological methods, and suggestions for the future, *Prog. Neurobiol.*, 37, 525, 1991.

151. Royet, J.P., Stereology: a method for analyzing images, *Prog. Neurobiol.*, 37, 433, 1991.

152. Mayhew, T.M., A review of recent advances in stereology for quantifying neural structure, *J. Neurocytol.*, 21, 313, 1992.

153. Gundersen, H.J.G., Stereology: the fast lane between neuroanatomy and brain function — or still only a tightrope? *Acta Neurol. Scand. Suppl.*, 137, 8, 1992.

154. Coggeshall, R.E. and Lekan, H.A., Methods for determining numbers of cells and synapses: a case for more uniform standards of review, *J. Comp. Neurol.*, 364, 6, 1996.

155. Mayhew, T.M. and Gundersen, H.J.G., 'If you assume, you can make an ass out of u and me': a decade of the disector for stereological counting of particles in 3D space, *J. Anat.*, 188, 1, 1996.

156. Coggeshall, R.E., Assaying structural changes after nerve damage, an essay on quantitative morphology, *Pain Suppl.*, 6, S21, 1999.

157. West, M.J., Stereological methods for estimating the total number of neurons and synapses: issues of precision and bias, *Trends Neurosci.*, 22, 51, 1999.
158. Glaser, J. and Glaser, E.M., Stereology, morphometry, and mapping: the whole is greater than the sum of its parts, *J. Chem. Neuroanat.*, 20, 115, 2000.
159. Geuna, S., Appreciating the difference between design-based and model-based sampling strategies in quantitative morphology of the nervous system, *J. Comp. Neurol.*, 427, 333, 2000.
160. Keuker, J.I., Vollmann-Honsdorf, G.K., and Fuchs, E., How to use the optical fractionator: an example based on the estimation of neurons in the hippocampal CA1 and CA3 regions of tree shrews, *Brain Res. Protoc.*, 7, 211, 2001.
161. West, M.J., Design based stereological methods for estimating the total number of objects in histological material, *Folia Morphol.*, 60, 11, 2001.
162. Weibel, E.R., *Stereological Methods, Vol. 1. Practical Methods for Biological Morphometry*, Academic Press, London, 1979.
163. Weibel, E.R., *Stereological Methods, Vol. 2. Theoretical Foundations*, Academic Press, London, 1980.
164. Elias, H. and Hyde, M.D., *Guide to Practical Stereology*, Karger, Basel, 1983.
165. Reith, A. and Mayhew, T.M., *Stereology and Morphometry in Electron Microscopy: Some Problems and Their Solutions (An Ultrastructural Pathology Publication)*, Taylor and Francis, London, 1988.
166. Howard, C.V. and Reed, M.G., *Unbiased Stereology: Three-Dimensional Measurement in Microscopy*, Springer, Berlin, 1998.
167. Vedel Jensen, E.B., *Local Stereology*, World Scientific Publishing, London, 1998.
168. Nurcombe, V., Wreford, N., and Bertram, J.F., *Stereological Methods for Biology*, Chapman & Hall, Boston, 1999.
169. Russ, J.C. and Dehoff, R.T., *Practical Stereology*, 2nd ed., Plenum Publishers, New York, 2000.
170. Mouton, P.R., *Principles and Practices of Unbiased Stereology: An Introduction for Bioscientists*, Johns Hopkins University Press, Baltimore, 2002.
171. Howell, K., Hopkins, N., and Mcloughlin, P., Combined confocal microscopy and stereology: a highly efficient and unbiased approach to quantitative structural measurement in tissues, *Exp. Physiol.*, 87, 747, 2002.

5 The Effects of Normal Aging on Nerve Fibers and Neuroglia in the Central Nervous System

Alan Peters

CONTENTS

I.   INTRODUCTION

For the past several years, this laboratory has been involved in examining the effects of age on the brains of rhesus monkeys (*Macaca mulatta*). This species was chosen because these monkeys have a lifespan of about 35 years [1], so that one monkey year is equivalent to about one human year of life. Furthermore, although some senile plaques may be present in the brains of the older monkeys, there are no neurofibrillary tangles and the monkeys show no signs of developing Alzheimer's disease as they become older. They do, however, exhibit cognitive decline with age, similar to the cognitive decline that occurs in normally aging humans, and the extent of the cognitive decline can be assessed in monkeys by psychological tests that are adapted from those used on humans (e.g., [2–4], see also Chapter 2). Taken together, these attributes make the rhesus monkey an excellent model in which to study the effects of normal aging on the brain.

It is now generally accepted that there is no significant overall loss of neurons from the cerebral cortex of rhesus monkeys and other primates during normal aging (see [5–7]). Moreover, when one examines sections of cerebral cortex from old monkeys by either light or electron microscopy, there are few indications that neurons undergo morphological changes with age, beyond some accumulation of lipofuscin in their cell bodies and a loss of dendritic spines. However, Smith et al. [8] have recently asserted that when they compared the prefrontal cortex of young and aging monkeys, they found a 32% loss of neurons from area 8A of old monkeys. In contrast, they found that the numbers of neurons in the adjacent area 46 remained unchanged, as reported earlier by Peters et al. [9]. Smith et al. [8] suggest that their finding demonstrates that neuronal loss from the aging cerebral cortex may be localized.

The cells that do show obvious alterations with age are the neuroglial cells. All three classical types of neuroglial cells in old monkeys show accumulations of material in their perikarya and, in addition, there are obvious changes in the morphology of the myelin sheaths and axons of some nerve fibers.

II. MYELIN SHEATHS

The first hints that there are alterations in nerve fibers with age came from light microscope studies. Thus, Lintl and Braak [10] found that when the myelinated nerve fibers in sections of visual cortex from human brains are stained with hematoxylin, from the third decade of life onward there is a reduction in the staining intensity of the myelin in the line of Gennari, and they suggested that this is because the amount of myelin in this intracortical plexus is reduced. Similarly, Kemper [11] showed that with increasing age there a decrease in the staining intensity of nerve fibers in the human cortex, especially in the association cortices, which are the last areas of the cortex to myelinate. At present, however, it is not clear whether the age-associated decrease in myelin staining intensity is due to loss of nerve fibers or to changes in the dye-binding properties of myelin. Indeed, the effects of age on nerve fibers are complex because there are several events taking place at the same time. Some changes affect only the myelin sheaths and others affect both the axons and their myelin sheaths. For present purposes, these changes can be defined as alterations causing the breakdown or degeneration of myelin sheaths, degeneration and loss of nerve fibers, continued production of myelin, and remyelination.

A.   DEGENERATIVE CHANGES IN MYELIN SHEATHS

The most common age-related morphological alteration in myelin sheaths is the accumulation of pockets of dense cytoplasm between splits of the lamellae at the major dense line (Figure 5.1). These pockets of dense cytoplasm become more frequent with increasing age (e.g., [12, 13]). Because the major dense line is formed

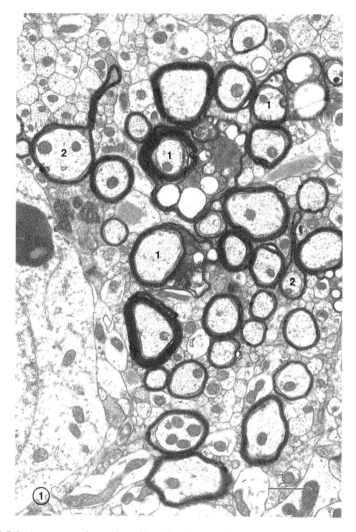

FIGURE 5.1 A transversely sectioned bundle of nerve fibers in layer 4C of the visual cortex of a 29-year-old monkey. Three of the nerve fibers (1) have disrupted myelin sheaths with splits between the lamellae that contain dense, vacuolated cytoplasm. Two other nerve fibers (2) have sheaths with redundant myelin. (Scale bar = 1 μm.)

by the apposition of the cytoplasmic faces of successive lamellae of the oligoden-droglial cell plasma membrane that forms the sheath, it can be concluded that the dense cytoplasm must belong to the parent oligodendroglial cell. Sometimes, there is only one pocket of dense cytoplasm but it is not uncommon for several pockets of dense cytoplasm to occur in the same segment of the sheath, between adjacent turns of the spiraling myelin lamellae, which results in an obvious bulging of the sheath. Also, several loci containing pockets of dense cytoplasm may occur along an individual internodal length of myelin.

Based on the fact that the cytoplasm in the pockets is dense, it is assumed that its presence is a sign of degeneration, and this conclusion is supported by the fact that Cuprizone toxicity can also lead to the formation of dense cytoplasm in the inner tongue process of degenerating sheaths (e.g., [14, 15]), and that similar dense cytoplasm occurs in the sheaths of mice with myelin-associated glycoprotein deficiency (e.g., [16]). It should also be pointed out that anti-ubiquitin antibodies immunostain dense inclusions within focal swellings of myelin sheaths in the white matter of old humans [17] and dogs [18], suggesting that the electron-dense material between the lamellae of sheaths in old animals contains proteins that are not being degraded by proteosomes. Interestingly, Wang et al. [19] have shown that in humans there is no correlation between the amount of soluble and insoluble ubiquitinated material in white matter and the cognitive scores of the humans from which the tissue was derived, but there is a correlation between decreased levels of myelin basic protein and decreased cognitive scores. These results lead the authors to conclude that white matter pathology may contribute to age-associated decline in cognition.

In examining the ultrastructure of degenerative changes in myelin during normal aging, it is important to recognize that myelin in white matter is often poorly preserved, largely due to the fact that white matter has many fewer capillaries than gray matter. Consequently, the nerve fibers in white matter are less accessible to fixatives that are introduced by perfusion fixation, and this can result in defects in the preservation of myelin sheaths, However, the most common change brought about by poor preservation of myelin is focal splitting or shearing of the myelin lamellae, and the frequency of this shearing increases as the quality of preservation of the tissue is diminished. There is no indication that such shearing of myelin lamellae occurs as a result of normal aging, and it does not seem to occur even in myelin sheaths altered by experimental interventions. Nevertheless, fixation defects must not be misconstrued as age changes.

An age change less common than the occurrence of pockets of dense cytoplasm is the formation of myelin balloons (Figure 5.2). These balloons can be spectacular because they can be 10 μm or more in diameter, so that in light microscopic preparations they appear as holes in the neuropil [20]. When the balloons are examined by electron microscopy, it becomes evident that they are fluid-filled cavities that occupy splits in the intraperiod line of the sheath. Although myelin balloons often appear as isolated circular profiles bounded by several lamellae of compact myelin, appropriate sections through balloons show that they bulge from the sides of myelin sheaths, leaving the axon flattened against the opposite side sheath from where the balloon protrudes (Figure 5.2). Consequently, the isolated circular profiles are generated by sections that pass to one side of the connection between the balloon and its parent sheath. Because there is no decrease in the widths of the myelin lamellae surrounding the balloons, and because there is no indication that myelin is elastic in nature, the generation of these balloons must require the parent oligodendrocyte to produce large amounts of additional myelin. It should be added that sometimes small pockets of dense cytoplasm can occur at the base of a balloon, and that the nature of the fluid contained in balloons is not known.

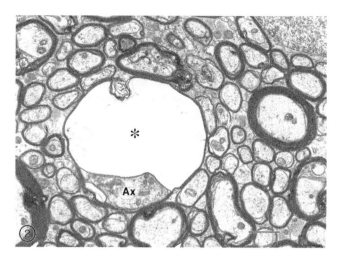

FIGURE 5.2 A ballooned nerve fiber in the anterior commissure of a 25-year-old monkey. Ballooning of the sheath results in a fluid-filled space (asterisk) and causes the axon (Ax) to be pushed to one side of the expanded sheath. (Scale bar = 1 μm.)

In monkeys, alterations to myelin sheaths are not common in animals less than about 10 years old but they become noticeable in middle-aged monkeys; and in monkeys over 25 years of age, as many as 5 to 6% of profiles on myelinated nerve fibers show some morphological changes.

Although we have only examined the monkey central nervous system, similar myelin balloons have been reported by Faddis and McGinn [21] in the cochlear nucleus of normally aging gerbils. It is assumed that ballooning of myelin is a degenerative change because it can occur in the early stages of Wallerian degeneration in the dorsal funiculus of the spinal cord following section of dorsal roots [22] and also can occur in rats with severe diabetes [23]. In addition, myelin balloons can be generated by Cuprizone poisoning [24], by experimental toxicity produced by triethyl tin (e.g., [25]), by chronic copper poisoning [26], and by lysolecithin [27].

It has been shown that with age the composition of myelin changes, as reported by Malone and Szoke [28]. They found that in aging rats there are changes in the cholesterol:phospholipid ratios in myelin and an increased saturation of the long acyl chains of myelin glycosphingolipids, and they suggest that these changes may cause an increased fluidity and decreased stability of myelin. Sloane et al. [29] also found the composition of myelin to alter with age, because there is a decrease in the amount of associated glycoprotein. On the other hand, with increasing age, levels of the oligodendrocyte-specific proteins CNPase and myelin/oligodendrocyte specific protein (MOSP) increase dramatically in white matter homogenates and in myelin, suggesting that there is new formation of myelin by oligodendrocytes, perhaps in response to myelin degradation and injury caused by proteolitic enzymes such as calpain, which increases in white matter with age.

In a study using microarrays to determine alterations in gene expression in the hippocampus of aging rats, Blalock et al. [30] found that the genes for myelin-associated oligodendroglial basic protein (MOSP) and myelin-associated glycoprotein (S-MAG) are among those that are upregulated. And in another study in which the effects of aging on the frontal cortex of the human brain were assessed, Lu et al. [31] found that the genes that are upregulated after the age of 40 include those for proteolipid protein and oligodendrocyte lineage transcription factor 2. Blalock et al. [30] suggest that upregulation of these genes is related to myelin degeneration with increasing age, although the upregulation might also be associated with remyelination, which, as will be shown later, is also known to occur during aging.

B.   DEGENERATION AND LOSS OF NERVE FIBERS

For a nerve fiber to completely degenerate, it is necessary for the ensheathed axon to degenerate, and in turn this causes the myelin sheath surrounding the axon to also degenerate. Classically, these events were first described in experimental Wallerian degeneration, in which sectioning of a nerve fiber leads to degeneration of the portion of the nerve fiber isolated from its parent neuron. When nerve fibers caused to degenerate following experimental lesions are examined by electron microscopy, it is found that the cytoplasm of the degenerating axon can show accumulations of mitochondria and lysosomes before it eventually becomes dense. Axons with these features are sometimes encountered in the normally aging brain, but to show that there is nerve fiber degeneration and loss during aging requires quantitative analyses.

Among the earliest quantitative studies to show that there is loss of nerve fibers with age are the stereological analyses carried out by Pakkenberg and Gundersen [32]. They examined a total of 94 normal human brains, from individuals ranging in age from 20 to 95 years, and concluded that there is a 12% decrease in the overall volume of the cerebral hemispheres, accompanied by a 28% decrease in the volume of the white matter. This study was followed by a report by Tang et al. [33] that focused on the nerve fibers of white matter in the cerebral hemispheres and concluded that the loss of white matter volume is due to a 27% overall loss in the total length of nerve fibers in the white matter. Later, Marner et al. [34] extended this study by examining a total of 26 brains and concluded that the loss of white matter from the normally aging human cerebral hemispheres is almost 23% between the ages of 20 and 80 years, and that the overall loss of nerve fiber length is 45%. They suggest that this is produced by a loss of the thinner fibers, and that there is a relative preservation of larger-diameter fibers.

The conclusion from these studies is that there is a an overall loss of some nerve fibers from the human brain during normal aging; a similar conclusion was reached previously by Meier-Ruge et al. [35], who examined autopsied brains from cognitively normal humans. Meier-Ruge et al. [35] examined semithick sections in which nerve fibers were stained for light microscopy and, on the basis of counts, they concluded that with age there is a 16% nerve fiber loss from the white matter of the precentral gyrus and a 10.5% loss of nerve fibers from the corpus callosum.

There is also MRI data from humans (e.g., [36, 37]) and from monkeys ([38]; see also [39]) supporting the conclusion that there is a loss of white matter from the cerebral hemispheres with increasing age, and especially from the frontal lobes (e.g.,

[40, 41]). In addition, there are MRI studies that show that the signal characteristics of white matter alter in normal human aging. These changes are considered to indicate that white matter is undergoing degenerative changes, which result in disconnections between parts of the brain (e.g., [42, 43]). The study by De Groot et al. [44] indicates that the most common locations for white matter lesions in the aging human brain are the subcortical and periventricular white matter. The subcortical fibers mainly consist of short U-fibers that connect adjacent areas of the cortex while the periventricular fibers are mainly long association fibers. After analyzing the frequency of occurrence of lesions and correlating the data with the cognitive status of the subjects examined, De Groot et al. [44] conclude that it is the lesions of the long association fibers that play a dominant role in bringing about cognitive decline.

It is suggested by Bartzokis et al. [45] that the deterioration of myelin sheaths with age is related to the sequence in which fiber tracts myelinate during development, such that the tracts that myelinate last are the ones most severely affected during aging. It is those same association fiber tracts that Kemper [11] has shown to exhibit staining pallor with age. Kemper [11] has also shown that, in the human brain, the primary cortices, in which myelination is completed earliest, show little change in myelin staining intensity with increasing age, while the association cortices show a distinct loss of staining intensity. But in contrast to these studies emphasizing white matter, there are other studies on monkeys (e.g., [46]) and humans (e.g., [47–49]) that suggest there is cortical thinning during normal aging, such that gray matter loss exceeds white matter loss (e.g., [50]) and, moreover, that the portion of the brain most affected by aging is the frontal lobes (e.g., [51]).

To obtain direct evidence that nerve fibers are lost from white matter with age, we have examined well-circumscribed fiber tracts in the monkey brain using design-based stereology. One of the first tracts we examined was the optic nerve. The cross-sectional area of the optic nerve does not alter much with age, but it was found that while the average total number of nerve fibers in the optic nerves of young monkeys is 16×10^5, in monkeys over 25 years of age the number of nerve fibers is reduced to an average of 9×10^5. Some old monkeys lose only a small percentage of their nerve fibers, but in extreme cases the number of nerve fibers is reduced to 4×10^5, which represents a 75% loss of nerve fibers [52]. In the optic nerves showing such extreme loss, almost every nerve fiber has myelin sheath defects and, while some nerve fibers have degenerating axons, other myelin sheaths are empty (Figure 5.3). Correlated with the loss of nerve fibers there is hypertrophy of astrocytes, which develop abundant glial filaments and fill spaces vacated by degenerated nerve fibers. Oligodendrocytes and microglial cells also increase in number with age, and many of the microglial cells became engorged with phagocytosed debris, much of which can be recognized as degenerating myelin [53]. Cavallotti et al. [54] also found a loss of nerve fibers from the optic nerve of the aging rat, accompanied by an increase in the numbers of astrocytes and an increase in GFAP reactivity.

The anterior commissure is another well-circumscribed bundle of white matter in which the total numbers of nerve fibers can be accurately determined [55]. In the anterior commissures of young monkeys, the mean number of nerve fibers is 2.2×10^6, while in monkeys over 25 years of age the mean number is reduced to

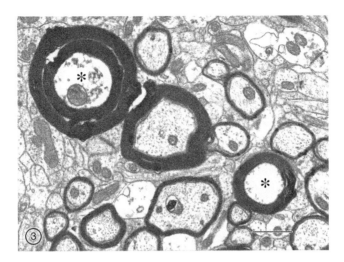

FIGURE 5.3 This micrograph from the primary visual cortex of a 13-year-old monkey shows two nerve fibers (asterisks) in which the axon has degenerated, leaving empty myelin sheaths behind. (Scale bar = 1 μm.)

1.2×10^6. This loss of fibers is accompanied by a 25% reduction in the cross-sectional area of the anterior commissure. Some middle-aged monkeys, 12 to 20 years of age, also were available for study and it became evident that, in terms of the total numbers of nerve fibers, middle-aged monkeys resemble young ones, so most of the loss of nerve fibers appears to occur after middle age. Nerve fibers with abnormal myelin sheaths are evident at all ages, but there is a progressive, age-related increase in their frequency, such that in young monkeys only 0.4% of profiles of nerve fibers show alterations in myelin, while the number increases to 1.8% in middle-aged monkeys, and reaches 5.4% in old monkeys. Similarly, as would be expected from the loss of nerve fibers, there is a significant increase in the numbers of axons that show degenerative changes with age. Because most of the monkeys used in this study had been behaviorally tested, it was possible to correlate the data with a decline in their cognitive status. A positive correlation was found between the reduction in the total numbers of nerve fibers and cognitive impairment, but there was not a strong correlation between myelin sheath abnormalities and cognitive status.

In rats, Fujisawa [56] examined the effects of age on the nerve fibers in the posterior funiculus of the spinal cord and found that degenerating axons begin to appear long before the posterior funiculus has finished growing and has acquired its full complement of nerve fibers. Fujisawa [56] also showed that axonal degeneration occurs simultaneously at all levels of the spinal cord and that it involves nerve fibers of all sizes.

Our conclusion is that there is a loss of myelinated nerve fibers from white matter with age; and it is probably ubiquitous because we also found loss of nerve fibers from the splenium of the corpus callosum [57], as well as from the fornix of monkeys (unpublished data).

C. Continued Production of Myelin

In the primary visual cortex of the monkey, there are vertical bundles of myelinated nerve fibers that are most prominent in layer 4C. It was noticed that with age some of the myelin sheaths around the larger-diameter fibers in the bundles become appreciably thicker. Consequently, electron micrographs were taken of these bundles of nerve fibers in both young and old monkeys, and the diameters of the axons and the thickness of their myelin sheaths were measured [58]. The analysis indicated that no change is evident in the diameters of the axons with age, and there is no change in the width of individual myelin lamellae. Nevertheless, the mean numbers of lamellae in the myelin sheaths increase from 5.6 in young monkeys to 7.0 in old monkeys, and much of this increase in the mean thickness of myelin sheaths is due to an increase in the numbers of larger nerve fibers that have more than ten lamellae. In young monkeys, few nerve fibers have sheaths with more than 10 lamellae; but in the old monkeys it is not uncommon to encounter sheaths with as many as 20 lamellae, and in many cases such sheaths show circumferential splits, so that the sheaths appear to consist of an inner set of compact lamellae surrounded by an outer, separate set. A consequence of this increase in the thickness of myelin sheaths with age is evident at the paranodes of some of the thickened nerve fibers in the central nervous systems of aging monkeys. In longitudinal sectioned nerve fibers, the para-nodal loops of myelin normally terminate in a regular sequence, and all of them are in contact with the underlying membrane of the axon. However, at the paranodes formed by many of these thickened sheaths, the paranodal loops pile up on one another and become disarrayed, so that there is only space enough for some of the loops to reach the underlying axon (unpublished data). Earlier, Sugiyama et al. [59] reported this same phenomenon in the thickened nerve fibers of old rats.

As far as can be determined, there are no other studies of the effects of age on the thickness of myelin sheaths in primates, but there have been a number of such studies in rodents. The authors have reached various conclusions. For example, Sturrock [60] examined the anterior and posterior limbs of the anterior commissure in the brains of 5- and 18-month-old mice and concluded that there is no change in the numbers of lamellae with age. In contrast, Godlewski [61] found that the myelin sheaths in the corpus callosum and optic nerves of 2.5-year-old rats were thicker than those of 4-month-old rats. In the peripheral nervous system of rodents, Caselli et al. [62] found no change in the numbers of lamellae in the sciatic nerves of rats with age, while Cebellos et al. [63] reported that in the tibial nerve of mice, myelin sheaths become thicker between 6 and 33 months of age, with some sheaths becoming very thick, as we have found in monkey visual cortex [58]. With such variations in the data, it is difficult to know the true situation in rodents. Obviously, more studies are necessary.

Another morphological alteration that occurs with age is an increase in the frequency of nerve fibers with redundant myelin, that is, sheaths that are overly large for the size of the enclosed axon, so that in cross sections the axon is at one end of a large loop of myelin (see Figure 5.1). Sheaths with redundant myelin were first described by Rosenbluth [64] in the cerebellum of the toad. In a study of the effects of age on myelin sheath in the white matter of mice, Sturrock [60] found such redundant sheaths to be common in old mice. As far as the monkey is concerned, redundant sheaths can be found even in young monkeys, although their frequency of occurrence increases with age.

On the basis of these observations, it can be concluded that — at least in the monkey — oligodendrocytes continue to produce myelin throughout life, and that this continued myelin production is occurring even as some sheaths are degenerating.

D.   REMYELINATION AND AGING

As we continued to examine the effects of aging on nerve fibers, it was noticed that in cross sections of the vertically oriented bundles of nerve fibers in both the primary visual and prefrontal cortices of older monkeys examined by electron microscopy, there is an increase in the frequency of occurrence of profiles of paranodes [65]. Paranodes occur at both ends of a length of myelin, adjacent to the nodes of Ranvier, and they are the sites where the lamellae of myelin gradually terminate. In visual cortex, there is a 57% increase in the frequency of cross-sectioned paranodal profiles with age and in area 46 of prefrontal cortex the increase is of the order of 90%. Such an increase in the frequency of profiles of paranodes could be due to either an increase in the lengths of paranodes with age, or to a real increase in the numbers of paranodes. Examination of the lengths of paranodes in primary visual cortex shows that with age there is an 11% increase in the lengths of paranodes, but this is insufficient to account for the large 57% increase in the frequency of paranodal profiles. This suggests that most of the increase in the frequency of paranodal profiles with age must be due to an increase in the total number of paranodes, and hence in the total number of internodal lengths of myelin. The implication is that some shorter internodal lengths of myelin are generated with increasing age, as would occur if the initially formed long internodal lengths of myelin degenerate and the resulting lengths of bare axons are remyelinated by a series of shorter internodal lengths.

In support of the proposal that remyelination occurs in the cerebral cortices of older monkeys, in the vertical bundles of nerve fibers in the visual cortices of old monkeys, we have found inappropriately thin myelin sheaths around some axons, as well as some short internodes that are only 3 to 6 μm long. Both of these features are considered the hallmarks of remyelination and support the contention that during normal aging some myelin sheaths break down, and that the resulting bare lengths of axons are then remyelinated by shorter lengths of new myelin. To determine that some myelin sheaths are completely degenerated, leaving the axon bare, is difficult to prove. However, in support of the concept that some myelin sheaths degenerate with age, it has been found that astrocytes in the cerebral cortices of old monkeys sometimes contain phagocytosed myelin lamellae and that some of the more amorphous phagocytosed inclusions in astrocytes label with antibodies to myelin basic protein [65].

Because an increase in the frequency of internodes can be expected to slow the rate of conduction along a nerve fiber, the correlation between the frequency of paranodal profiles in the vertical bundles of nerve fibers and the decline in cognition was examined. In prefrontal area 46, there is a significant correlation between these measures, but not in primary visual cortex (area 17). The reason why a correlation only exists for area 46 may be because prefrontal cortex plays a much greater role in cognition than area 17.

In a subsequent study, it was found that there is also an increase in the frequency of paranodal profiles in the anterior commissures of old monkeys [55]. In the anterior commissure, the increase is on the order 60%. However, when the frequency of occurrence of paranodal profiles in the anterior commissures of young monkeys, 5 to 10 years of age, is compared to that of middle-aged monkeys, 12 to 20 years of age, there is no difference between them. The increase in frequency of paranodal profiles only occurs in monkeys over 25 years of age. As stated earlier, there is a loss of nerve fibers from the anterior commissure with age, and it might be suggested that the increase in the frequency of occurrence of paranodal profiles is brought about by a preferential loss of the large-diameter fibers with the longest internodes and paranodes. However, this is not the case because the fiber diameter spectrum of nerve fibers is similar in young and old monkeys. So again, the most logical explanation is that there is some degeneration of internodal lengths of myelin, followed by remyelination of the affected axons by shorter internodal lengths of myelin.

Ibanez et al. [66] have reviewed the affects of aging on the remyelination of nerve fibers and the regenerative capacity of myelin sheaths to be restored in conditions such as multiple sclerosis. They cite data to show that as animals grow older, their capacity for remyelination declines. They suggest that the capacity for remyelination can be partially reversed by steroid hormones and their derivatives.

E. CORRELATIONS WITH COGNITION

Most of the monkeys in which we have examined the effects of age on nerve fibers have been behaviorally tested and an index of their cognitive impairment (CII) has been generated (see [4, 12, 67,68]; see also Chapter 2). Consequently, it has been possible to ascertain what age-related alterations in nerve fibers might result in cognitive impairment. In area 17 [12], in prefrontal area 46 [57], and in corpus callosum [57], the increase in the frequency of profiles of altered myelin sheaths correlates significantly with cognitive impairment. In area 46 there is also a correlation with the increased frequency of paranodal profiles, but there is no such correlation in other structures examined. This raises the question of what brings about such behavioral correlations. Myelin is known to provide insulation around nerve fibers, so that saltatory conduction is possible. Consequently, it is likely that defects in myelin might lead to some breakdown in the insulation and affect conduction.

Although correlations between the age-related defects in the structure of the myelin and conduction velocity have not been examined, there have been several studies of the effects of age on conduction velocity in old animals. For example, Aston-Jones [69] examined the conduction velocity along nerve fibers connecting nucleus basalis to frontal cortex in rats and found a significant reduction in conduction velocity in old animals. Similarly, Morales et al. [70] have shown a reduction in conduction velocity of lumbar motor neurons in the spinal cords of cats, and Xi et al. [71] have shown a reduction in conduction velocity along nerve fibers in the pyramidal tracts of old cats. Interestingly, in proteolipid deficient mice, in which there is decompaction of the myelin, there is also a reduction in conduction velocity [72], and a reduction also occurs in demyelinating diseases (see [73, 74]). Attention should also be drawn to a recent study by Wang et al. [75] on the visual system of old monkeys. This study shows that the neurons in layer 4 of primary visual cortex in old monkeys exhibit normal visual response latencies, but in other parts of V1, and throughout secondary visual area V2, hyperactivity (increased firing frequency) of neurons is accompanied by delays in both intracortical and intercortical transfer of information. In part this may be explained by delays in the transfer of information along nerve fibers due to alterations in their myelin sheaths. In addition, Chang et al. [76] recently demonstrated a similar increase in the firing rates of rhesus monkey prefrontal cortical pyramidal cells with normal aging. These workers have hypothesized that this "hyperactivity" may represent a compensatory response to increased action potential conduction failures along the axon due to the extensive myelin dystrophy that occurs with age.

F.　Summary of Aging-Related Myelin Changes

In summary, in the monkey, the process of myelin formation appears to continue throughout life in the central nervous system and results in the formation of thicker myelin sheaths and in the formation of redundant myelin. Beginning in middle age, some myelin sheaths begin to degenerate, and subsequently some of the resulting bare axons become remyelinated by shorter internodal lengths. This conclusion is supported by the finding that some short internodes do indeed exist, and that some axons have inappropriately thin myelin sheaths. In addition, it is evident that with age there is an increase in the frequency of occurrence of profiles of paranodes, as would occur with an overall increase in the numbers of internodes with increasing age. At the same time that these changes are taking place in myelin, some axons degenerate; this leads to complete degeneration of the affected nerve fibers and results in a reduction in the total number of nerve fibers in the white matter.

It is proposed that these alterations in the structure of myelin sheaths, coupled with an increase in the numbers of internodal lengths along nerves, bring about a reduction in the conduction velocity of affected nerve fibers. This would result in a change in the timing of sequential events in neuronal circuits, and it is suggested that this change in timing is at least partially responsible for the cognitive decline exhibited by old primates. In addition, the loss of some nerve fibers from white matter tracts with age would lead to some disconnection between groups of neurons in the brain, which could also adversely affect cognition.

III.　NEUROGLIAL CELLS

The three classically defined types of neuroglial cells — oligodendrocytes, astrocytes, and microglial cells — all show distinct and unique alterations in their morphology with age. According to Pakkenberg et al. [77], however, there seems to be little change in the overall numbers of neuroglial cells with age in the human neocortex. They found that in the neocortex of young humans, with a mean age of 26.2 years, there are some 39 billion neuroglial cells, which does not differ significantly from the 36 billion neuroglial cells they found in the brains of individuals with a mean age of 89.2 years. However, other studies suggest that there are some alterations in the frequency of neuroglia with age, and the neuroglial cells that seem to be most affected in specific portions of the brain are oligodendrocytes and microglial cells.

A. OLIGODENDROCYTES

Oligodendrocytes are the neuroglial cells that form the myelin sheaths in the central nervous system. As far as is known, this is their only function. As their name suggests, these cells have few visible processes, so that in light microscopic preparations of young animals stained by one of the silver stains or by Perl's reaction for ferric iron (which is relatively abundant in oligodendrocytes, along with ferritin and transferrin [78, 79]), a few wispy, undulating processes can be seen leaving the cell body. However, when Perl's stain is used on old monkeys, it becomes apparent that some of the processes of oligodendrocytes have acquired bulbous enlargements (Figure 5.4). These enlargements are of various sizes, with the largest ones reaching diameters of 5 μm. Another age-related change is that, whereas most oligodendrocytes in young monkeys occur individually, in old monkeys it is common to find oligodendrocytes in pairs, groups, or in rows (Figure 5.5). There is a significant correlation between the increased incidence of pairs, groups, and rows of oligodendrocytes and increasing age [80, 81].

These age-related changes in oligodendrocytes are also evident in electron microscopic preparations. In young monkeys, oligodendrocytes are encountered throughout the gray and white matter, and they are recognized by having a dark nucleus with clumped chromatin. In general, the nucleus has a rounded or oval profile, but sometimes it may have a more irregular shape. The nucleus is surrounded by an electron-dense cytoplasm with short and rather dilated cisternae of granular endoplasmic reticulum, polyribosomes, rather stubby mitochondria, and profiles of the Golgi apparatus. Microtubules occur throughout the cytoplasm but they can be difficult to discern due to the density of the cytoplasmic matrix. However, the microtubules become more evident at the bases of processes into which they funnel, and become closely packed.

In old monkeys, the oligodendrocytes have these same basic features but a difference is that many of them have dense inclusions in their perikaryal cytoplasm. These dense inclusions are irregular in shape and come in various sizes [82, 80]. Furthermore, most of the inclusions are composed of both pale and dense components that sometimes appear to form layers. Vaughan and Peters [83] reported the existence of similar inclusions in the oligodendrocytes within the auditory cortex of aging rats, and Rees [84] reported dense inclusions in oligodendrocytes in the cerebral cortex of aged human brains. At present, the origins of these inclusions are not known and their morphology gives no clues as to the sources of their contents. However, because they are not membrane bound, it is assumed that they are not phagocytic inclusions. Rather, they might be derived from the degeneration of some component of the aging myelin sheath attached to the oligodendrocyte. This possibility is reinforced by the fact that, in addition to the ones in the perikarya, other

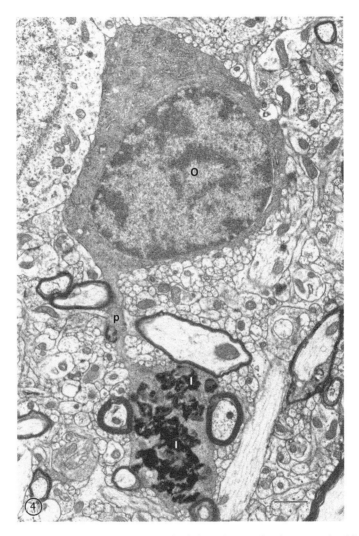

FIGURE 5.4 An oligodendrocyte in layer 3 of the primary visual cortex of a 29-year-old monkey. The oligodendrocyte (O) has a long process (p) that expands into a large bulge containing dense inclusions (I). (Scale bar = 1 μm.)

inclusions are present in the swellings that occur along the process of oligodendrocytes in older monkeys. It has been reported that similar swellings also occur along the processes of oligodendrocytes in the twitcher mouse, which is a model for globoid cell leukodystrophy. Using Perl's reaction, LeVine and Torres [85] reported that in these animals some of the oligodendrocytes have large swellings in the portions of their processes extending from the outsides of the myelin sheaths, and other swellings along the lengths of the processes. As a consequence, LeVine and Torres [85] suggested that the material in the swellings comes from components in the sheaths that are being turned over or replaced, so that the material originates in

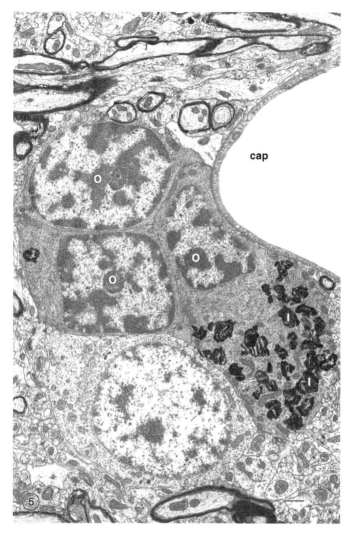

FIGURE 5.5 A nest of three oligodendrocytes (O) lying next to a capillary (cap) in the primary visual cortex of a 28-year-old monkey. One of the oligodendrocytes has an aggregate of dense inclusions (I) in its cytoplasm. (Scale bar = 1 μm.)

the myelin sheaths and is then moved to the cell body of the oligodendrocyte, where it forms the dense inclusions found there.

The fact that there is an age-related increase in the numbers of oligodendrocytes in pairs, rows, and groups suggests that oligodendrocytes are proliferating with age and that there is an increase in their numbers [81]. Such an increase was first suggested when a comparison was made between the mean numbers of neuroglial cells in the primary visual cortex of young and old monkeys [82]. It was found that oligodendrocytes comprised 35% of the total population of neuroglial cells in young monkeys and 40% in the cortices of the neuroglia in old monkeys. For this study, only a few monkeys were available; but in a later study that involved seven young, six middle-aged, and eleven old monkeys, counts were made of the numbers of neuroglial cells in layer 4C of the primary visual cortex and, when young and old monkeys are compared, it was found that there is a 50% increase in the numbers of oligodendrocytes with age in this cortical layer. This increase begins in middle age but, interestingly, there seems to be no parallel increase in the numbers of astrocytes or of microglial cells in layer 4C [81].

There is also an increase in the numbers of oligodendrocytes in the monkey optic nerve with age. This is accompanied by an increase in the numbers of microglial cells, but not of astrocytes [53]. In contrast, there is no increase in the total numbers of any of the neuroglial cell types in the aging anterior commissure [55].

When there is an increase in the number of oligodendrocytes with age, questions arise as to where they come from and why they are needed. The answer to the second part of the question is that they are probably needed to form the increased numbers of internodal lengths of myelin that are generated with age [65]. As to the origins of the increased numbers of oligodendrocytes, the age-related increase in the frequency of oligodendrocytes in pairs, rows, and groups in some parts of the brain suggests that some of the oligodendrocytes might be dividing. However, the prevailing view is that there is little evidence that mature oligodendrocytes divide (see [14, 86, 87]) and that new oligodendrocytes are generated from oligodendroglial precursor cells (see [86, 88–90]), which can be visualized using antibodies to NG2 chondroitin proteoglycan and to platelet derived growth factor alpha receptor (e.g., [91–93]). These NG2+ cells are relatively common in the central nervous system and, as considered in a later section of this chapter, there is good reason to consider that they comprise a fourth and distinct type of neuroglial cell.

B.   ASTROCYTES

As their name might suggest, astrocytes are star-shaped neuroglial cells that have numerous processes radiating from their cell bodies. Under the electron microscope, these cells have pale nuclei with very little clumping of the chromatin. The cytoplasm is also pale, which distinguishes these cells from oligodendrocytes and microglial cells, both of which have dark cytoplasm. A unique component of the cytoplasm of astrocytes is the 9-nm-thick intermediate filaments, which occur throughout the perikaryon and aggregate into bundles that pass into the processes. Because of the richness of the bundles of filaments in their cytoplasm, the astrocytes of white matter are often referred to as filamentous astrocytes, while the astrocytes in gray matter, which has fewer filaments, are referred to as protoplasmic astrocytes. Another feature of astrocytes is that they are extensively coupled by gap junctions. The study by Cotrina et al. [94] shows that in mice, gap junction proteins are maintained at high levels during aging, although there is some reorganization in terms of the number and sizes of the junctions labeled by antibodies to various connexins. What effect this has on the function of the aging brain is not known.

Antibodies to the glial fibrillary acid protein (GFAP) often are used to visualize astrocytes in light microscopic preparations. Such preparations show the cell bodies and radiating processes of astrocytes to good advantage, and give the impression that the processes are smooth. Essentially, this is true of the astrocytes in white matter, which have processes that tend to pass at right angles to the orientation of the nerve fibers, but it is not true of the astrocytes in gray matter. The filaments in these protoplasmic astrocytes extend along the axes of the larger-diameter processes but they do not usually enter and reveal the presence of the many thin and irregularly shaped excrescences that emanate from the thicker processes. And indeed, when astrocytes in gray matter are examined under the electron microscope, they are seen to have very irregular shapes and the fine, irregular processes mold themselves to the components of the surrounding neuropil.

As stated in the above section dealing with oligodendrocytes, astrocytes do not appear to increase in number during normal aging of the monkey. Most reports suggest that the same is true for rodents (e.g., [95–98]) and humans [99]. However, Peinado et al. [100] have reported that in the parietal cortex of the aging rat, there is a 20% increase in the numbers of astrocytes with age; and in the frontal cortex, Peinado et al. [101] found a 10 to 20% increase in neuroglial cells with age, depending on the cortical layer being examined. Similarly, Mouton et al. [102] have reported that the hippocampi of young female mice have about 20% more astrocytes and microglia than the hippocampi of old female mice. They also report that in the dentate gyrus and CA1 regions of the hippocampus, female mice have 25 to 40% more astrocytes and microglia than age-matched males. However, as pointed out, in their study of the total numbers of glial cells in human neocortex, Pakkenberg et al. [77] concluded that there is no significant increase in the total numbers of neuroglia with age.

There is general agreement that astrocytes undergo hypertrophy with age. They both increase in size and become more filamentous. Thus, when nerve fibers are lost with age, the astrocytes undergo hypertrophy and fill up the space vacated by the degenerated nerve fibers, as has been seen in the optic nerves [53] and in the corpus callosum (unpublished data). The hypertrophy also is evident in layer 1 of the cerebral cortex. In monkeys, layer 1 becomes thinner with age, largely because of the loss of some of the branches of the apical dendritic tufts of pyramidal cells [6, 103]. This leads to an impressive thickening of the glial limiting membrane on the outside of the cortex. However, there is no increase in the number of astrocytes. The thickening is brought about by an increase in the number of layers of astrocytic processes forming the glial limiting membrane, and this is accompanied by an increase in the numbers of intermediate filaments in these processes. This hypertrophy of astrocytes with age has also been noted by Hansen et al. [99], who found a strong increase in GFAP labeling in layer 1 of aging human brains. Simultaneous with the thickening of the glial limiting membrane, the processes of the astrocytes in layer 1 become more profuse and more filamentous as they undergo hypertrophy to fill the spaces vacated by the loss of apical dendritic branches of neurons [104]. Overall, the effect is somewhat similar to the response of astrocytes to a lesion when they form a glial scar.

Other studies have also recorded an increase in the amount of GFAP and an increase in the intensity of GFAP labeling with age in the brains of rats and mice [105–107] and in monkeys [108–110]. Consistent with this, Nichols et al. [111] have shown that there is an increase in GFAP mRNA with age in rats and humans.

Consequently, hypertrophy of astrocytes with age, but not an increase in their numbers, seems to be a ubiquitous event.

In addition to undergoing hypertrophy, astrocytes in both white and gray matter undertake phagocytosis in the aging brain. Indeed, astrocytes with inclusions in their cell bodies (Figure 5.6) have been encountered in all parts of the brain we have examined, including the cerebral cortex of both the rat [83] and monkey [9, 65, 82], as well as the optic nerves [53] and anterior commissure [55] of the monkey. The inclusions can be quite massive and most commonly consist of an electron-dense, sometimes granular, component intermixed with a paler component that appears to derive from lipid. In addition, we have encountered lamellar inclusions that are obviously the remains of phagocytosed myelin sheaths, because they have a periodic structure with major dense and intraperiod lines that match those in normal myelin. The presence of phagocytosed myelin in astrocytes is consistent with the fact that myelin degeneration occurs throughout the central nervous system of the aging monkey. The degenerating myelin that is phagocytosed by astrocytes is probably then degraded by them and incorporated into the more amorphous inclusions because when an antibody to myelin basic protein is used, labeling can be found over some of the amorphous inclusions [65]. The sources of the other material phagocytosed by astrocytes are not known.

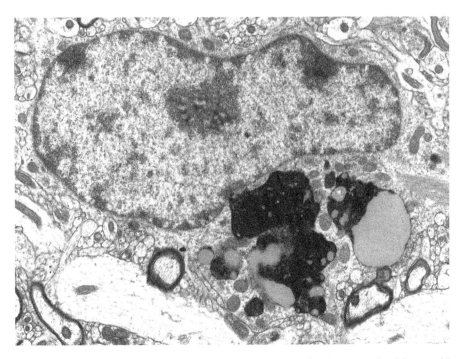

FIGURE 5.6 An astrocyte (As) in layer 5 of the primary visual cortex of a 35-year-old monkey. The cytoplasm of the astrocyte contains bundles of filaments (f), as well as inclusions (I) with dense and pale components. (Scale bar = 1 μm.)

C.   MICROGLIAL CELLS

Microglial cells have dark nuclei, similar in appearance to those of oligodendrocytes, although the nuclei tend to be rather smaller and either oval or bean shaped. The cytoplasm of microglial cells is electron dense, but somewhat paler than that of oligodendrocytes. However, the similarities between microglial cells and oligodendrocytes can make it difficult in light microscopic preparations to distinguish between the two cell types. The differences between them are more obvious in electron microscopic preparations because, in contrast to the short stubby cisternae present in oligodendrocytes, microglial cells have long cisternae of granular endoplasmic reticulum. Moreover, microglial cell bodies have more irregular shapes because they tend to mold themselves to the outlines of the components in the surrounding neuropil. Another interesting difference between these two cell types is that when microglial cells are adjacent to the cell bodies of neurons, there is usually a thin astrocytic process interposed between the cell bodies of the microglial cells and the neurons, whereas the plasma membranes of oligodendrocytes lie immediately adjacent to those of neurons without an intervening astrocytic process. Another important difference between these two cell types is that in old animals it is common to find large inclusions of phagocytosed material in the cell bodies of microglial cells (Figure 5.7).

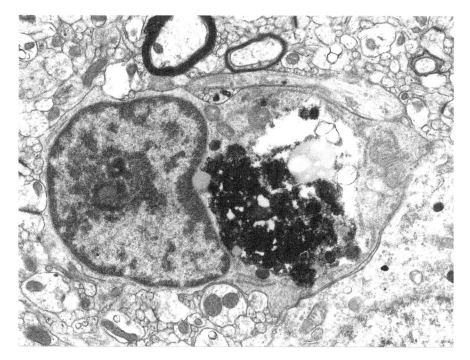

FIGURE 5.7 A microglial cell in the primary visual cortex of a 27-year-old monkey. The microglial cell has a dark, rounded nucleus (N) and its dark cytoplasm contains a large clump of electron-dense debris (D). (Scale bar = 1 μm.)

Microglial cells are generally regarded as the phagocytes of the central nervous system. Immunolabeling with antibodies to HLA-DRm, an MHC class antigen, and other antibodies shows that microglial cells become activated with age. This activation is evident in the white matter of the cerebral hemispheres of old rats [112], old monkeys (e.g., [113, 114]), and humans (e.g., [115]); and it is of interest that Sloane et al. [114] show that the extent of microglial cell activation in white matter is related to the degree of cognitive impairment in old monkeys. In contrast to white matter, gray matter shows few activated microglial cells and yet when tissue from old animals is examined by electron microscopy, microglial cells containing inclusions of phagocytosed material are encountered in both white and gray matter. The appearance of these inclusions is highly variable. In general, there are both electron-dense and pale components and, while some inclusions are small, others may be so large that the cytoplasm of the microglial cell is distended and confined to a thin rim that surrounds the inclusions. As a consequence, the nucleus is flattened against one side of the cell body. Typically, it is not possible to determine the origins of the phago-cytosed material in microglial cells. The one exception we have encountered is in the optic nerves of old monkeys, in which some of the microglial cells can be seen to contain phagocytosed myelin sheaths [53]. In the optic nerves of old monkeys, the degeneration of nerve fibers can be very extensive and may require increased numbers of microglial cells to deal with the removal of this debris. This is probably the reason that the optic nerve is the only structure in which we have so far encountered a significant increase in the numbers of microglial cells with age. Thus, in the optic nerves of monkeys, the numbers of microglial cells increase from about 5% of the total population of neuroglial cells in young monkeys to about 10% of the total in old monkeys. In all other parts of the monkey brain that we have examined, the percentage of microglial cells is between about 5 to 7% of the total population of neuroglial cells and increases little, if at all, with age. Long et al. [98] found the same to be true in the hippocampus of the mouse, although Mouton et al. [102] have reported that in female mice there are about 20% more astrocytes and microglia in the dentate gyrus and CA1 regions of the hippocampus in old mice than in young ones. As pointed out in the section on astrocytes, Mouton et al. [102] find that when males and females are compared, there are 25 to 40% more astrocytes and microglia in females than in males in these same regions of the hippocampus. They suggest than because astrocytes and microglial cells are thought to be targets of gonadal hormones, the effects of sex hormones and of reproductive aging may be at the root of this difference.

Although it has not been studied in detail, it can be presumed that as they become phagocytes, the microglia of the brain undergo morphological transformations from the ramified, resting microglial cell with many branching processes to an activated form in which the branches are withdrawn to enable the cell to become motile and to move to locations where it is needed for phagocytosis. These stages of transfor-mation have been nicely shown by Stence et al. [116] in a study in which they cut tissue slices of rat hippocampus, labeled the microglial cells with a fluorescent label, and followed the activation of the microglial cells that is induced by slicing the tissue. However, Streit et al. [117] suggest that with age, microglial cells undergo morphological alterations that are different from activation, and they designate the changes as microglial dystrophy. Streit et al. [117] examined microglial cells that had been labeled with an antibody, LN-3, in the cerebral cortices of two non-demented humans, one 38 years old and the other 68 years old. They found most of the microglial cells in the younger brain to have a typical ramified morphology, although they also encountered other dystrophic microglia with short, gnarled processes. Such dystrophic cells, which had lost their finely branched processes and had some processes that showed beading and the formation of spheroids were described as being more common in the older brain. Streit et al. [117] suggest that such microglial dystrophy is a sign that the cells are undergoing senescent changes. However, it would be prudent to undertake further studies before accepting this concept.

D.   A FOURTH NEUROGLIAL CELL TYPE

As pointed out when oligodendrocytes were considered, there is a fourth type of neuroglial cell present in the central nervous system. Until recently, this type of neuroglial cell has been largely overlooked in most studies of the normal adult nervous system because superficially they resemble protoplasmic astrocytes. When antibodies to NG2 chondroitin sulfate proteoglycan are used to label these cells, it becomes apparent that the NG2-labeled cells make up some 5% of the total number of neuroglial cells in the central nervous system (e.g., [88]). NG2-labeled cells in gray matter have a variety of shapes. They are generally characterized by small cell bodies from which extend irregular, branched processes with thin protrusions decorating them, while the cells in white matter have processes that pass parallel to the nerve fibers (e.g., [92]). There is general agreement that at least some of the NG2-labeled cells in the mature central nervous system are oligodendroglial progenitors (e.g., [88, 118]), but they may also have other functions that are presently unclear. It is also generally agreed that the cells that label with NG2 antibodies are distinct from the three classical types of neuroglial cells because they do not label with antibodies specific for the classical neuroglia. For example, they do not label with antibodies to GFAP, vimentin, or S-100, which are specific markers for astrocytes (e.g., [91, 119–121]), and Ye et al. [122] have shown that laser dissection captured NG2+ cells do not react with antibodies that are specific for astrocytes, microglial cells, or neurons. However, they do express mRNAs for myelin basic protein and for proteolipid protein, showing that at least some of the NG2+ cells can be precursors for oligodendroglia.

In electron microscopic preparations, the NG2+ cells bear a resemblance to astrocytes [123], in that they have pale nuclei and pale cytoplasm (Figure 5.8). However, the NG2+ cells have more irregular nuclei than typical astrocytes. The chromatin is dispersed and the cells have a thin layer of heterochromatin beneath the nuclear envelope, a layer that is generally more marked than that of astrocytes. The cell bodies of the NG2+ cells have a rather thin layer of cytoplasm around the nucleus, but there is usually abundant cytoplasm at the poles of the cells. It is evident that the cytoplasm contains free polyribosomes, a few cisternae of rough endoplasmic reticulum with a concentration of ribosomes on their surfaces, and some profiles of the Golgi apparatus. However, the mitochondria are generally smaller than those of

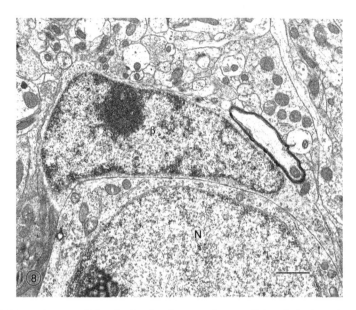

FIGURE 5.8 A β neuroglial cell, the fourth type of neuroglial cell, in the primary visual cortex of a 16-year-old monkey. The neuroglial cell (β) is lying next to a neuron (N). The neuroglial cell has a pale nucleus and sparse cytoplasm that contains few organelles. (Scale bar = 1 μm.)

astrocytes and intermediate filaments are not found in the cytoplasm. Other differences are that the NG2+ cells have more regular outlines than astrocytes; they are often seen to contain centrioles; and although the NG2+ cells can be found throughout the central nervous system, when they are adjacent to capillaries, there is always a thin astrocytic process separating the NG2+ cells from the basal lamina of the capillary.

There seems little doubt that these NG2+ cells are neuroglial cells that were earlier included in the category of protoplasmic astrocytes. The first ones to recognize the existence of this fourth type of glial cell were Reyners et al. [124, 125] and, because of their resemblance to astrocytes, they called them "β astrocytes." But in the light of the newer information about these cells, it is evident that this name is no longer appropriate and even misleading. Consequently, it is suggested that they might be called "β neuroglial cells" in acknowledgment of the fact that Reyners and colleagues were the first ones to give a clear description of these cells.

To date it is not clear whether these neuroglial cells play any definitive role in aging, although they might be the source of the increased numbers of oligodendrocytes that occur in some parts of the normally aging brain.

IV. CONCLUSIONS

It is obvious that there are profound alterations in myelin sheaths and in neuroglial cells with increasing age. The age-dependent alterations in oligodendrocytes are obviously related to the complex morphological changes exhibited by myelin sheaths, some of which undergo degenerative changes, even as the production of myelin continues in an endeavor to repair the ravages brought about by age. There seems little doubt that the myelin changes affect conduction velocity and the transfer of information from one part of the brain to another, and this may well be the source of much of the cognitive decline exhibited by aging mammals. The role of the astrocytes in aging appears to be twofold: (1) to repair damage by filling spaces left by the degeneration of parts of nerve fibers and neurons and other parts of neurons, such as the loss of apical dendrites from layer 1 of neocortex with age, and (2) to act as phagocytes. The role of astrocytes as phagocytes in the aging brain has been largely overlooked. It is known that they phagocytose some degenerating myelin, but what other components they might ingest is not known. The same is true of microglial cells. They can also ingest degenerating myelin but the origins of all the material these two neuroglial cell types phagocytose in the aging brain are not yet known. If the origins of the material could be identified, it would provide important clues as to what components of the central nervous system are breaking down and being removed from the aging brain.

ACKNOWLEDGMENTS

This work was supported by National Institutes of Health-National Institute on Aging Grant number 2P01 AG 00001.

REFERENCES

1. Tigges, J., Gordon, T.P., McClure, H.M., Hall., E.C., and Peters, A. Survival rate and life span of the rhesus monkey. *Neurobiol. Aging*, 11, 201, 1988.
2. Bachevalier, J., Landis, L.S., Walker, L.C., Brickso, M., Mishkin, M., and Price, D.L. Aged monkeys exhibit behavioral deficits indicative of widespread cerebral dysfunction. *Neurobiol. Aging*, 12, 99, 1991.
3. Albert, M. and Moss, M.B. Neuropychology of aging: finding in humans and monkeys, in *Handbook of the Biology of Aging, 4th ed.*, Schneider, E., Rowe, J.W., and Morris, J.H., Eds., Academic Press, San Diego, 1996, 217.
4. Herndon, J., Moss. M.B., Killiany, R.J., and Rosene, D.L. Patterns of cognitive decline in early, advanced and oldest of the old aged rhesus monkeys. *Behav. Res.*, 87, 25, 1997.
5. Morrison, J.H. and Hof, P.R. Life and death of neurons in the aging brain. *Nature*, 278, 412, 1997.
6. Peters, A., Morrison, J.H., Rosene, D.L., and Hyman, B.T. Are neurons lost from the primate cerebral cortex during aging? *Cerebr. Cortex*, 8, 295, 1998.
7. Merrill, D.A., Roberts, J.A.S., and Tuszynski, M.H. Conservation of neuron number and size in entorhinal cortex layers II, III, and V/VI of aged primates. *J. Comp. Neurol.*, 422, 396, 2000.
8. Smith, D. E., Rapp, P.R., McKay, H.M., Roberts, J.A., and Tuszynski, M.H. Memory impairment in aged primates is associated with focal death of cortical neurons and atrophy of subcortical neurons. *J. Neurosci.*, 24, 4373, 2004.

9. Peters, A., Leahu, D., Moss, M.B., and McNally, K.J. The effects of aging on area 46 of the frontal cortex of the rhesus monkey. *Cerebr. Cortex,* 6, 621, 1994.

10. Lintl, P. and Braak, H. Loss of intracortical myelinated fibers: a distinctive age-related alteration in the human striate area. *Acta Neuropathol.,* 61, 178, 1983.

11. Kemper, T.L. Neuroanatomical and neuropathological changes during aging and dementia, in *Clinical Neurology of Aging,* Albert M.L. and Knoefel. J.E., Eds., Oxford University Press, New York, 1994, 3.

12. Peters, A. Moss, M.B., and Sethares, C. Effects of aging on myelinated nerve fibers in monkey primary visual cortex. *J. Comp. Neurol.,* 419, 364, 2000a.

13. Peters, A. and Sethares, C. Aging and the myelinated fibers in prefrontal cortex and corpus callosum of the monkey. *J. Comp. Neurol.,* 442, 277, 2002b.

14. Ludwin, S.K. Pathology of the myelin sheath, in *The Axon: Structure, Function, and Pathophysiology,* Waxman, S.G., Kocsis, J.D., and Stys, P.K., Eds., Oxford University Press, New York, 1995, 412.

15. Ludwin, S.K. The pathobiology of the oligodendrocyte. *J. Neuropathol. Exp. Neurol.,* 56, 111, 1997.

16. Lassmann, H., Bartsch, U., Mantag, D., and Schaschner, M. Dying-back oligodendrogliopathy: a late sequel of myelin-associated glyocoprotein deficiency. *Glia,* 19, 104, 1997.

17. Dickson, D.W., Crystal, H.A., Mattiace, L.A., Masur, D.M., Blau, A.D., Davies, P., Yen, S.H., and Aronson, M.K. Identification of normal and pathological aging in prospectively studied nondemented elderly humans. *Neurobiol. Aging,* 13, 179, 1990.

18. Uchida, K., Nakayama, H., Tateyama, S., and Goto, N. Immunohistochemical analysis of constituents of senile plaques and cerebro-vascular amyloid in aged dogs. *J. Vet. Med. Sci.,* 54, 1023, 1992.

19. Wang, D.-S.D., Bennett, D.A., Mufson, E.J., Mattila,P., Cochran, E., and Dickson, D.W. Contribution of changes in ubiquitin and myelin basic protein to age-related cognitive decline. *Neurosci. Res.,* 48, 93, 2004.

20. Feldman, M.L. and Peters, A. Ballooning of myelin sheaths in normally aged macaques. *J. Neurocytol.,* 27, 605, 1998.

21. Faddis, B.T. and McGinn, M.D. Spongiform degeneration of the gerbil cochlear nucleus: an ultrastructural and immunohistochemical evaluation. *J. Neurocytol.,* 26, 625, 1997.

22. Franson, P. and Ronnevi, L.-O. Myelin breakdown in the posterior funiculus of the kitten after dorsal rhizotomy: a qualitative and quantitative light and electron microscopic study. *Anat. Embrol.,* 180, 273, 1989.

23. Tamura, E. and Parry, G.J. 1994 Severe radicular pathology in rats with long-standing diabetes. *J. Neurol. Sci.,* 127, 29, 1994.

24. Ludwin, S.K. Central nervous system demyelination and remyelination in the mouse: an ultrastructural study of Cuprizone toxicity. *Lab Invest.,* 39, 597, 1978.

25. Malamud, N. and Hirano, A. *Atlas of Neuropathology,* University of California Press, Berkeley, 1973.

26. Hull, J. M. and Blakemore W.F. Chronic copper poisoning and changes in the central nervous system of sheep. *Acta Neuropathol.,* 29, 9, 1974.

27. Blakemore, W.F. Observations of remyelination in the rabbit spinal cord following demyelination induced by lysolecithin. *Neuropathol. Appl. Neurobiol.,* 4, 47, 1978.

28. Malone, M.J. and Szoke, M.C. Neurochemical studies in aging brain. 1. Structural changes in myelin lipids. *J. Gerontol.,* 37, 262, 1982.

29. Sloane, J.A., Hinman, J.D., Lubonia, M., Hollander, W., and Abraham, C.R. Age-dependent myelin degeneration and proteolysis of oligodendrocyte proteins is associated with the activation of calpain-1 in the rhesus monkey. *J. Neurochem.*, 84, 157, 2003.

30. Blalock, E.M., Chen, K.-C., Sharrow, K., Herman, J.P., Porter, N.M., Foster, T.C., and Landfield, P.W. Gene microarrrays in hippocampal aging: statistical profiling identifies novel processes correlated with cognitive impairment. *J. Neurosci.*, 23, 3801, 2003.

31. Lu, T., Pan, Y., Kao, S.-Y., Li, C., Kohane, I., Chan, J., and Yankner, B.A. Gene regulation and DNA damage in the ageing human brain. *Nature*, 429, 883, 2004.

32. Pakkenberg, B. and Gundersen, H.J.G. Neocortical neuron number in humans: effects of age and sex. *J. Comp. Neurol.*, 384, 312, 1997.

33. Tang, Y., Nyengaard, J.R., Pakkenberg, B., and Gundersen, H.J.G. Age-induced white matter changes in the human brain: a stereological investigation. *Neurobiol. Aging*, 18, 609, 1997.

34. Marner, L., Nyengaard, J.R., Tang, Y., and Pakkenberg, B. Marked loss of myelinated nerve fibers in the human brain with age. *J. Comp. Neurol.*, 462, 144, 2003.

35. Meier-Ruge A., Ulrich, J., Bruhlmann, M., and Meier, E. Age-related white matter atrophy in the human brain. *Ann. N.Y. Acad. Sci.*, 673, 260, 1992.

36. Albert, A. Neuropsychological and neurophysiological changes in healthy adult humans across the age range. *Neurobiol. Aging*, 14, 623, 1993.

37. Guttman, C.R.G., Jolesz, F.A., Kikinis, R., Killiany, R.J., Moss, M.B., Sandor, T., and Albert, M.S. White mater changes in normal aging. *Neurology*, 50, 972, 1998.

38. Lai, Z.C., Rosene, D.L., Killiany, R.J., Pugliese, D, Albert, M.S., and Moss, M.B. Age-related changes in the brain of the rhesus monkey: MRI changes in white matter but not gray matter. *Soc. Neurosci. Abstracts*, 21, 1564, 1995.

39. Peters, A. and Rosene, D.L. In aging, is it gray or white? *J. Comp. Neurol.*, 462, 139, 2003.

40. Jernigan, T.L., Archibald, S.L., Fennema-Notestine, C., Gamst, A.C., Stout, J.C., Bonner, J., and Hesselink, J.R. Effects of age on tissues and regions of the cerebrum and cerebellum. *Neurobiol. Aging*, 22, 581, 2001.

41. Takahashi, T., Murata, T., Omori, M., Kosaka, H., Takahashi, K., Yonekura, Y., and Wada, Y. Quantitative evaluation of age-related white matter microstructural changes on MRI by multifractal analysis. *J. Neurol. Sci.*, 225, 33, 2004.

42. O'Sullivan, M., Jones, D.K., Summers, P.E., Morris, R.G., Williams, S.C.R., and Markus, H.S. Evidence for cortical "disconnection" as a mechanism of age-related cognitive decline. *Neurology*, 57, 632, 2001.

43. Davatzikos C. and Resnick, S.M. Degenerative age changes in white matter connectivity visualized in vivo using magnetic resonance imaging. *Cerbr. Cortex*, 12, 767, 2002.

44. De Groot, J.C., de Leeuw, F.-E., Oudkerk, M., van Gijn, J., Hofman, A., Jolles, J., and Bretler, M.B. Cerebral white matter lesions and cognitive function: the Rotterdam scan study. *Ann. Neurol.*, 47, 145, 2000.

45. Bartzokis, G., Cummings, J.L. Sultzer, D., Hendersen, V.W., Nuechterlein K.H., and Mintz, J. White matter structural integrity in healthy aging adults and patients with Alzheimer disease. *Arch Neurol.*, 60, 393, 2004.

46. Andersen, A.H., Zhang, Z., Gash, D.M., and Avison, M.J. Age-associated changes in CNS composition identified by MRI. *Brain Res.*, 829, 90, 1999.

47. Pfefferbaum, A., Mathalon, D.H., Rawles, J.M., Zipursky, R.B., and Lim, K.O. A quantitative magnetic resonance study of changes in brain morphology from infancy to late adulthood. *Arch. Neurol.*, 9, 874, 1994.

49. Resnick, S.M., Pham, D.L., Kraut, M.A., Zonderman, A.B., and Davatzikos, C. Longitudinal magnetic resonance imaging studies of older adults: a shrinking brain. *J. Neurosci.*, 23, 3295, 2003.

49. Sullivan, E.V., Rosenbloom, M., Serventi, K.L., and Pfefferbaum, A. Effects of age and sex on volumes of the thalamus, pons, and cortex. *Neurobiol. Aging*, 25, 185, 2004.

50. Salat, D.H., Buckner, R.L. Snyder, A.Z., Greve, D.N., Desikan, R.S.R, Busa, E., Morris, J.C., Dale, A.M., and Fischl, B. Thinning of the cerebral cortex in aging. *Cerebr. Cortex*, 14, 721, 2004.

51. Raz, N., Gunning-Dixon, F., Head, D., Rodrigue, K.M., Williamson, A., and Acker, J.D. Aging, sexual dimorphism, and hemispheric asymmetry of the cerebral cortex: replicability of regional differences in volume. *Neurobiol. Aging*, 25, 377, 2004.

52. Sandell, J.H. and Peters, A. Effects of age on nerve fibers in the rhesus monkey optic nerve. *J. Comp. Neurol.*, 429, 541, 2001.

53. Sandell, J.H. and Peters, A. Effects of age on the glial cells in the rhesus monkey optic nerve. *J. Comp. Neurol.*, 445, 13, 2002.

54. Cavallotti, D., Cavallotti, C., Pescosolido, N., Iannetti, G.D., and Pacella E. A morphometric study of age changes in the rat optic nerve. *Ophthalmologica*, 215, 366, 2001.

55. Sandell, J.H. and Peters, A. Disrupted myelin and axon loss in the anterior commissure of the aged rhesus monkey. *J. Comp. Neurol.*, 466, 14, 2003.

56. Fujisawa, K. Study of axonal dystrophy. III. Posterior funiculus and posterior column of ageing and old rats. *Acta Neuropathol.*, 76, 115, 1988.

57. Peters, A. and Sethares, C. Aging and the myelinated fibers in prefrontal cortex and corpus callosum of the monkey. *J. Comp. Neurol.*, 442, 277, 2002b.

58. Peters, A., Sethares, C., and Killiany, R.J. Effects of age on the thickness of myelin sheaths in monkey primary visual cortex. *J. Comp. Neurol.*, 435, 241, 2001b.

59. Sugiyama, I., Tanaka, K., Akita, M., Yoshida, K., Kawase, T., and Asou, H. Ultrastructural analysis of the paranodal junctions of myelinated fibers in 31-month-old-rats. *J. Neurosci. Res.*, 70, 309, 2002.

60. Sturrock, R.R. Changes in neuroglia and myelination in the white matter of aging mice. *J. Gerontol.*, 31, 513, 1976.

61. Godlewski, A. Morphometry of myelin fibers in the corpus callosum and optic nerve of aging rats. *J. Hirnforsch.*, 32, 39, 1991.

62. Caselli, U., Bertoni-Freddari, C., Paolini, R., Fattoretti, P., Casoli, T., and Meier-Ruge, W. Morphometry of axon cytoskeleton at internodal regions of rat sciatic nerve during aging. *Gerontology*, 45, 307, 1999.

63. Cebellos, D., Cuadras, J., Verdu, E., and Navarro, X. Morphometric and ultrastructural changes with ageing in mouse peripheral nerve. *J. Anat.*, 195, 563, 1999.

64. Rosenbluth, J. Redundant myelin sheaths and other ultrastructural features of the toad cerebellum. *J. Cell Biol.*, 28, 73, 1966.

65. Peters, A. and Sethares, C. Is there remyelination during aging of the primate central nervous system? *J. Comp. Neurol.*, 460, 238, 2003.

66. Ibanez, C., Shields, S.A., El-Etr, M., Leonelli, E., Lia, W.-W., Sim, F.J., Baulieu, E.-E., Melcangi, R.C., Schumacher, M., and Franklin, R.J.M. Steroids and the reversal of age-associated changes in myelination and remyelination. *Progr. Neurobiol.*, 71, 49, 2003.

67. Moss, M.B., Killiany, R.J., and Herndon, J.G. Age-related cognitive decline in rhesus monkey, in *Neurodegenerative and Age-Related Changes in Structure and Function of the Cerebral Cortex. Cerebral Cortex Vol. 14*, Peters, A. and Morrison, J.H., Eds., Kluwer Academic/Plenum Publishers, New York, 1999, 21.

68. Killiany, R.J., Moss, M.B., Rosene, D.L., and Herndon. J. Recognition memory function in early senescent rhesus monkeys. *Psychobiology,* 28, 45, 2000.

69. Aston-Jones, G., Rogers, J., Shaver, R.D., Dinan, T.G., and Moss. D.E. Age-impaired impulse flow from nucleus basalis to cortex. *Nature,* 318, 462, 1985.

70. Morales, F.R., Boxer, P.A., Fung, S.J., and Chase, M.H. Basic electrophysiological properties of spinal cord motoneurons during old age in the cat. *J. Neurophysiol.,* 58, 180, 1987.

71. Xi, M.-C., Liu, R.-H., Engelhardt, K.K., Morales, F.R., and Chase, M.H. Changes in the axonal conduction velocity of pyramidal tract neurons in the aged cat. *Neuroscience,* 92, 219, 1999.

72. Gutiérrez, R., Bioson, D., Heinenmann, U., and Stoffel, W. Decompaction of CNS myelin leads to a reduction of the conduction velocity of action potentials in optic nerve. *Neurosci. Lett.,* 195, 93, 1995.

73. Waxman, S.G., Kocsis, J.D. and Black. J.A. Pathophysiology of demyelinated axons, in *The Axon: Structure, Function and Pathophysiology,* Waxman, S.G., Kocsis, J.D., and Stys, P.K., Eds., Oxford University Press, New York, 1995, 438.

74. Felts, P.A., Baker, T.A., and Smith, K.J. Conduction along segmentally demyelinated mammalian central axons. *J. Neurosci.,* 17, 7267, 1997.

75. Wang, Y., Zhou, Y., Ma, Y., and Leventhal, A.G. Degradation of signal timing in cortical area V1 and V2 of senescent monkeys. *Cerebr. Cortex,* 15, 403, 2005.

76. Chang, Y-. M., Rosene, D.L., Killiany, R.J., Mangiamele, L.A., and Luebke, J.I. Increased action potential firing rates of layer 2/3 pyramidal cells in the prefrontal cortex are significantly related to cognitive performance in aged monkeys. *Cerebr. Cortex,* 15, 409, 2005.

77. Pakkenberg, B., Pelvig, D., Marner, L., Bundgaard, M.J., Gundersen, H.J.G., Nyengaard, J.R., and Regeur, L. Aging and the human neocortex. *Exp. Gerontol.,* 38, 95, 2003.

78. Benkovic, S.A. and Connor, J.R. Ferritin, transferrin, and iron in selected regions of the adult and aged rat brain. *J. Comp. Neurol.,* 338, 97, 1993.

79. Connor, J.R., Pavlick, G., Karli, D, Menzies, S.L., and Palmer, C. 1995 A histochemical study of iron-positive cells in the developing rat brain. *J. Comp. Neurol.,* 355, 111, 1995.

80. Peters, A. Age-related changes in oligodendrocytes in monkey cerebral cortex. *J. Comp. Neurol.,* 371, 153, 1996.

81. Peters, A. and Sethares, C. Oligodendrocytes, their progenitors and other neuroglial cells in the aging primate cerebral cortex. *Cerebr. Cortex,* 14, 995, 2004a.

82. Peters, A., Josephson, K., and Vincent, S.L. Effects of aging on the neuroglial cells and pericytes within area 17 of the rhesus monkey cerebral cortex. *Anat. Rec.,* 229, 384, 1991.

83. Vaughan, D.W. and Peters, A. Neuroglial cells in the cerebral cortex of rats from young aldulthood to old age: an electron microscope study. *J. Neurocytol.,* 3, 404, 1974.

84. Rees, S. A quantitative electron microscope study of the ageing human cerebral cortex. *Acta Neuropathol.,* 36, 347, 1976.

85. LeVine, S.M. and Torres, M.V. Morphological features of degenerating oligodendrocytes in twitcher mice. *Brain Res.,* 587, 348, 1992.

86. Norton, W.T. Do oligodendrocytes divide? *Neurochem. Res.*, 21, 295, 1996.

87. Keirstead, H.S. and Blakemore, W.F. Identification of post-mitotic oligodendrocytes incapable of remyelination within demyelinated adult spinal cord. *J. Neuropathol. Exp. Neurol.*, 56, 1191, 1997.

88. Levine, J.M., Reynolds, R., and Fawcett, J.W., The oligodendrocyte precursor cell in health and disease. *Trends Neurosci.*, 24, 2001.

89. Chen, Z.J., Negra, M., Levine, A., Ughrin, Y., and Levine, J.M. Oligodendrocyte precursor cells; reactive cells that inhibit axon growth and regeneration. *J. Neurocytol.*, 31, 481, 2002.

90. Watanabe, M., Toyama, Y., and Nishiyama, A. Differentiation of proliferating NG2-positive glial progenitor cells in a remyelinating lesion. *J. Neurosci. Res.*, 69, 826, 2002.

91. Levine, J.M., Stincone, F., and Lee, Y.S., Development and differentiation of glial precursor cells in rat cerebellum. *Glia,* 7, 307, 1993.

92. Nishiyama, A., Yu, M., Drazba, J.A., and Tuohy, V.K. Normal and reactive NG2+ cells are distinct from resting and activated microglia. *J. Neurosci. Res.*, 48, 299, 1997.

93. Stallcup, W.B. The NG2 proteoglycan: past insights and future prospects. *J. Neurocytol.*, 31, 423, 2002.

94. Cotrina, M.L., Gao, Q., Lin, J.H.C., and Nedergaaard, M. Expression and function of astrocytic gap junctions in aging. *Brain Res.,* 901, 55, 2001.

95. Diamond, M.C., Johnson, R.E., and Gold, M.W. Changes in neuron number and size and glial number in the young, adult and aging rat medial occipital cortex. *Behav. Biol.*, 20, 409, 1977.

96. Vaughn, J.E. and Peters, A. Electron microscopy of the early postnatal development of fibrous astrocytes. *Am. J. Anat.,* 121, 131, 1967.

97. Berciano, M.T., Andres, M.A., Calle, E., and Lafarga, M. Age-induced hypertrophy of astrocytes in rat supraoptic nucleus: a cytological, morphometric, and immunocytochemical study. *Anat. Rec.,* 243, 129, 1995.

98. Long, J.M., Kalehua, A.N., Muth, N.J., Calhoun, M.E., Jucker, M., Hengemihle, J.M., Ingram, D.K., and Mouton, P.R. Stereological analysis of astrocyte and microglia in aging mouse hippocampus. *Neurobiol. Aging,* 19, 497, 1998.

99. Hansen, L.A., Armstrong, D.M., and Terry, R.D. An immunohistochemical quantification of fibrous astrocytes in the aging human cerebral cortex. *Neurobiol. Aging,* 8, 1, 1987.

100. Peinado, M.A., Quesada, A., Pedrosa, J.A., Torres, M.I., Esteban, F.J., De Moral, M.L., Hernandez, R., Rodrigo, J., and Peinado, J.M. Quantitative and ultrastructural changes in glia and pericytes in the parietal cortex of the aging rat. *Microsc. Res. Tech.,* 43, 34, 1998.

101. Peinado, M.A., Martinez, M., Pedrosa, J.A., Quesada, A., and Peinado, J.M. Quantitative morphological changes in neurons and glia in frontal cortex of the aging rat. *Anat Rec.*, 237, 104, 1993.

102. Mouton, P.R., Long, J.M., Lei, D.L., Howard, V., Jucker, M., Calhoun, M.E., and Ingram, D.K. Age and gender effects on microglia and astrocyte numbers in brains of mice. *Brain Res.,* 956, 30, 2002.

103. Peters, A., Moss, M.B., and Sethares, C. The effects of aging on layer 1 of primary visual cortex in the rhesus monkey. *Cerebr. Cortex,* 11, 93, 2001a.

104. Peters, A. and Sethares, C. The effects of age on the cells in layer 1 of primate cerebral cortex. *Cerebr. Cortex,* 12, 27, 2002a.

105. O'Callaghan, J.P. and Miller, D.B. The concentration of glial fibrillary acidic protein increases with age in the mouse and rat brain. *Neurobiol. Aging,* 12, 171. 1991.

106. Kohama, S.G., Goss, J.R., Finch, C.E., and McNeill, T.H. Increases in glial fibrillary protein in the aging female mouse brain. *Neurobiol. Aging,* 16, 59, 1995.

107. Amenta, F., Bronzetti, E., Sabbatini, M., and Vega, J.A. Astrocyte changes in aging cerebral cortex and hippocampus: a quantitative immunohistochemical study. *Microsc. Res. Tech.,* 43, 29, 1998.

108. Colombo, J.A. Interlaminar astroglial processes in the cerebral cortex of adult monkeys but not in adult rats. *Acta Anat.,* 155, 57, 1996.

109. Colombo, J.A., Yáñez, A., Puissant, V., and Lipina, S. Long, interlaminar astroglial processes in the cortex of adult monkeys. *J. Neurosci. Res.,* 40, 551, 1995.

110. Sloane, J.A., Hollander, W., Rosene, D.L., Moss, M.B., Kemper, T., and Abraham, C.R. Astrocytic hypertrophy and altered GFAP degradation with age in subcortical white matter of the rhesus monkey. *Brain Res.,* 862, 1, 2000.

111. Nichols, N.R., Day, J.R., Laping, N.J., Johnson, S.A., and Finch, C.E. GFAP mRNA increases with age in rat and human brain. *Neurobiol. Aging,* 14, 421, 1993.

112. Ogura, K., Ogawa, M., and Yoshida, M. Effects of ageing on microglia in the normal rat brain: immunohistochemical observations. *Neuroreport,* 5, 1224. 1994.

113. Sheffield, L.G. and Berman, N.E.J. Microglial expression of MHC class II increases in normal aging of nonhuman primates. *Neurobiol. Aging,* 19, 47, 1998.

114. Sloane, J.A., Hollander, W., Moss, M.B., Rosene, D.L., and Abraham, C.R. Increased microglial activation and protein nitration in white matter of the aging monkey. *Neurobiol. Aging,* 20, 395, 1999.

115. Mattiace, L.A., Davies, P., and Dickson, D.W. Detection of HLA-DR on microglia in the human brain is a function of both clinical and technical factors. *Am. J. Pathol.,* 136, 1101, 1990.

116. Stence, N., Waite, M., and Dailey, M.E. Dynamics of microglial activation: a confocal time-lapse analysis in hippocampal slices. *Glia,* 33, 256, 2001.

117. Streit, W.J., Sammons, N.W., Kuhns, A.J., and Sparks, D.L. Dystrophic microglia in the aging human brain. *Glia,* 45, 208, 2004.

118. Levison, S.W., Young, G.M., and Goldman, J.E. Cycling cells in the adult rat neocortex preferentially generate oligodendroglia. *J. Neurosci. Res.,* 57,435, 1999.

119. Levine. J.M. and Card, J.P. Light and electron microscopic localization of a cell surface antigen (NG2) in the rat cerebellum. *J. Neurosci.,* 7, 2711, 1987.

120. Ong, W.Y. and Levine, J.M. A light and electron microscopic study of NG2 chondroitin sulfate proteoglycan-positive oligodendrocyte precursor cells in normal and kianate-lesioned rat hippocampus. *J. Neurosci.,* 92, 83, 1999.

121. Bu, J., Akhtar, N., and Nishiyama, A. Transient expresson of NG2 proteoglycan by a subpopulation of activated macrophages in an excitotoxic hippocampal lesion. *Glia,* 34, 296, 2001.

122. Ye, P., Bagnell, R., and D'Ercole, A.J. Mouse NG2+ oligodendrocyte precursors express mRNA for proteolipid protein but not its DM-20 variant. a study of laser microdissection-captured NG+ cells. *J. Neurosci.,* 23, 4401, 2003.

123. Peters, A. and Sethares, C. A fourth type of neuroglial cell in the adult central nervous system. *J. Neurocytol.,* 33, 345, 2004b.

124. Reyners, H., Gianfelici de Reyners, E., and Maisin, J.-R. A newly recognized radiosensitive glial cell type in the cerebral cortex. *J. Neurocytol.,* 11, 967, 1982.

125. Reyners, H., Gianfelici de Reyners, E, Regniers, L., and Maisin. J.-R. A glial progenitor cell in the cerebral cortex of the adult rat. *J. Neurocytol.,* 15, 53, 1986.

6 Neurogenesis in the Adult and Aging Brain

David R. Riddle and Robin J. Lichtenwalner

CONTENTS

I.   OVERVIEW OF NEUROGENESIS IN THE ADULT BRAIN

A.   HISTORICAL CONTEXT

Long past the publication of evidence to the contrary, it was widely held that neurons were produced in the brain only during a discrete period of development. Ramon y Cajal's contention that "in adult centers, the nerve paths are something fixed and immutable: everything may die, nothing may be regenerated" held sway even after studies by Altman in the 1960s [1–4], followed by Kaplan and Hinds in the 1970s [5], provided evidence for the birth of new neurons in the adult brain. Despite electron microscopic and morphological evidence that some adult-born cells (identified by the incorporation of tritiated thymidine into their DNA) were neurons, the concept of ongoing adult neurogenesis was slow to reach acceptance because there were no definitive phenotypic markers of neurons that could be combined with autoradiographic birth dating and no concept of adult stem cells in the brain. Moreover, the earliest attempts to demonstrate neurogenesis in primates did not provide convincing evidence for new neurons, so the rodent studies appeared to have little relevance for humans.

Interest in adult neurogenesis increased tremendously in the 1980s after Nottebohm demonstrated seasonally regulated neurogenesis in the song nuclei of songbirds and provided evidence that adult neurogenesis subserved a neural function (reviewed in [6, 7]). Nottebohm's analyses left no doubt that tritiated thymidine labeled cells in the adult bird brain were neurons, and evidence that the production of new neurons peaks at the time birds acquire new songs provided a compelling indication that adult neurogenesis is functionally significant, at least in birds. Subsequent studies demonstrated that neurogenesis also was ongoing in the hippocampus of adult birds and that the extent of hippocampal neurogenesis correlated both seasonally and across species with seed-storing, a behavior that depends on hippocampally dependent spatial learning [8–10]. Spurred in part by the dramatic findings in avian species, interest in adult neurogenesis in mammals increased precipitously into the 1990s, with several laboratories publishing seminal investigations of the nature and extent of neurogenesis in the adult mammalian brain (e.g., [11–15]). In addition to critical studies assessing adult neurogenesis *in vivo* using radioactive thymidine and the thymidine analog bromodeoxyuridine (BrdU), demonstrations that cells with stem cell properties could be isolated from the adult brain established a source for new neurons in the adult brain (e.g., [16–19]). Although the debate continues regarding the extent of adult neurogenesis across brain regions and across species [20–23], clearly new neurons are continually produced in some regions of the adult mammalian brain, even in humans [24], new neurons are integrated into functional circuits, and the ongoing neuronal turnover is significant for some functions.

B. REGIONAL DISTRIBUTION OF ADULT NEUROGENESIS

That the reality of adult neurogenesis was neither easily demonstrated nor quickly accepted was a function of its limited representation with the brain. Although there is evidence that new neurons may be added to several other neural regions under some conditions, in the normal adult brain, neurogenesis appears to be restricted to three areas, each with a focal population of progenitor cells and a characteristic pattern of differentiation and migration of new neurons.

1. Neurogenesis in the Hippocampus

Neural progenitor cells in the hippocampus are located in the subgranular zone (SGZ) at the border between the granule cell layer (GCL) and hilus of the dentate gyrus (DG; see [25–29] for reviews). Some of the daughter cells produced by division of those precursor cells differentiate into neurons and develop the prominent apical dendrite that characterizes dentate granule neurons as they move into the GCL. Adult-born neurons project axons to the primary target of dentate granule neurons, the stratum lucidum of area CA3, as early as 4 to 10 days after their final mitosis [30, 31], are integrated into the hippocampal circuitry, and are electrophysiologically comparable to earlier born granule neurons within several weeks [32]. The structural [31] and functional [33] development of adult-born granule neurons is slightly slowed, however, compared to the development of those born at the developmental peak of genesis.

2. Neurogenesis in the Subventricular Zone and Rostral Migratory Stream

Quantitatively, the extent of adult neurogenesis in the hippocampus is only a fraction of that in the anterior portion of the adult subventricular zone (SVZ), a thin, persistent remnant of the secondary proliferative zone of the developing brain. Although not readily identifiable by cell-type specific markers, neural stem cells can be isolated from the adult SVZ and shown in culture to be both self-renewing and multipotent, capable of generating both neurons and glia. Studies indicate that the neural stem cells have some characteristics of astrocytes, but clearly not all astrocytes in the region are neural stem cells [34–36]. Extensive analysis of the adult SVZ indicates that the region comprises several cell types in addition to the slowly dividing stem cells, including a more rapidly dividing population of transit amplifying progenitor (TAP) cells, neuroblasts, glial cells, and a monolayer of ependymal cells lining the ventricle [35]. Neuroblasts born in the SVZ maintain the ability to proliferate as they migrate through the SVZ, into the rostral migratory stream (RMS), and anteriorly to the olfactory bulb (OB), finally differentiating into interneurons (e.g., [37–40]). Throughout their migration, chains of neuroblasts are ensheathed by slowly proliferating astrocytes, which presumably help maintain an appropriate microenvironment for migration and cell division. The division of neuroblasts within the RMS, far from the SVZ, demonstrates that the environment that supports the division of neuronal progenitors is much more extensive in the SVZ/RMS than in the DG, where the division of progenitor cells is spatially restricted. It also is important to note that the stem/progenitor cell populations differ between the SVZ and the SGZ [41], and that the progenitor population in the adult hippocampus lacks true stem cells, containing only more restricted progenitor cells [42, 43].

3.   Neurogenesis in the Olfactory Epithelium

Concurrent with the early demonstrations of neuronal addition in the adult hippocampus and OB, several laboratories described the birth of new olfactory receptor neurons (ORNs) within the adult olfactory epithelium (OE; reviewed in [44]). Progenitor cells in the basal layer of the olfactory epithelium give rise to new receptor neurons that migrate superficially as they develop their characteristic apical dendrite and project an axon to the glomerular layer of the OB. Quantitative studies indicate that ORNs may have lifespans as short as a few weeks or months (influenced in part by ongoing damage to the exposed olfactory mucosa); thus, neurogenesis in the adult olfactory epithelium supports a process of wholesale turnover, compared to the more selective replacement of new neurons within the granule cell and interneuron populations of the DG and OB. Although less extensively studied than the RMS/SVZ and hippocampus, the mechanisms of regulation on neurogenesis in the peripheral olfactory system are beginning to be elucidated [44]. Because olfactory loss may be an early indicator of age-related neural decline and Alzheimer's disease pathogenesis (discussed in [45]), understanding aging-related changes in the peripheral olfactory system may provide particularly important translational and clinical benefits.

4.   Neurogenesis in Other Neural Regions?

Although it generally is agreed that the three regions above are the only sites of (relatively) large-scale, ongoing neuronal replacement in the normal adult brain, there is evidence that at least the potential for adult neurogenesis is more widespread. Cells with properties similar to the stem cells obtained from the hippocampus and anterior SVZ have been isolated from other brain regions, including the striatum, cerebral cortex, septum, spinal cord, hypothalamus, and even white matter (reviewed in [46]). These cells show at least some capacity for self-renewal in culture, as well as the ability to give rise to both neuronal and glial lineages. Despite the apparently wide distribution of such progenitor cells, however, evidence for constitutive neuronal replacement in areas other than the three regions above remains controversial, in part because of methodological challenges in analyzing cells that divide slowly or seldom and critical questions of what constitutes adequate proof that a particular cell is newly born and that a cell identified as newly born is a neuron [22, 47]. Such debates notwithstanding, it is clear that if neurogenesis does occur in the cerebral cortex [20, 23, 48], amygdala [49], spinal cord [50], or other regions, it is at a level that is orders of magnitude below that in the DG and SVZ/RMS.

There is more compelling evidence that neurogenesis may be induced in normally nonneurogenic regions of the adult brain in response to injury and neuronal death. There are reports of both injury-induced activation of local precursor cells to generate new neurons and migration of precursor cells from neurogenic to nonneurogenic regions, upon injury to the latter. Regions of the brain exhibiting such induced neurogenesis include the cerebral cortex, striatum, and CA1 region of the hippocampus, with neurogenesis occurring in response to focal neuronal degeneration and ischemia [51–54]. Whether such induced neurogenesis is or can be made sufficient to facilitate functional recovery remains to be established, but it offers exciting translational and clinical possibilities [46].

The isolation of progenitor cells from, and presence of "inducible" neurogenesis within, normally nonneurogenic regions of the adult brain illustrates that the characteristically neurogenic regions differ from the remainder of the brain primarily in their permissiveness for neurogenesis, rather than simply representing the sole repositories of neuronal progenitor cells. Elucidating the aspects of the cellular microenvironment that are critical for permitting or promoting the generation of new neurons is a fundamental challenge in understanding the regulation of neurogenesis and how that regulation is affected under a variety of physiological conditions, including aging. This task is made particularly challenging by the recognition that the neurogenic microenvironment reflects a complex and dynamic molecular state, rather than a fixed cellular environment (discussed in [46]). Changes in the neurogenic environment represent one possible contributor to the profound decrease in neurogenesis that occurs with brain aging.

II.   DECREASED NEUROGENESIS IN THE AGING BRAIN

A.   EXTENT OF AGING-RELATED CHANGES

Evidence that neurogenesis is sustained in the senescent brain, albeit at a lower level than in young adults, was provided among early studies of adult neurogenesis using thymidine labeling and electron microscopy [55]. Recent and more quantitative studies revealed the extent of the aging-related decline in neuronal production in each neurogenic region and provide a foundation for ongoing studies of the mechanisms of regulation of aging-related changes.

1.   Hippocampus

Since the mid-1990s, several laboratories have demonstrated that the level of hippocampal neurogenesis in aging and aged animals is only a fraction of that seen in young adults. Experiments using a variety of BrdU labeling paradigms, supplemented with immunolabeling for markers of immature neurons, have revealed the extent and time course of aging-related changes in rats and mice (e.g., [12, 13, 56–59]. The reduction in production of new neurons is profound, consistently on the order of 80% or more, and occurs relatively early in the aging process, with the greatest decline occurring by middle age and only a modest, if any, additional decline during later senescence [13, 58, 60]. Although detailed quantitative studies are limited to rodent models, limited data indicate that the effects of aging on hippocampal neurogenesis are similar in primates. The temporal pattern may differ, however, because one study of macaques revealed a large (approximately 70%) decrease in neurogenesis between young adulthood and middle age, as well as a substantial and additional decrease between middle and old age [14]. Comparisons across species must be made carefully, of course, given the limited sampling in most primate studies and the challenge of determining comparable life stages in species with very different lifespans.

2.   SVZ/RMS

The aging SVZ has not been studied as extensively or quantitatively as the aging hippocampus but undergoes a similar decline in proliferation. In mice, the number of BrdU-labeled cells present in the SVZ a few hours after labeling is lower by about a factor of 2 in 20- to 25-month-old vs. 2- to 4-month-old mice [61, 62] and in 24-month-old vs. 3-month-old Fisher-344 rats [63]. As in the hippocampus, the greatest reduction in cell genesis within the SVZ occurs between young adulthood and middle age, with a more modest additional decline with further aging [64]. The aging-related reduction in the appearance of newborn neurons in the OB is somewhat greater than the decline in proliferation within the SVZ; at 1 month after labeling, only 30% as many BrdU-labeled cells are apparent in the OB of older animals [61]. Thus, it appears that the aging-related decrease in progenitor proliferation in the SVZ is compounded by an additional deficit in the division of neuroblasts as they migrate through the RMS, and/or by decreased survival of migrating neuroblasts in older animals. Detailed light and electron microscopic studies indicate that, with aging, neurogenesis in the SVZ becomes restricted to the dorsolateral aspect of the lateral ventricle and increased numbers of astrocytes become interposed among the ependymal cells [64]. Thus, in the case of the SVZ, both the size and cellular makeup of the neurogenic environment are reduced during aging. Notably, the aging-related decline in the neurogenic activity of the SVZ/RMS is not limited to rodents; both the size of the SVZ and the number of migrating neuroblasts are reduced in old macaques compared to young adults [65].

3.   Olfactory Epithelium

Data on aging-related changes in the genesis of olfactory receptor neurons are limited and analysis of changes is complicated by the fact that the olfactory epithelium, by virtue of its exposed location within the nasal cavity, is uniquely vulnerable to damage from a variety of insults. There are substantial aging-related changes in the organization of the olfactory epithelium, including a decrease in the number of ORNs and patchy replacement of the sensory epithelium by respiratory epithelium (e.g., [66, 67]. It cannot be assumed, however, that loss of ORNs is the result of decreased genesis. A short report that noted decreased generation of ORNs in the olfactory epithelium of aged mice [68] was followed by a detailed study of Fisher-344 × Brown Norway rats from 7 to 32 months of age [69]. Significantly, in the latter study, the animals were maintained in a barrier facility to minimize the possible impact of rhinitis and other disease on the olfactory epithelium. Although the anterior olfactory epithelium exhibited evidence of degeneration and gross morphological changes, the posterior region was well preserved, and BrdU labeling demonstrated that progenitor cells were dividing and new ORNs were produced even in the oldest animals. The generation of new neurons in the olfactory epithelium still was significantly reduced in older individuals; the number of BrdU-labeled basal cells and immature (GAP43-positive) neurons was approximately 40% lower in 32-month-old rats compared to 7-month-old young adults. Other investigators demonstrated a similar decrease between young adulthood and middle age in Sprague Dawley rats [70]. In addition to such evidence for decreased proliferation of progenitor cells, expression of NeuroD, a basic helix-loop-helix transcription factor that is thought to function in neuronal differentiation, is reduced in the aged olfactory epithelium [71].

B.   MECHANISMS OF AGING-RELATED CHANGES

Although the aging-related decline in neurogenesis is profound, the neurobiological changes that contribute to that change are not yet understood. To understand how and why neurogenesis changes in the aging brain, one must consider several processes that influence the rate of neuronal turnover and establish which processes change with aging. The control of adult neurogenesis involves multiple points of regulation, including the size of the progenitor cell population and the rate of division of progenitors cells, the survival of daughter cells, the commitment of daughter cells to a specific (neuronal or glial) lineage, and the rate of neuronal growth and differentiation. In principle, alterations in the regulation of any or all of these processes might contribute to aging-related changes in neuronal replacement. Recent studies have begun to reveal the specificity of aging effects, despite still limited data and occasionally conflicting results.

1.   Number and Proliferation Rate of Progenitor Cells

Much of the aging-related decline in neurogenesis in both the DG and SVZ is the result of a dramatic decline in the division of progenitor cells. Quantitative analyses of cell division in the SGZ and SVZ of young adult and older animals, utilizing S-phase labeling with BrdU, have consistently demonstrated 50 to 90% declines in the number of BrdU-labeled cells present in the neurogenic regions immediately or shortly after BrdU injection (e.g., [12, 13, 57, 58, 60–62,72–74]). Stem cells divide so slowly that changes in their rate of division are unlikely to contribute detectably to *in vivo* measurements of proliferation in adults; thus, the reported changes likely reflect a decrease in the division of more restricted and more rapidly dividing progenitor populations. Although many studies used BrdU labeling protocols that included injections over several days and survival periods of up to a week, which may conflate changes in cell division with changes in survival, recent studies using discrete labeling periods and short survival times (1 hour or less) leave no doubt that there is less cell division in older animals. Consistent with the analysis of more general measures of neurogenesis, most of the aging-related decline in the division of progenitor cells occurs by middle age, with only modest additional declines during later senescence [64]. Both the temporal pattern and the magnitudes of decline are similar in mice and rats, the only species for which there are extensive quantitative data. When examined in the same individuals, the magnitude of the decline is greater in the SGZ than in the SVZ (90 and 50% declines, respectively, comparing 3-month-old and 20-month-old mice [62]).

In principle, the decrease in BrdU labeling could reflect a smaller population of progenitor cells, slower and/or less frequent division of a constant population of progenitors, and/or changes in cell cycle kinetics. At least two studies of the SVZ indicate that the cell cycle of progenitors in the SVZ lengthens in older animals [61, 64]. It should be noted, however, that the change in cell cycle length appears to occur between middle and old age, later than most of the decline in proliferation [64]. In addition to lengthening of the cell cycle, more progenitor cells leave the cell cycle in older animals [64], raising the possibility that the age-related change in cell division includes deviations from steady-state kinetics (which are assumed by most analytical methods). Testing empirically for changes in the length of the S-phase or other components of the cell cycle and for changes in check-point regulation is critical [75, 76], but these difficult and resource-intensive experiments have not been completed for aging animals.

Determining whether the size of the population of stem and progenitor cells declines with aging is as challenging as quantifying cell cycle changes, and recent attempts to answer the question have provided intriguing but somewhat conflicting results. Tropepe et al. [61] reported that progenitor cells isolated from young adult and aged mice formed comparable numbers of, and similarly sized, neurospheres *in vitro*, leading the authors to conclude that both the number and proliferative potential of progenitor cells is maintained during aging, and that the aging-related decline in proliferation *in vivo* is due solely to changes in the microenvironment in which progenitor cells proliferate. A more recent study, however, demonstrated a twofold reduction in the number of neurospheres recovered in culture from old relative to young adult mice [77]. Consistent with that study, Luo and colleagues [64] combined BrdU labeling, immunolabeling for Ki-67 (a nuclear protein expressed by dividing cells), and ultrastructural analysis to analyze the number of neuroblasts and TAP cells and reported that both decrease by middle age. Quantifying the population of slowly cycling stem cells is more difficult than analyzing the "later" progenitor cells, but there also is evidence for an aging-related decrease in the number of neural stem cells in the SVZ, based on labeling for the G1-phase cell cycle marker Mcm2 and labeling with nucleoside analogs [77, 78]. The magnitude of the reported declines in stem cells, neuroblasts, and TAP cells is similar to the decline in BrdU labeling (approximately 50%) and, like the decline in cell division, most of the decrease in progenitor cell number occurs by middle age. In considering these and similar studies, it is important to remember that there are no definitive, state-independent markers for neural progenitor cells, and that a "loss" of cells based on immunolabeling or morphological criteria could simply reflect loss of expression of specific phenotypic traits. The ability of progenitor cells in aged animals to respond to a variety of stimuli and return neurogenesis to levels at or near that seen in young adults [56–58, 62, 72, 79–82] demonstrates that even in the aged brain there is a population of neural progenitor cells that is adequate to maintain neuro-genesis at a youthful level, given the proper conditions.

2. Cell Survival

Because, at all ages, many of the newborn cells in the adult DG and SVZ/RMS die before reaching full maturity, changes in cell survival could contribute to the aging-related decline in neurogenesis. In young adult rats, 50% of newborn (BrdU-labeled) cells in the DG die within 28 days after labeling; those that survive past the first month live for at least 5 additional months and replace granule cells that were born during development or earlier in adulthood [83]. It has proved difficult to assess directly the survival of newborn neurons in the neurogenic regions. Common markers of apoptosis (e.g., terminal transferase-mediated dUTP nick-end-labeling, TUNEL) generally do not reveal a large enough population of dying cells in the adult DG to account for the extent of cell birth and the fact that the total number of dentate granule cells remains stable throughout adulthood, suggesting either the window during which dying cells can be detected is too short to permit accurate assessment of their number or many cells are dying by a mechanism that is not recognized by current detection methods. Studies using BrdU labeling support the conclusion that aging does not diminish the survival of newborn cells, and that most of the decline in neurogenesis is accounted for by decreased proliferation (e.g., [13, 56, 58]). Using the ratio of the number of BrdU-labeled cells present at 4 weeks after labeling to the number present immediately after labeling as an index of survival, studies of aging mice [56] and rats [58] revealed no decrease in the survival of newborn cells in young adult, middle-aged, and old animals. Aging may, however, alter the balance of cell death among undifferentiated, differentiating, and mature cells in a manner that is not apparent with currently available methods.

3. Neuronal Commitment and Differentiation

Although the survival of newborn cells in neurogenic regions appears to be unaffected by age, the percentage of newborn cells that become neurons is much lower in middle-aged and old animals than in young adults (e.g., [12, 56, 58, 60, 84]). When examined approximately 4 weeks after BrdU labeling, the percentage of newborn cells in the DG that express neuronal markers is reduced by about 60% between young adulthood and middle-age in rats [58, 84], and by 40% or more in mice [56, 60]. Thus, in aged animals, the overall reduction in the proliferation of progenitor cells is compounded by a decrease in the fraction of cells that are produced that become neurons. The aging-related decrease in the development of newborn neurons may not reflect a decrease in initial commitment to a neuronal lineage, however, because a comparable percentage of newborn cells expresses the neuroblast marker doublecortin (Dcx) 24 hours after BrdU labeling [84]. The subsequent development of new neurons is compromised in older animals, however, because both the rate of migration into the granule cell layer and the rate of structural maturation are slowed in middle-aged and old rats, compared to young adults [84].

Just as one might describe the population of many countries as "graying," with older individuals representing an increasing percentage of the population, there is a significant "graying" of the population of dentate granule neurons and OB interneurons during the transition from young adulthood into middle and old age. As the rate of addition of new neurons declines, the population of young, developing neurons, which are thought to play a unique role in hippocampal and olfactory function (Section IV.A), decreases relative to the population of older, less plastic neurons. Moreover, the differentiation of newborn neurons is slowed in older animals [84], presumably impacting their integration into neural circuits and their influence on the neural processes that depend on neuronal turnover. Given evidence that adult neurogenesis is important for some functions of the hippocampus and OB (Section IV.B), amelioration of the aging-related decline in neurogenesis represents an attractive target for reducing aging-related cognitive dysfunction. Any attempt to prevent or diminish the effects of aging on neurogenesis depends, however, on understanding the molecular mechanisms that control neurogenesis and mediate the aging-related changes.

III. REGULATORS OF NEUROGENESIS IN THE ADULT AND AGING BRAIN

The list of intrinsic factors (e.g., transcription factors and cell cycle regulators) and extracellular growth factors, hormones, and neurotransmitters that influence neurogenesis in the adult neurogenic zones is large, diverse, and ever-growing (see [85, 86] for reviews). Intrinsic cell cycle regulators have been studied primarily in the developing nervous system, only recently in adults [85], and not at all in the aging brain; they are not discussed here. Importantly, many recent studies indicate that the aging-related decline in neurogenesis develops primarily from changes in the neurogenic microenvironment and in the factors that control the division of stem and progenitor cells, not from loss of, or changes intrinsic to, those precursors. Among the most striking recent advances in the understanding of adult neurogenesis was the observation that proliferation does not occur randomly or homogeneously throughout the neurogenic regions, but rather that dividing progenitor cells are found in close association with the microvasculature, in a "vascular niche," and that neurogenesis is associated with a process of active vasculogenesis and remodeling (e.g., [87–90]). This view provides hope that aging-related changes may be reversed by experimental modulation of the microenvironment if the critical cellular and molecular factors that define that environment can be identified. A complete discussion of the neurogenic niche and of all the extrinsic factors that might influence adult neurogenesis is beyond the scope of this chapter; the discussion here focuses on factors for which there is evidence of an important role in mediating aging-related changes in neurogenesis in the hippocampus and SVZ (see [44] for an excellent review of the regulation of neurogenesis in the OE).

A.   HORMONES AND GROWTH FACTORS

1.   Stress Hormones

Stress and corticosteroids were among the first studied regulators of adult neurogenesis [91, 92]. The idea that stress and glucocorticoids contribute to the aging-related decline in neurogenesis is particularly attractive, given widespread evidence that stress influences brain aging and cognitive function (e.g., [93–95]; see Chapter 13), and that aging is associated with elevated levels of corticosteroids [96]. Stress-induced depression of proliferation in the DG has been demonstrated in several species (shrews and marmosets, as well as rats and mice) and in response to a wide variety of stressors (reviewed in [97]) but there are, as yet, no studies of stress effects specifically in old animals. The effects of stress on neurogenesis overall are more complex than the effects on proliferation. Some studies indicate that stress-induced depression of proliferation is accompanied by a decrease in neuronal production, as one would predict [90, 99]. Others, however, have shown that the stress-induced reduction in proliferation is followed, after a short period, by an increase in cell survival, such that the overall addition of new neurons remains largely unchanged [100, 101]. Whatever the complexity of stress-induced changes, clearly they are mediated, at least in part, by glucocorticoids. Depletion of glucocorticoids by adrenalectomy increases the number of BrdU-labeled cells in the DG in both young adult and old rats (e.g., [57]), and increasing glucocorticoid activity decreases proliferation [92, 102]. The relationship between glucocorticoid levels and neurogenesis is not simple, however, because physical activity, living in an enriched environment, and training on learning paradigms all increase glucocorticoids but also increase neurogenesis (see [97]). Moreover, despite the profound effects of glucocorticoids on neurogenesis in the DG, proliferation in the SVZ remains unchanged following adrenalectomy [103]. Progress in investigating the expression of glucocorticoid and mineralocorticoid receptors on neural precursor cell populations [104] is beginning to clarify the cellular targets of stress hormones within neurogenic regions and offers promise that the specific role of those factors in aging-related changes in neurogenesis soon will be clearer.

2. Growth Hormone/Insulin-Like Growth Factor-1 Axis

Interest in the growth hormone/insulin-like growth factor-1 (GH/IGF-1) axis as a mediator of aging-related changes in the brain and other organ systems developed from the recognition that a substantial decline in serum GH and IGF-1 levels is one of the most robust hallmarks of mammalian aging (reviewed in [105–107]. Given the pleiotropic effects of IGF-1 in the brain and increasing evidence that GH has direct effects in the brain, as well as regulating IGF-1 levels, it is reasonable to expect that the aging-related decline in GH/IGF-1 activity is significant for brain structure and function. There is experimental evidence that restoring GH and/or IGF-1 in older animals ameliorates many aging-related neural changes (105, 107). With respect to neurogenesis, several lines of evidence implicate the GH/IGF-1 axis in aging-related changes. The regulation of adult neurogenesis appears to be linked to the regulation of angiogenesis (e.g., [87, 90, 108]), which is modulated in the aging brain by the GH/IGF-1 axis [109]. In addition, several laboratories have demonstrated that modulating IGF-1 levels in adult rodents alters hippocampal neurogenesis (see [107, 110] for reviews). Neurogenesis is decreased by hypophysectomy (Hx), which decreases levels of GH (and other pituitary hormones) and IGF-1, and neurogenesis in Hx animals is restored by peripheral infusion of IGF-1 [111]. IGF-1 also mediates the ability of physical exercise to increase neurogenesis [112]. Finally, direct intracerebral ventricular (icv) infusion of IGF-1 into aged rats ameliorates the aging-related decline in neurogenesis [58].

Although the evidence that the GH/IGF-1 axis plays some role in the regulation of adult neurogenesis and contributes to aging-related changes is intriguing, the mechanisms of such regulation remain poorly understood, particularly with respect to which endogenous source or sources of IGF-1 are most important for regulating adult neurogenesis and which aspects of neurogenesis are regulated by the GH/IGF-1 axis. IGF-1 is available to cells in the CNS from at least three sources: from the plasma across the blood-brain barrier [113, 114], following production by cells of the cerebral vasculature [115, 116], and from local production by neurons and glia within the brain parenchyma [115–117]. Teasing apart the endocrine, paracrine, and autocrine effects of IGF-1 on neurogenesis remains a significant challenge, but some insight was provided by the initially paradoxical observation that hippocampal neurogenesis increases in Ames dwarf mice, a model of GH/IGF-1 deficiency. Although Ames mice have profound deficits in circulating GH and IGF-1, analysis revealed greatly increased IGF-1 levels in the hippocampus, presumably accounting for the increase in neurogenesis [118]. Thus, at least for the regulation of adult neurogenesis, local production of IGF-1 may be more important than endocrine levels. Quantitative data on levels and production of IGF-1 within the brain parenchyma are limited, but IGF-1 levels within the rat hippocampus decline significantly by middle age and then only slightly, if at all, during later senescence [119], a temporal pattern that correlates with the aging-related change in neurogenesis.

Even as the regional regulation of IGF-1 production and activity becomes clearer, it is not yet established that IGF-1 modulates the same aspects of neurogenesis that are most affected by aging, and one must consider the possibility that changes in neurogenesis in response to experimental modulation of IGF-1 levels reflect a pharmacological effect rather than normal physiological regulation. As discussed, the aging-related changes in neurogenesis include both decreased proliferation and changes in commitment and/or differentiation, whereas effects on survival are less clear. The reported increase in the number of BrdU-labeled cells in the SGZ following restoration of IGF-1 by icv infusion in aged rats appears to involve increased proliferation [58], but because BrdU was injected over several days in that study, one cannot exclude the possibility that IGF-1 affected survival. Significantly, icv infusion of IGF-1 has no effect on the percentage of newborn cells that committed to neuronal differentiation; thus, it is unlikely that decreased GH/IGF-1 activity accounts for the aging-related decline in neuronal commitment in the DG. A recent study of neurogenesis in a model of adult-onset GH/IGF-1 deficiency indicates that IGF-1 modulates the survival of newborn neurons [120] but, as noted above, the effects of aging on survival remain unclear. Taken together, the available data suggest that the aging-related decline in the activity of the GH/IGF-1 axis contributes to, but cannot fully account for, aging-related changes in neurogenesis. Additional factors clearly are involved.

3.   Fibroblast Growth Factor

Fibroblast growth factor 2 (FGF-2), also known as basic fibroblast growth factor (bFGF), declines in the aging hippocampus and, like the declines in IGF-1 and in neurogenesis, the decrease in FGF-2 occurs by middle age [119]. The aging-related decline in FGF-2 appears to be due, at least in part, to decreased local production, because both the number of FGF-positive cells and the intensity of immunolabeling is reduced in middle-aged and old mice compared to young adults [119]. There is more than correlative evidence that FGF-2 contributes to the aging-related decline in neurogenesis; infusion (icv) of FGF-2 into old mice partially ameliorates the aging-related decline in BrdU labeling [62]. In the SGZ, the number of BrdU-labeled cells in FGF-2 infused old mice is 20% of that seen in normal, young adults, compared to the 10% seen in control aged mice. The effects of FGF-2 infusion are greater in the SVZ, where the number of BrdU-labeled cells in FGF-treated aged animals approaches the level seen in normal, young adults. The effects of FGF-2 treatment of aged animals, like the effects of IGF-1, not only suggest the factors may mediate (in part) the aging-related decline in neurogenesis, but they also demonstrate that the aged brain retains the capacity to respond to growth factors with increased neurogenesis, an important consideration as one contemplates the therapeutic potential of modulating neurogenesis to ameliorate aging-related cognitive deficits or neurodegeneration.

4.   Vascular Endothelial Growth Factor

Vascular endothelial growth factor (VEGF) shows the same pattern of aging-related decline in the hippocampus as IGF-1 and FGF-2; levels of VEGF in middle-aged and aged animals are only about half that in young adults [119]. VEGF is of particular interest with respect to aging-dependent regulation of neurogenesis because adult neurogenesis and angiogenesis may be linked (e.g., [87–90]), but there are multiple mechanisms by which VEGF might influence neurogenesis, some of which need not involve the vasculature. Reports that VEGF receptors are expressed by neurons, as well as by vascular endothelial cells (discussed in [121, 122], and that neurogenesis is increased in response to doses of VEGF that are too low to induce endothelial proliferation, indicate that VEGF may influence neurogenesis independently of its ability to promote angiogenesis [123]. Although the ability of VEGF to restore neurogenesis in aged animals has not been tested directly, there is evidence that modulating VEGF activity in young adults alters neurogenesis in both the DG and SVZ/RMS. VEGF knockout mice show reduced neurogenesis in both neurogenic regions and icv infusion of VEGF increases neurogenesis [124]. Significantly, there is accumulating evidence that VEGF mediates some of the effects of stress [125], of exercise [126, 127], and of complex environments and learning on adult neurogenesis [128, 129].

5.   Brain-Derived Neurotrophic Factor

Brain-derived neurotrophic factor (BDNF) is expressed at high levels in the adult hippocampus, including the DG [130], and a variety of evidence implicates BDNF as an important mediator of aging-related neural changes in the brain (reviewed in [131]). The effects of aging on hippocampal BDNF levels remain controversial, with some laboratories reporting an aging-related decrease (e.g., [132, 133]) but others finding little or no change [134, 135]. The specific role of BDNF in modulating neurogenesis in the normal adult and aging brain also remains unclear. Consistent with the hypothesis that BDNF is a proneurogenic factor is evidence that neurogenesis decreases in BDNF knockout mice [136] and that increasing BDNF levels in the SVZ by adenovirus [137] or icv infusion [138, 139] increases the number of neuroblasts and new neurons in the SVZ and OB. Direct unilateral intrahippocampal infusion of BDNF increases neurogenesis in the DG, but the effect must be indirect and not by direct stimulation of progenitor cells because increased neurogenesis is evident bilaterally while exogenous BDNF appears to remain restricted to the infused hemisphere [140]. The effects of BDNF on proliferation and neurogenesis also are influenced by other factors. In apparent contrast to the evidence that BDNF promotes neurogenesis in the normal adult brain, infusion of the factor following an ischemic event reduces the increase in neurogenesis that usually follows ischemia [141]. Moreover, reducing endogenous BDNF following ischemia promotes, rather than decreases, neurogenesis [142]. Additional evidence for complex, differential regulation of BDNF and its effects comes from reports that one form of dietary restriction, every-other-day feeding, increases adult neurogenesis by increasing BDNF [143, 144], whereas another form of dietary restriction, 40% calorie reduction, does not affect BDNF levels and does not increase neurogenesis [60, 135].

6.   Epidermal Growth Factor Family

Members of the epidermal growth factor (EGF) family of growth factors and receptors have been implicated in the regulation of both embryonic and adult neurogenesis (e.g., [61, 145–148]). Adult TGF-α knockout mice show decreased proliferation in the SVZ and fewer new neurons migrating to the OB [61]. Aged mice show reduced EGF receptor signaling in the SVZ and decreased neuronal replacement in the OB, along with deficits in olfactory discrimination [149]. Infusion of EGF increases proliferation in the SVZ, but also reduces neuronal replacement in the OB [145, 146]. Thus, EGF not only promotes proliferation of precursors but also directs differentiating cells away from differentiation as neurons. The capacity to respond to EGF with increased proliferation in the SVZ is retained in old animals [150], in which increased proliferation is associated with improved performance in a passive avoidance learning task [151]. EGF does not promote proliferation in the adult hippocampus as it does in the SVZ [146], but another family member, heparin-binding EGF (HB-EGF), increases both BrdU labeling and the number of doublecortin-positive cells in the SVZ and the SGZ [62]. As with all the growth factors discussed above, the roles of EGF family members in regulating neurogenesis in the adult and aging brain are only beginning to be elucidated.

7.   Transforming Growth Factor-β Family

Members of the Transforming Growth Factor-β family of growth factors, particularly TGF-β and bone morphogenetic proteins (BMPs), are powerful regulators of neural stem cells and of neurogenesis in both developing and adult brains. Much like BDNF, the effects of TGF-β on neurogenesis appear to be context dependent. Intracerebroventricular infusion of TGF-β reduces proliferation of progenitor cells in both the DG and SVZ of adult mice [152], and chronic overexpression of TGF-β in aged transgenic mice virtually eliminates neurogenesis [153], but TGF-β mediates pro-neurogenic effects of microglia following adrenalectomy (see below). The question of whether changes in TGF-β signaling contribute to changes in neurogenesis in normally aging mice has not yet been addressed. Whether changes in BMP signaling contribute to aging-related changes in neurogenesis similarly is unknown, but BMPs influence adult neural stem cells in much the same way that they influence stem cells in the developing brain. In the adult SVZ, in the absence of other factors, BMPs direct stem cells toward a glial fate, but that gliogenic signal is blocked by the BMP inhibitor noggin, which is expressed by ependymal cells [154, 155]. Thus, a change in the balance of BMP signaling and inhibitors could contribute to the aging-related decrease in the percentage of newborn cells that differentiate as neurons (Section II.B.3).

8.   Retinoic Acid

Retinoic acid (RA), a member of the steroid/thyroid hormone super family, is an essential growth factor and regulates many aspects of embryonic neural development. Recent evidence indicates that RA continues to influence plasticity and regeneration in the adult brain and may influence neurogenesis in the olfactory epithelium, SVZ, and hippocampus, with possible effects on both proliferation of progenitor cells and differentiation of newborn neurons [156, 157]. Changes in RA signaling may be particularly important in the aging olfactory system, with effects in both the OE and the SVZ [45]. RA critically regulates the initial development of the peripheral olfactory system and continues to influence olfactory progenitor cells in the adult [158–160]. In addition to activating basal stem cells in the OE, RA influences a small population of cells in the SVZ that appear to be stem cells (i.e., they are slowly dividing, express GFAP, and form neurospheres when isolated in culture). A variety of studies in humans and animal models suggest that RA promotes recovery of olfactory function in aged individuals and following injury to the peripheral olfactory system [45]. Moreover, RA improves performance on an odor-mediated learning task when administered to senescent mice [161]. Perhaps most intriguingly, because dietary vitamin A is the primary source of retinoids, RA could play the central role in a feed-forward cycle in which a modest aging-related decline in olfactory function contributes to reduced appetite, which leads to reduced food intake and sub-optimal vitamin A levels, resulting in decreased RA signaling and thereby to further deficits in olfactory neurogenesis (discussed in [45]). Further investigation may establish RA as an important therapeutic target for ameliorating the age-related decline in olfactory function.

B.   NEUROTRANSMITTERS

Several neurotransmitters have been implicated in the regulation of adult neurogen-esis, consistent with the growing awareness that neurotransmitters can act as trophic factors as well as synaptic messengers and with evidence that activity within the adult hippocampus and olfactory system influences the production and integration of new neurons. In the OB, centrifugal projections of cholinergic, serotonergic, and catecholaminergic inputs each can influence the differentiation and survival of new neurons [155]. Cholinergic neurons in the basal forebrain project to both the DG and the OB, and the number of newborn granule neurons decreases in both regions following lesion of that cholinergic projection [162, 163]. GABA plays a key role in the integration of newborn neurons in the adult brain [164], and additional influences of serotonin may link changes in neurogenesis to the development of depression [165, 166]. Few studies have investigated neurotransmitter-dependent regulation of neurogenesis in aged animals, but loss of dopaminergic projections from the substantia nigra to the SVZ further decreases the number of proliferating progenitors and developing neurons in the SVZ of aged primates [65], and treatment with antagonists to the NMDA type glutamate receptor increases neurogenesis in aged rats [59], the latter suggesting that the decline in neurogenesis may be one of several deficits influenced by aging-related changes in glutamate signaling (see Chapter 8).

C. INFLAMMATORY MEDIATORS

Evidence from many laboratories and studies suggests that aging-related increases in inflammatory processes contribute to the development of neural deficits (e.g., [167–170]). This hypothesis is based on evidence that (1) basal levels of many pro-inflammatory cytokines increase in older brains and (2) those cytokines affect the function, and even the survival, of neurons, glia, and progenitor cells. Although not yet established, it is reasonable to suspect that aging-related activation of microglia suppresses neurogenesis (and thereby cognitive function), because neurogenesis is profoundly affected by changes in the neurogenic microenvironment that are mediated by reactive microglia and inflammatory cytokines. Inducing an inflammatory response by infusion of the bacterial toxin lipopolysaccharide (LPS) virtually eliminates neurogenesis in the adult brain, with the extent of reduction in individuals well correlated with the number of activated microglia [171]. Neurogenesis is restored in LPS-infused animals by treatment with minocycline, a tetracycline derivative that inhibits the activation of microglia. Studies using brain irradiation to induce microglia activation and a sustained inflammatory response demonstrate that inflammatory-induced changes in neurogenesis arise as a result changes in the neurogenic environment, rather than intrinsic changes in progenitor cells. Hippocampal progenitor cells can be cultured from irradiated brains, divide normally, and produce a normal array of cell types in culture, but hippocampal progenitor cells from non-irradiated brains do not divide and produce neurons when transplanted into an irradiated brain, as they do when transplanted into a nonirradiated brain [108]. Significantly, these deleterious changes in the progenitor cell niche arise, at least in part, from the radiation-induced inflammatory response, because treatment with non-steroidal anti-inflammatory drugs (NSAIDs) ameliorates the deleterious effects of whole-brain irradiation on hippocampal neurogenesis [172].

Thus, to the extent that microglial activation and a chronic inflammatory response accompany brain aging (e.g., [168, 173, 174]), one would expect they contribute to the aging-related decline in neurogenesis, and possibly to cognitive deficits. It must be recognized, however, that the "activation" of microglial cells and their relationship to other cell types is significantly more complex than previously appreciated (e.g., [175]), and that activated microglia are not always antineurogenic. Following adrenalectomy, microglia increase neurogenesis via TGF-β [176] and microglia activated by anti-inflammatory cytokines associated with T-helper cells also increase neurogenesis [177, 178], in contrast to endotoxin-activated microglia, which inhibit neurogenesis [179]. The balance of pro- and anti-inflammatory factors produced by microglial cells under specific conditions determines their effect on the neurogenic microenvironment, and clarification of the role of inflammation in aging-related changes in neurogenesis awaits a clearer understanding of aging and aged microglia (see [180] for a recent discussion of aging-related changes in microglia).

IV. FUNCTIONAL SIGNIFICANCE OF ADULT NEUROGENESIS

Since the initial demonstrations that neurogenesis continues in the adult brain, it has been a major challenge to understand the functional significance of the ongoing production of new neurons in the mammalian brain (function is better understood in avian species [6, 181, 182]). It has been demonstrated repeatedly in rodents that adult-born neurons become functional; that is, they develop synaptic and electro-physiological properties characteristic of mature neurons and are integrated into synaptic networks. The current challenge is establishing the importance of neuro-genesis at the systems and cognitive levels. There is compelling evidence that newborn neurons have distinct electrophysiological properties that endow them with greater plasticity, which may permit them to play a unique role in hippocampal and olfactory circuits (discussed in [183] and below). Some investigators suggest that ongoing neuronal replacement provides more long-term and adaptive, rather than acute, benefits [182, 184, 185], perhaps permitting the hippocampus and OB to be optimized for particular environments [186]. Such long-term function might explain, in part, the difficulties in linking differences in neurogenesis to differences in cog-nitive ability. Further complicating the issue, it cannot be assumed that new neurons in the hippocampus have the same or even similar functional roles as new neurons in the OB. Even a cursory summary of the investigations addressing this issue is beyond the scope of this chapter, but many excellent reviews and discussions are available (e.g., [7, 182–193]). It is important here, however, to consider the exper-imental approaches that have been taken and to consider the limited number of studies that have examined the issue in aging animals.

A. CELL PHYSIOLOGY OF NEWBORN NEURONS

Many laboratories are studying adult-born neurons at the cellular level, using elec-trophysiological methods to compare the membrane and synaptic properties of newborn neurons to those of older neurons and to assess the integration of the new neurons into neural circuits. Such studies are critical to understanding what capacities are added by the constant addition of new neurons. Although the questions of whether and when adult-born neurons send projections into target regions was answered soon after the rediscovery of adult neurogenesis (e.g., [30, 194, 195]), investigations of the electrophysiological development of adult-born neurons and their functional integration required the development of methods for identifying newborn neurons in living tissue. In recent years, adult-born neurons have been labeled with fluorescent proteins controlled by viral vectors or developmentally regulated promoters, so that one can identify and record from the neurons in living preparations (e.g., [32, 33, 196–198]. Such studies have provided detailed descriptions of the development of cell physiological and synaptic properties of dentate granule neurons and granule and periglomerular neurons in the OB, both in normal adults and under a variety of clinically relevant experimental conditions (reviewed in [186]). Evidence that long-term potentiation (LTP) can be induced more readily in newborn dentate granule neurons than in older granule neurons [199, 200] suggests that unique mechanisms for synaptic plasticity may underlie the contributions of newborn neurons to hippocampal and olfactory function. To date, electrophysiological studies of newborn neurons have not been done in aged animals, as most experiments are done using brain slices, which are more difficult to prepare from old animals, and it is unknown whether the functional maturation of new neurons is altered in older individuals. Evidence that the dendritic maturation of newborn dentate granule neurons is slowed in older animals [84] suggests, however, that the development of mature functional properties by newborn neurons also may be altered in senescent animals.

B.   ADULT NEUROGENESIS AND COGNITIVE FUNCTION

Systems-level studies of the significance of adult neurogenesis have taken three general approaches: (1) experimentally decreasing or stopping neurogenesis and testing for changes in performance in some cognitive task, (2) testing whether training in a cognitive task alters neurogenesis, and (3) testing whether individual performance in a cognitive task correlates with individual differences in ongoing neurogenesis. Numerous such studies have addressed the role of neurogenesis in hippocampal-dependent learning (see [193] for a recent review); investigations of the contributions of neurogenesis to olfactory function are more limited but indicate a strong relationship between the number of newborn neurons and olfactory performance (see, e.g., [198, 201–203]). Several broad conclusions can be drawn from the available literature. First, some, but not all, functions of the hippocampus and OB depend on ongoing neurogenesis. Second, some cognitive functions appear to be linked to newborn cell proliferation, whereas others are linked to survival. Third, demonstrated associations between neurogenesis and performance in a given cognitive task are complex and dependent upon specific stages and aspects of learning and specific stages of maturity of newborn cells (e.g., [204]). Finally, it is difficult to demonstrate direct and causal links between neurogenesis and neural function since manipulations that alter neurogenesis (brain irradiation and treatment with antimitotic agents commonly are used) generally have broader and non-specific effects; moreover, training in cognitive tasks may produce neural changes that influence neurogenesis secondarily (e.g., changes in the vasculature or in the production of growth factors).

C.   NEUROGENESIS AND COGNITIVE FUNCTION IN AGED ANIMALS

Attempts to link aging-related changes in neurogenesis to aging-related changes in neural and cognitive function are largely limited to correlative analyses. Enwere and colleagues [149] demonstrated that aged (24 months old) mice are less capable than young adult (2 months old) mice in making fine olfactory discriminations, but are not impaired in discriminating more discrete odors. Because the same deficit in fine, but not gross, discrimination was evident in transgenic mice with deficits in olfactory neurogenesis that are similar to those seen in aging, the authors suggested that the impairment in fine olfactory discrimination that is seen with age results from the reduction in neurogenesis. Direct evidence of such a mechanistic link is not, as yet, available.

There have been several attempts to link changes in neurogenesis and aging-related deficits in hippocampal-dependent functions. A recent study of Fisher-344 × Brown Norway hybrid rats from the aging colony maintained by the National Institute on Aging demonstrated by correlation analysis that two measures of neurogenesis, immunolabeling for proliferating cells and for developing neurons in the DG, were among a subset of structural and histological changes that predict performance on hippocampal-dependent tasks [205]. In addition to such correlational evidence from normal animals, the reductions in aging-related cognitive deficits seen in long-lived Ames dwarf mice [118] and in rats treated with the neurosteroid pregnalone sulfate [206] or maintained on antioxidant-rich diets [79] all are associated with increased neurogenesis in the DG. Other investigations have taken advantage of the recognition that aging-related cognitive deficits are not homogenously represented among populations of aged rats; some individuals exhibit large impairments while others perform at levels comparable to young adults [207]. Critically, such individual variability in cognitive performance is consistent across cognitive domains [208]. Thus, to look for neurobiological changes that may underlie cognitive impairments, one can test for differences in specific anatomical, biochemical or electrophysiological endpoints comparing impaired and unimpaired senescent animals (e.g., [209, 210]. Using this approach, Drapeau and colleagues [211] reported that 20-month-old rats that exhibited better spatial memory performance in the Morris Water Maze (MWM) had higher levels of neurogenesis in the DG, as demonstrated by BrdU labeling and immunolabeling with a marker of dividing cells (anti-Ki-67) 3 weeks after the end of behavioral testing. No such correlation between performance and proliferation was evident in 3-month-old animals. The authors also reported that the commitment of newborn cells to a neuronal lineage (i.e., the percentage of BrdU-labeled cells co-labeled with a neuronal marker) was higher in better performing than poorer performing old rats, and that behavioral performance positively correlated with the survival of newborn neurons. Given the BrdU labeling protocol used in the study, however, it is not clear that the difference in "survival" did not simply reflect the difference in proliferation. A link between aging-related declines in hippocampal function and neuronal turnover also was suggested by a report that decreased survival of newborn cells in the DG of 28-month-old rats is associated with a deficit in contextual fear conditioning ([212], but see also [190] for evidence that trace fear conditioning, but not contextual fear conditioning, is compromised by reduction of neurogenesis in young rats).

Although the idea that decreased cognitive performance in aged rodents is strongly correlated with decreased cognitive performance is intuitively appealing, several studies found no such connection. Merrill and colleagues [213] tested young adult and aged Fisher-344 rats in the MWM and then assessed neurogenesis by BrdU labeling for several days after the completion of behavioral testing. Although the number of BrdU-labeled cells in the SGZ of the DG was reduced in old rats compared to young adults, there was no difference in this measure of proliferation between aged rats that were impaired in the MWM and those that performed at a level comparable to young animals. A similar study of Long-Evans rats, in which proliferation was measured by BrdU labeling 1 week after completion of behavioral testing, also found no correlation between cognitive performance and neurogenesis [214]. Surprisingly, in a subsequent study, the latter investigators examined the survival of newborn neurons approximately 1 month after BrdU labeling (and the completion of testing in the MWM) and found that survival was greater in the aged rats with impaired cognitive function than in aged animals that were not impaired [215]; that is, hippocampal function was worse in those rats in which neurogenesis was greater. At this point, one must conclude that elucidating the functional links between aging-related changes in neurogenesis and aging-related cognitive deficits will require reconsideration of intuitive biases, assessment of a broader array of cognitive tasks, better measures of neurogenesis that differentiate among mechanisms of regulation, and new approaches that move beyond the limitations of correlational studies.

V.   CONCLUSIONS

Given that neurogenesis is regionally restricted in the adult brain, the direct contribution of changes in neurogenesis to the development of aging-related cognitive decline is likely limited, perhaps accounting for the difficulty thus far in linking the decline in neurogenesis to specific neural deficits. As investigations of the contributions of adult neurogenesis to neural function continue, however, it is reasonable to expect they will demonstrate that the aging-related loss of the plasticity afforded by the continued addition of new neurons contributes to functional decline in senescence. Moreover, the interest of experimental gerontologists in the regulation of neurogenesis in the adult and aging brain extends beyond direct roles in hippocampal and olfactory function. It is reasonable to expect that the changes in neuronal microenvironment that lead to the decline in neurogenesis in older individuals may contribute to functional changes in established neurons and glial cells as well. In addition, the ability to isolate and expand neural stem cells from healthy brains, along with a rapidly growing capacity to regulate those cells and their progeny, keeps alive a vision of using transplanted stem cells to treat neurodegenerative diseases [216–221]. Even more appealing is that every advance in understanding the regulation of neurogenesis *in vivo* is a step toward therapeutic manipulation of endogenous progenitors to replace lost neurons or compensate for lost function [222], whether that occurring with normal aging or as a result of neurodegenerative disease.

Although neuronal turnover is reduced in every neurogenic region of the aged brain, neuronal precursor cells clearly survive, remain responsive to growth factors and other physiological stimuli (e.g., [56, 58, 72, 81, 223]), and can increase their activity in response to damage (e.g., [63, 80]). Continued exploration of the regulation of neural progenitor cells in the adult and aging brain is critical not only for understanding normal, aging-related cognitive deficits, but also for progress toward the goal of using the brain's regenerative potential to restore function lost to injury or neurodegenerative disease.

ACKNOWLEDGMENTS

Preparation of this chapter was supported in part by the National Institute on Aging, Grant No. AG11370.

REFERENCES

1. Altman, J., Autoradiographic investigation of cell proliferation in the brains of rats and cats, *Anat. Rec.*, 145, 573, 1963.
2. Altman, J., Postnatal growth and differentiation of the mammalian brain, with implications for a morphological theory of memory, in *The Neurosciences, First Program Study*, Quarton, G.C., Melnechuck, T., and Schmitt, F.O., Eds., Rockefeller University Press, New York, 1967, 723.
3. Altman, J., DNA metabolism and cell proliferation, in *Handbook of Neurochemistry, Vol. 2: Structural Neurochemistry*, Lajtha, A., Ed., Plenum Press, New York, 1969, 137.
4. Altman, J. and Das, G.D., Autoradiographic and histological evidence of postnatal hippocampal neurogenesis in rats, *J. Comp. Neurol.*, 124, 319, 1965.
5. Kaplan, M.S. and Hinds, J.W., Neurogenesis in the adult rat: electron microscopic analysis of light radioautographs, *Science*, 197, 1092, 1977.
6. Nottebohm, F., Neuronal replacement in adult brain, *Brain Res. Bull.*, 57, 737, 2002.
7. Nottebohm, F., The road we travelled: discovery, choreography, and significance of brain replaceable neurons, *Ann. N.Y. Acad. Sci.*, 1016, 628, 2004.
8. Barnea, A. and Nottebohm, F., Seasonal recruitment of hippocampal neurons in adult free-ranging black-capped chickadees, *Proc. Natl. Acad. Sci. U.S.A.*, 91, 11217, 1994.
9. Patel, S.N., Clayton, N.S., and Krebs, J.R., Spatial learning induces neurogenesis in the avian brain, *Behav. Brain Res.*, 89, 115, 1997.
10. Lee, D.W., Miyasato, L.E., and Clayton, N.S., Neurobiological bases of spatial learning in the natural environment: neurogenesis and growth in the avian and mammalian hippocampus, *Neuroreport*, 9, R15, 1998.
11. Cameron, H.A. et al., Differentiation of newly born neurons and glia in the dentate gyrus of the adult rat, *Neuroscience*, 56, 337, 1993.
12. Seki, T. and Arai, Y., Age-related production of new granule cells in the adult dentate gyrus, *Neuroreport*, 6, 2479, 1995.
13. Kuhn, H.G., Dickinson-Anson, H., and Gage, F.H., Neurogenesis in the dentate gyrus of the adult rat: age-related decreases of neuronal progenitor proliferation, *J. Neurosci.*, 16, 2027, 1996.

14. Gould, E. et al., Hippocampal neurogenesis in adult Old World primates, *Proc. Natl. Acad. Sci. U.S.A.*, 96, 5263, 1999.
15. Van Praag, H., Kempermann, G., and Gage, F.H., Running increases cell proliferation and neurogenesis in the adult mouse dentate gyrus, *Nat. Neurosci.*, 2, 266, 1999.
16. Gage, F.H., Ray, J., and Fisher, L.J., Isolation, characterization, and use of stem cells from the CNS, *Annu. Rev. Neurosci.*, 18, 159, 1995.
17. McKay, R., Stem cells in the central nervous system, *Science*, 276, 66, 1997.
18. Gage, F.H., Mammalian neural stem cells, *Science*, 287, 1433, 2000.
19. Temple, S., The development of neural stem cells, *Nature*, 414, 112, 2001.
20. Gould, E. et al., Neurogenesis in the neocortex of adult primates, *Science*, 286, 548, 1999.
21. Kornack, D.R. and Rakic, P., Cell proliferation without neurogenesis in adult primate neocortex, *Science*, 294, 2127, 2001.
22. Rakic, P., Neurogenesis in adult primate neocortex: an evaluation of the evidence, *Nat. Rev. Neurosci.*, 3, 65, 2002.
23. Dayer, A.G. et al., New GABAergic interneurons in the adult neocortex and striatum are generated from different precursors, *J. Cell Biol.*, 168, 415, 2005.
24. Eriksson, P.S. et al., Neurogenesis in the adult human hippocampus, *Nat. Med.*, 4, 1313, 1998.
25. Gage, F.H. et al., Multipotent progenitor cells in the adult dentate gyrus, *J. Neurobiol.*, 36, 249, 1998.
26. Kempermann, G. and Gage, F.H., Neurogenesis in the adult hippocampus, *Novartis Found. Symp.*, 231, 220, 2000.
27. Gould, E. and Gross, C.G., Neurogenesis in adult mammals: some progress and problems, *J. Neurosci.*, 22, 619, 2002.
28. Ming, G.L. and Song, H., Adult neurogenesis in the mammalian central nervous system, *Annu. Rev. Neurosci.*, 28, 223, 2005.
29. Christie, B.R. and Cameron, H.A., Neurogenesis in the adult hippocampus, *Hippocampus*, 16, 199, 2006.
30. Hastings, N.B. and Gould, E., Rapid extension of axons into the CA3 region by adult-generated granule cells, *J. Comp. Neurol.*, 413, 146, 1999.
31. Zhao, C. et al., Distinct morphological stages of dentate granule neuron maturation in the adult mouse hippocampus, *J. Neurosci.*, 26, 3, 2006.
32. Van Praag, H. et al., Functional neurogenesis in the adult hippocampus, *Nature*, 415, 1030, 2002.
33. Overstreet-Wadiche, L.S., Bensen, A.L., and Westbrook, G.L., Delayed development of adult-generated granule cells in dentate gyrus, *J. Neurosci.*, 26, 2326, 2006.
34. Morshead, C.M. et al., Neural stem cells in the adult mammalian forebrain: a relatively quiescent subpopulation of subependymal cells, *Neuron*, 13, 1071, 1994.
35. Doetsch, F., Garcia-Verdugo, J.M., and Alvarez-Buylla, A., Cellular composition and three-dimensional organization of the subventricular germinal zone in the adult mammalian brain, *J. Neurosci.*, 17, 5046, 1997.
36. Doetsch, F. et al., Subventricular zone astrocytes are neural stem cells in the adult mammalian brain, *Cell*, 97, 703, 1999.
37. Luskin, M.B., Restricted proliferation and migration of postnatally generated neurons derived from the forebrain subventricular zone, *Neuron*, 11, 173, 1993.
38. Luskin, M.B. et al., Neuronal progenitor cells derived from the anterior subventricular zone of the neonatal rat forebrain continue to proliferate *in vitro* and express a neuronal phenotype, *Mol. Cell. Neurosci.*, 8, 351, 1997.

39. Pencea, V. et al., Neurogenesis in the subventricular zone and rostral migratory stream of the neonatal and adult primate forebrain, *Exp. Neurol.*, 172, 1, 2001.

40. Coskun, V. and Luskin, M.B., Intrinsic and extrinsic regulation of the proliferation and differentiation of cells in the rodent rostral migratory stream, *J. Neurosci. Res.*, 69, 795, 2002.

41. Ray, J. and Gage, F.H., Differential properties of adult rat and mouse brain-derived neural stem/progenitor cells, *Mol. Cell. Neurosci.*, 31, 560, 2006.

42. Seaberg, R.M. and van der Kooy, D., Adult rodent neurogenic regions: the ventricular subependyma contains neural stem cells, but the dentate gyrus contains restricted progenitors, *J. Neurosci.*, 22, 1784, 2002.

43. Bull, N.D. and Bartlett, P.F., The adult mouse hippocampal progenitor is neurogenic but not a stem cell, *J. Neurosci.*, 25, 10815, 2005.

44. Schwob, J.E., Neural regeneration and the peripheral olfactory system, *Anat. Rec.*, 269, 33, 2002.

45. Rawson, N.E. and LaMantia, A.-S., A speculative essay on retinoic acid regulation of neural stem cells in the developing and aging olfactory system, *Exp. Gerontol.*, 42, 46, 2007.

46. Emsley, J.G. et al., Adult neurogenesis and repair of the adult CNS with neural progenitors, precursors, and stem cells, *Prog. Neurobiol.*, 75, 321, 2005.

47. Nowakowski, R.S. and Hayes, N.L., New neurons: extraordinary evidence or extraordinary conclusion? *Science*, 288, 771, 2000.

48. Gould, E. et al., Adult-generated hippocampal and neocortical neurons in macaques have a transient existence, *Proc. Natl. Acad. Sci. U.S.A.*, 98, 10910, 2001.

49. Bernier, P.J. et al., Newly generated neurons in the amygdala and adjoining cortex of adult primates, *Proc. Natl. Acad. Sci. U.S.A.*, 99, 11464, 2002.

50. Yamamoto, S. et al., Proliferation of parenchymal neural progenitors in response to injury in the adult rat spinal cord, *Exp. Neurol.*, 172, 115, 2001.

51. Magavi, S.S., Leavitt, B.R., and Macklis, J.D., Induction of neurogenesis in the neocortex of adult mice, *Nature*, 405, 951, 2000.

52. Arvidsson, A. et al., Neuronal replacement from endogenous precursors in the adult brain after stroke, *Nat. Med.*, 8, 963, 2002.

53. Nakatomi, H. et al., Regeneration of hippocampal pyramidal neurons after ischemic brain injury by recruitment of endogenous neural progenitors, *Cell*, 110, 429, 2002.

54. Parent, J.M. et al., Rat forebrain neurogenesis and striatal neuron replacement after focal stroke, *Ann. Neurol.*, 52, 802, 2002.

55. Kaplan, M.S., Formation and turnover of neurons in young and senescent animals: and electronmicroscopic and morphometric analysis, *Ann. N.Y. Acad. Sci.*, 457, 173, 1985.

56. Kempermann, G., Kuhn, H.G., and Gage, F.H., Experience-induced neurogenesis in the senescent dentate gyrus, *J. Neurosci.*, 18, 3206, 1998.

57. Cameron, H.A. and McKay, R.D., Restoring production of hippocampal neurons in old age, *Nat. Neurosci.*, 2, 894, 1999.

58. Lichtenwalner, R.J. et al., Intracerebroventricular infusion of insulin-like growth factor-I ameliorates the age-related decline in hippocampal neurogenesis, *Neuroscience*, 107, 603, 2001.

59. Nacher, J. et al., NMDA receptor antagonist treatment increases the production of new neurons in the aged rat hippocampus, *Neurobiol. Aging*, 24, 273, 2003.

60. Bondolfi, L. et al., Impact of age and caloric restriction on neurogenesis in the dentate gyrus of C57BL/6 mice, *Neurobiol. Aging*, 25, 333, 2004.

61. Tropepe, V. et al., Transforming growth factor-alpha null and senescent mice show decreased neural progenitor cell proliferation in the forebrain subependyma, *J. Neurosci.*, 17, 7850, 1997.
62. Jin, K. et al., Neurogenesis and aging: FGF-2 and HB-EGF restore neurogenesis in hippocampus and subventricular zone of aged mice, *Aging Cell*, 2, 175, 2003.
63. Jin, K. et al., Ischemia-induced neurogenesis is preserved but reduced in the aged rodent brain, *Aging Cell*, 3, 373, 2004.
64. Luo, J. et al., The aging neurogenic subventricular zone, *Aging Cell*, 5, 139, 2006.
65. Freundlieb, N. et al., Dopaminergic substantia nigra neurons project topographically organized to the subventricular zone and stimulate precursor cell proliferation in aged primates, *J. Neurosci.*, 26, 2321, 2006.
66. Naessen, R., An enquiry on the morphological characteristics and possible changes with age in the olfactory region of man, *Acta Otolaryngol.*, 71, 49, 1971.
67. Paik, S.I. et al., Human olfactory biopsy. The influence of age and receptor distribution, *Arch. Otolaryngol. Head Neck Surg.*, 118, 731, 1992.
68. Dodson, H.C. and Bannister, L.H., Structural aspects of ageing in the olfactory and vomeronasal epithelia in mice, in *Olfaction and Taste, Vol. VII*, van der Starre, H., Ed., IRL Press, London, 1980, 151.
69. Loo, A.T. et al., The aging olfactory epithelium: neurogenesis, response to damage, and odorant-induced activity, *Int. J. Dev. Neurosci.*, 14, 881, 1996.
70. Weiler, E. and Farbman, A.I., Proliferation in the rat olfactory epithelium: age-dependent changes, *J. Neurosci.*, 17, 3610, 1997.
71. Nibu, K. et al., Expression of NeuroD and TrkB in developing and aged mouse olfactory epithelium, *Neuroreport*, 12, 1615, 2001.
72. Kempermann, G., Gast, D., and Gage, F.H., Neuroplasticity in old age: sustained fivefold induction of hippocampal neurogenesis by long-term environmental enrichment, *Ann. Neurol.*, 52, 135, 2002.
73. Heine, V.M., et al., Prominent decline of newborn cell proliferation, differentiation, and apoptosis in the aging dentate gyrus, in absence of an age-related hypothalamus-pituitary-adrenal axis activation, *Neurobiol. Aging*, 25, 361, 2004.
74. McDonald, H.Y. and Wojtowicz, J.M., Dynamics of neurogenesis in the dentate gyrus of adult rats, *Neurosci. Lett.*, 385, 70, 2005.
75. Cameron, H.A. and McKay, R.D., Adult neurogenesis produces a large pool of new granule cells in the dentate gyrus, *J. Comp. Neurol.*, 435, 406, 2001.
76. Hayes, N.L. and Nowakowski, R.S., Dynamics of cell proliferation in the adult dentate gyrus of two inbred strains of mice, *Brain Res. Dev. Brain Res.*, 134, 77, 2002.
77. Maslov, A.Y. et al., Neural stem cell detection, characterization, and age-related changes in the subventricular zone of mice, *J. Neurosci.*, 24, 1726, 2004.
78. Stoeber, K. et al., DNA replication licensing and human cell proliferation, *J. Cell. Sci.*, 114, 2027, 2001.
79. Casadesus, G. et al., Modulation of hippocampal plasticity and cognitive behavior by short-term blueberry supplementation in aged rats, *Nutr. Neurosci.*, 7, 309, 2004.
80. Darsalia, V. et al., Stroke-induced neurogenesis in aged brain, *Stroke*, 36, 1790, 2005.
81. Van Praag, H. et al., Exercise enhances learning and hippocampal neurogenesis in aged mice, *J. Neurosci.*, 25, 8680, 2005.
82. Zhang, R.L. et al., Delayed treatment with sildenafil enhances neurogenesis and improves functional recovery in aged rats after focal cerebral ischemia, *J. Neurosci. Res.*, 83, 1213, 2006.
83. Dayer, A.G. et al., Short-term and long-term survival of new neurons in the rat dentate gyrus, *J. Comp. Neurol.*, 460, 563, 2003.

84. Rao, M.S. et al., Newly born cells in the aging dentate gyrus display normal migration, survival and neuronal fate choice but endure retarded early maturation, *Eur. J. Neurosci.*, 21, 464, 2005.

85. Abrous, D.N., Koehl, M., and Le Moal, M., Adult neurogenesis: from precursors to network and physiology, *Physiol. Rev.*, 85, 523, 2005.

86. Hagg, T., Molecular regulation of adult CNS neurogenesis: an integrated view, *Trends Neurosci.*, 28, 549, 2005.

87. Palmer, T.D., Willhoite, A.R., and Gage, F.H., Vascular niche for adult hippocampal neurogenesis, *J. Comp. Neurol.*, 425, 479, 2000.

88. Doetsch, F., A niche for adult neural stem cells, *Curr. Opin. Genet. Dev.*, 13, 543, 2003.

89. Alvarez-Buylla, A. and Lim, D.A., For the long run: maintaining germinal niches in the adult brain, *Neuron*, 41, 683, 2004.

90. Ward, N.L. and LaManna, J.C., The neurovascular unit and its growth factors: coordinated response in the vascular and nervous systems, *Neurol. Res.*, 26, 870, 2004.

91. Gould, E. et al., Adrenal hormones suppress cell division in the adult rat dentate gyrus, *J. Neurosci.*, 12, 3642, 1992.

92. Cameron, H.A. and Gould, E., Adult neurogenesis is regulated by adrenal steroids in the dentate gyrus, *Neuroscience*, 61, 203, 1994.

93. McEwen, B.S., Sex, stress and the hippocampus: allostasis, allostatic load and the aging process, *Neurobiol. Aging*, 23, 921, 2002.

94. Miller, D.B. and O'Callaghan, J.P., Aging, stress and the hippocampus, *Ageing Res. Rev.*, 4, 123, 2005.

95. Lupien, S.J. et al., Stress hormones and human memory function across the lifespan, *Psychoneuroendocrinology*, 30, 225, 2005.

96. Sapolsky, R.M., Do glucocorticoid concentrations rise with age in the rat? *Neurobiol. Aging*, 13, 171, 1992.

97. Mirescu, C. and Gould, E., Stress and adult neurogenesis, *Hippocampus*, 16, 233, 2006.

98. Pham, K. et al., Repeated restraint stress suppresses neurogenesis and induces biphasic PSA-NCAM expression in the adult rat dentate gyrus, *Eur. J. Neurosci.*, 17, 879, 2003.

99. Westenbroek, C. et al., Chronic stress and social housing differentially affect neurogenesis in male and female rats, *Brain Res. Bull.*, 64, 303, 2004.

100. Tanapat, P. et al, Exposure to fox odor inhibits cell proliferation in the hippocampus of adult rats via an adrenal hormone-dependent mechanism, *J. Comp. Neurol.*, 437, 496, 2001.

101. Malberg, J.E. and Duman, R.S., Cell proliferation in adult hippocampus is decreased by inescapable stress: reversal by fluoxetine treatment, *Neuropsychopharmacology*, 28, 1562, 2003.

102. Gould, E. et al., Adrenal steroids regulate postnatal development of the rat dentate gyrus. II. Effects of glucocorticoids and mineralocorticoids on cell birth, *J. Comp. Neurol.*, 313, 486, 1991.

103. Rodríguez, J.J. et al., Complex regulation of the expression of the polysialylated form of the neuronal cell adhesion molecule by glucocorticoids in the rat hippocampus, *Eur. J. Neurosci.*, 10, 2994, 1998.

104. Garcia, A. et al., Age-dependent expression of gulcocorticoid- and mineralocorticoid receptors on neural precursor cell populations in the adult murine hippocampus, *Aging Cell*, 3, 363, 2004.

105. Carter, C.S., Ramsey, M.M., and Sonntag, W.E., A critical analysis of the role of growth hormone and IGF-1 in aging and lifespan, *Trends Genet.*, 18, 295, 2002.

106. Lanfranco, F. et al., Ageing, growth hormone and physical performance, *J. Endocrinol. Invest.*, 26, 861, 2003.

107. Trejo, J.L. et al., Role of serum insulin-like growth factor 1 in mammalian brain aging, *Growth Horm. IGF Res.*, 14, S39, 2004.

108. Monje, M.L. et al., Irradiation induces neural precursor-cell dysfunction, *Nat. Med.*, 8, 955, 2002.

109. Sonntag, W.E. et al., Decreases in cerebral microvasculature with age are associated with the decline in growth hormone and insulin-like growth factor 1, *Endocrinology*, 138, 3515, 1997.

110. Anderson, M.F. et al., Insulin-like growth factor-1 and neurogenesis in the adult mammalian brain, *Brain Res. Dev. Brain Res.*, 134, 115, 2002.

111. Aberg, M.A. et al., Peripheral infusion of IGF-1 selectively induces neurogenesis in the adult rat hippocampus, *J. Neurosci.*, 20, 2896, 2000.

112. Trejo, J.L., Carro, E., and Torres-Aleman, I., Circulating insulin-like growth factor I mediates exercise-induced increases in the number of new neurons in the adult hippocampus, *J. Neurosci.*, 21, 1628, 2001.

113. Coculescu, M, Blood-brain barrier for human growth hormone and insulin-like growth factor-I, *J. Pediatr. Endocrinol. Metab.*, 12, 113, 1999.

114. Armstrong, C.S., Wuarin, L., and Ishii, D.N., Uptake of circulating insulin-like growth factor-I into the cerebrospinal fluid of normal and diabetic rats and normalization of IGF-II mRNA content in diabetic rat brain, *J. Neurosci. Res.*, 59, 649, 2000.

115. Niblock, M.M. et al., Distribution and levels of insulin-like growth factor I mRNA across the life span in the Brown Norway x Fischer 344 rat brain, *Brain Res.*, 804, 79, 1998.

116. Sonntag, W.E. et al., Alterations in insulin-like growth factor-1 and protein expression and type 1 insulin-like growth factor receptors in the brains of ageing rats, *Neuroscience*, 88, 269, 1999.

117. Sun, L.Y. et al., Local expression of GH and IGF-I in the hippocampus of GH-deficient long-lived mice, *Neurobiol. Aging*, 26, 929, 2005.

118. Sun, L.Y. et al., Increased neurogenesis in dentate gyrus of long-lived Ames dwarf mice, *Endocrinology*, 146, 1138, 2005.

119. Shetty, A.K., Hattiangady, B., and Shetty, G.A., Stem/progenitor cell proliferation factors FGF-2, IGF-1, and VEGF exhibit early decline during the course of aging in the hippocampus: role of astrocytes, *Glia*, 51, 173, 2005.

120. Lichtenwalner, R.J. et al., Adult-onset deficiency in growth hormone and insulin-like growth factor-I decreases survival of dentate granule neurons: insights into the regulation of adult hippocampal neurogenesis, *J. Neurosci. Res.*, 83, 199, 2006.

121. Greenberg, D.A. and Jin, K., Experiencing VEGF, *Nat. Genet.*, 36, 792, 2004.

122. Galvan, V., Greenberg, D.A., and Jin, K., The role of vascular endothelial growth factor in neurogenesis in adult brain, *Mini Rev. Med. Chem.*, 6, 667, 2006.

123. Schanzer, A. et al., Direct stimulation of adult neural stem cells *in vitro* and neurogenesis *in vivo* by vascular endothelial growth factor, *Brain Pathol.*, 14, 237, 2004.

124. Sun, Y. et al., Vascular endothelial growth factor-B (VEGFB) stimulates neurogenesis: evidence from knockout mice and growth factor administration, *Dev. Biol.*, 289, 329, 2006.

125. Heine, V.M. et al., Chronic stress in the adult dentate gyrus reduces cell proliferation near the vasculature of VEGF and Flk-1 protein expression, *Eur. J. Neurosci.*, 21, 1304, 2005.

126. Fabel, K. et al., VEGF is necessary for exercise-induced adult hippocampal neurogenesis, *Eur. J. Neurosci.*, 18, 2803, 2003.

127. Ding, Y.H. et al., Cerebral angiogenesis and expression of angiogenic factors in aging rats after exercise, *Curr. Neurovasc. Res.*, 3, 15, 2006.

128. Cao, L. et al., VEGF links hippocampal activity with neurogenesis, learning and memory, *Nat. Genet.*, 36, 827, 2004.

129. During, M.J. and Cao, L., VEGF, a mediator of the effect of experience on hippocampal neurogenesis, *Curr. Alzheimer Res.*, 3, 29, 2006.

130. Yan, Q. et al., Expression of brain-derived neurotrophic factor protein in the adult rat central nervous system, *Neuroscience*, 78, 431, 1997.

131. Cotman, C.W., The role of neurotrophins in brain aging: a perspective in honor of Regino Perez-Polo, *Neurochem. Res.*, 30, 877, 2005.

132. Hayashi, M. et al., Changes in BDNF-immunoreactive structures in the hippocampal formation of the aged macaque monkey, *Brain Res.*, 918, 191, 2001.

133. Hattiangady, B. et al., Brain-derived neurotrophic factor, phosphorylated cyclic AMP response element binding protein and neuropeptide Y decline as early as middle age in the dentate gyrus and CA1 and CA3 subfields of the hippocampus, *Exp. Neurol.*, 195, 353, 2005.

134. Croll, S.D. et al., Expression of BDNF and trkB as a function of age and cognitive performance, *Brain Res.*, 812, 200, 1998.

135. Newton, I.G. et al., Caloric restriction does not reverse aging-related changes in hippocampal BDNF, *Neurobiol. Aging*, 26, 683, 2005.

136. Linnarsson, S., Willson, C.A., and Ernfors, P., Cell death in regenerating populations of neurons in BDNF mutant mice, *Brain Res. Mol. Brain Res.*, 75, 61, 2000.

137. Benraiss, A. et al., Adenoviral brain-derived neurotrophic factor induces both neostriatal and olfactory neuronal recruitment from endogenous progenitor cells in the adult forebrain, *J. Neurosci.*, 21, 6718, 2001.

138. Zigova, T. et al., Intraventricular administration of BDNF increases the number of newly generated neurons in the adult olfactory bulb, *Mol. Cell. Neurosci.*, 11, 234, 1998.

139. Pencea, V. et al., Infusion of brain-derived neurotrophic factor into the lateral ventricle of the adult rat leads to new neurons in the parenchyma of the striatum, septum, thalamus, and hypothalamus, *J. Neurosci.*, 21, 6706, 2001.

140. Scharfman, H. et al., Increased neurogenesis and the ectopic granule cells after intrahippocampal BDNF infusion in adult rats, *Exp. Neurol.*, 192, 348, 2005.

141. Larsson, E. et al., Suppression of insult-induced neurogenesis in adult rat brain by brain-derived neurotrophic factor, *Exp. Neurol.*, 177, 1, 2002.

142. Gustafsson, E., Lindvall, O., and Kakaia, Z., Intraventricular infusion of TrkB-Fc fusion protein promotes ischemia-induced neurogenesis in adult rat dentate gyrus, *Stroke*, 34, 2710, 2003.

143. Lee, J. et al., Dietary restriction increases the number of newly generated neural cells, and induces BDNF expression, in the dentate gyrus of rats, *J. Mol. Neurosci.*, 15, 99, 2000.

144. Mattson, M.P., Maudsley, S., and Martin, B., A neural signaling triumvirate that influences ageing and age-related disease: insulin/IGF-1, BDNF and serotonin, *Ageing Res. Rev.*, 3, 445, 2004.

145. Craig, C.G. et al., In vivo growth factor expansion of endogenous subependymal neural precursor cell populations in the adult mouse brain, *J. Neurosci.*, 16, 2649, 1996.

146. Kuhn, H.G. et al., Epidermal growth factor and fibroblast growth factor-2 have different effects on neural progenitors in the adult rat brain, *J. Neurosci.*, 17, 5820, 1997.

147. Tropepe, V. et al., Distinct neural stem cells proliferate in response to EGF and FGF in the developing mouse telencephalon, *Dev. Biol.*, 208, 166, 1999.

148. Arsenijevic, Y. et al., Insulin-like growth factor-I is necessary for neural stem cell proliferation and demonstrates distinct actions of epidermal growth factor and fibroblast growth factor-2, *J. Neurosci.*, 21, 7194, 2001.

149. Enwere, E. et al., Aging results in reduced epidermal growth factor receptor signaling, diminished olfactory neurogenesis, and deficits in fine olfactory discrimination, *J. Neurosci.*, 24, 8354, 2004.

150. Tirassa, P. et al., EGF and NGF injected into the brain of old mice enhance BDNF and ChAT in proliferating subventricular zone, *J. Neurosci. Res.*, 72, 557, 2003.

151. Fiore, M. et al., Brain NGF and EGF administration improves passive avoidance response and stimulates brain precursor cells in aged male mice, *Physiol. Behav.*, 77, 437, 2002.

152. Wachs, F.P. et al., Transforming growth factor-β1 is a negative modulator of adult neurogenesis, *J. Neuropathol. Exp. Neurol.*, 65, 358, 2006.

153. Buckwalter, M.S. et al., Chronically increased transforming growth factor-β1 strongly inhibits hippocampal neurogenesis in aged mice, *Am. J. Pathol.*, 169, 154, 2006.

154. Lim, D.A. et al., Noggin antagonizes BMP signaling to create a niche for adult neurogenesis, *Neuron*, 28, 713, 2000.

155. Lledo, P.M. and Saghatelyan, A., Integrating new neurons into the adult olfactory bulb: joining the network, life-death decisions, and the effects of sensory experience, *Trends Neurosci.*, 28, 248, 2005.

156. Mey, J. and McCaffery, P., Retinoic acid signaling in the nervous system of adult vertebrates, *Neuroscientist*, 10, 409, 2004.

157. McCaffery, P., Zhang, J., and Crandall, J.E., Retinoic acid signaling and function in the adult hippocampus, *J. Neurobiol.*, 66, 780, 2006.

158. Whitesides, J. et al., Retinoid signaling distinguishes a subpopulation of olfactory receptor neurons in the developing and adult mouse, *J. Comp. Neurol.*, 394, 445, 1998.

159. Thompson Haskell, G. et al., Retinoic acid signaling at sites of plasticity in the mature central nervous system, *J. Comp. Neurol.*, 452, 228, 2002.

160. Haskell, G.T. and Lamantia, A.S., Retinoic acid signaling identifies a distinct precursor population in the developing and adult forebrain, *J. Neurosci.*, 25, 7636, 2005.

161. Etchamendy, N. et al., Alleviation of a selective age-related relational memory deficit in mice by pharmacologically induced normalization of brain retinoid signaling, *J. Neurosci.*, 21, 6423, 2001.

162. Cooper-Kuhn, C.M., Winkler, J., and Kuhn, H.G., Decreased neurogenesis after cholinergic forebrain lesion in the adult rat, *J. Neurosci. Res.*, 77, 155, 2004.

163. Mohapel, P. et al., Forebrain acetylcholine regulates adult hippocampal neurogenesis and learning, *Neurobiol. Aging*, 26, 939, 2005.

164. Ge, S. et al., GABA regulates synaptic integration of newly generated neurons in the adult brain, *Nature*, 439, 589, 2006.

165. Kempermann, G., Regulation of adult hippocampal neurogenesis — implications for novel theories of major depression, *Bipolar Disord.*, 4, 17, 2002.

166. Malberg, J.E., Implications of adult hippocampal neurogenesis in antidepressant action, *J. Psychiatry Neurosci.*, 29, 196, 2004.

167. Murray, C.A. and Lynch, M.A., Evidence that increased hippocampal expression of the cytokine interleukin-1 β is a common trigger for age- and stress-induced impairments in long-term potentiation, *J. Neurosci.*, 18, 2974, 1998.

168. Bodles, A.M. and Barger, S.W., Cytokines and the aging brain — what we don't know might help us, *Trends Neurosci.*, 27, 621, 2004.

169. Nolan, Y. et al., Role of interleukin-4 in regulation of age-related inflammatory changes in the hippocampus, *J. Biol. Chem.*, 280, 9354, 2005.

170. Joseph, J.A. et al., Oxidative stress and inflammation in brain aging: nutritional considerations, *Neurochem. Res.*, 30, 927, 2005.

171. Ekdahl, C.T. et al., Inflammation is detrimental for neurogenesis in adult brain, *Proc. Natl. Acad. Sci. U.S.A.*, 100, 13632, 2003.

172. Monje, M.L., Toda, H., and Palmer, T.D., Inflammatory blockade restores adult hippocampal neurogenesis, *Science*, 302, 1760, 2003.

173. Wilson, C.J., Finch, C.E., and Cohen, H.J., Cytokines and cognition — the case for a head-to-toe inflammatory paradigm, *J. Am. Geriatr. Soc.*, 50, 2041, 2002.

174. Blalock, E.M. et al., Gene microarrays in hippocampal aging: statistical profiling identifies novel processes correlated with cognitive impairment, *J. Neurosci.*, 23, 3807, 2003.

175. Kim, S.U. and de Vellis, J., Microglia in health and disease, *J. Neurosci. Res.*, 81, 302, 2005.

176. Battista, D. et al., Neurogenic niche modulation by activated microglia; transforming growth factor β increases neurogenesis in the adult dentate gyrus, *Eur. J. Neurosci.*, 23, 83, 2006.

177. Butovsky, O. et al., Activation of microglia by aggregated beta-amyloid or lipopolysaccharide impairs MHC-II expression and renders them cytotoxic whereas IFN-gamma and IL-4 render them protective, *Mol. Cell. Neurosci.*, 29, 381, 2005.

178. Ziv, Y. et al., Immune cells contribute to the maintenance of neurogenesis and spatial learning abilities in adulthood, *Nat. Neurosci.*, 9, 268, 2006.

179. Butovsky, O. et al., Microglia activated by IL-4 or IFN-gamma differentially induce neurogenesis and oligodendrogenesis from adult stem/progenitor cells, *Mol. Cell. Neurosci.*, 31, 149, 2006.

180. Conde, J.R. and Streit, W.J., Microglia in the aging brain, *J. Neuropathol. Exp. Neurol.*, 65, 199, 2006.

181. Gahr, M. et al., What is the adaptive role of neurogenesis in adult birds? *Prog. Brain Res.*, 138, 233, 2002.

182. Kempermann, G., Why new neurons? Possible functions for adult hippocampal neurogenesis, *J. Neurosci.*, 22, 635, 2002.

183. Doetsch, F. and Hen, R., Young and excitable: the function of new neurons in the adult mammalian brain, *Curr. Opin. Neurobiol.*, 15, 121, 2005.

184. Kempermann, G., Wiskott, L., and Gage, F.H., Functional significance of adult neurogenesis, *Curr. Opin. Neurobiol.*, 14, 186, 2004.

185. Wiskott, L., Rasch, M.J., and Kempermann, G., A functional hypothesis for adult hippocampal neurogenesis: avoidance of catastrophic interference in the dentate gyrus, *Hippocampus*, 16, 329, 2006.

186. Lledo, P.-M., Alonso, M., and Grubb, M.S., Adult neurogenesis and functional plasticity in neuronal circuits, *Neuroscience*, 7, 179, 2006.

187. Alvarez-Buylla, A., Neurogenesis and plasticity in the CNS of adult birds, *Exp. Neurol.*, 115, 110, 1992.

188. Gould, E. et al., Neurogenesis in adulthood: a possible role in learning, *Trends. Cogn. Sci.*, 3, 186, 1999.

189. Shors, T.J. et al., Neurogenesis in the adult is involved in the formation of trace memories, *Nature*, 410, 372, 2001.

190. Shors, T.J. et al., Neurogenesis may relate to some but not all types of hippocampal-dependent learning, *Hippocampus*, 12, 578, 2002.

191. Carleton, A. et al., Making scents of olfactory neurogenesis, *J. Physiol. Paris*, 96, 115, 2002.

192. Meltzer, L.A., Yabaluri, R., and Deisseroth, K., A role for circuit homeostasis in adult neurogenesis, *Trends Neurosci.*, 28, 653, 2005.

193. Leuner, B., Gould, E., and Shors, T.J., Is there a link between adult neurogenesis and learning? *Hippocampus*, 16, 216, 2006.

194. Standfield, B.B. and Trice, J.E., Evidence that granule cells generated in the dentate gyrus of adult rats extend axonal projections, *Exp. Brain Res.*, 72, 399, 1988.

195. Markakis, E.A. and Gage, F.H., Adult-generated neurons in the dentate gyrus send axonal projections to field CA3 and are surrounded by synaptic vesicles, *J. Comp. Neurol.*, 406, 449, 1999.

196. Petreanu, L. and Alvarez-Buylla, A., Maturation and death of adult-born olfactory bulb granule neurons: role of olfaction, *J. Neurosci.*, 22, 6106, 2002.

197. Belluzzi, O. et al., Electrophysiological differentiation of new neurons in the olfactory bulb, *J. Neurosci.*, 23, 10411, 2003.

198. Carleton, A. et al., Becoming a new neuron in the adult olfactory bulb, *Nat. Neurosci.*, 6, 507, 2003.

199. Wang, S., Scott, B.W., and Wojtowicz, J.M., Heterogenous properties of dentate granule neurons in the adult rat, *J. Neurobiol.*, 42, 248, 2000.

200. Schmidt-Hieber, C., Jones, P., and Bischofberger, J., Enhanced synaptic plasticity in newly generated granule cells of the adult hippocampus, *Nature*, 429, 184, 2004.

201. Gheusi, G. et al., Importance of newly generated neurons in the adult olfactory bulb for odor discrimination, *Proc. Natl. Acad. Sci. U.S.A.*, 97, 1823, 2000.

202. Rochefort, C. et al., Enriched odor exposure increases the number of newborn neurons in the adult olfactory bulb and improves odor memory, *J. Neurosci.*, 22, 2679, 2002.

203. Magavi, S.S. et al., Adult-born and preexisting olfactory granule neurons undergo distinct experience-dependent modifications of their olfactory responses in vivo, *J. Neurosci.*, 25, 10729, 2005.

204. Dobrossy, M.D. et al., Differential effects of learning on neurogenesis: learning increases or decreases the number of newly born cells depending on their birth date, *Mol. Psychiatry*, 8, 974, 2003.

205. Driscoll, I. et al., The aging hippocampus: a multi-level analysis in the rat, *Neuroscience*, 139, 1173, 2006.

206. Mayo, W. et al., Individual differences in cognitive aging: implication of pregnenolone sulfate, *Prog. Neurobiol.*, 71, 43, 2003.

207. Gallagher, M. et al., Effects of aging on hippocampal formation in a naturally occurring animal model of mild cognitive impairment, *Exp. Gerontol.*, 38, 71, 2003.

208. Lasarge, C.L. et al., Deficits across multiple cognitive domains in a subset of ages Fischer 344 rats, *Neurobiol. Aging*, in press, 2007.

209. Nicolle, M.M. et al., Metabotropic glutamate receptor-mediated hippocampal phosphoinositide turnover is blunted in spatial learning-impaired aged rats, *J. Neurosci.*, 19, 9604, 1999.

210. Colombo, P.J. and Gallagher, M., Individual differences in spatial memory among aged rats are related to hippocampal PKC gamma immunoreactivity, *Hippocampus*, 12, 285, 2002.

211. Drapeau, E. et al., Spatial memory performances of aged rats in the water maze predict levels of hippocampal neurogenesis, *Proc. Natl. Acad. Sci. U.S.A.*, 100, 14385, 2003.

212. Wati, H. et al., A decreased survival of proliferated cells in the hippocampus is associated with a decline in spatial memory in aged rats, *Neurosci. Lett.*, 399, 171, 2006.

213. Merrill, D.A. et al., Hippocampal cell genesis does not correlate with spatial learning ability in aged rats, *J. Comp. Neurol.*, 439, 201, 2003.

214. Bizon, J.L. and Gallagher, M., Production of new cells in the rat dentate gyrus over the lifespan: relation to cognitive decline, *Eur. J. Neurosci.*, 18, 215, 2003.

215. Bizon, J.L., Lee, H.J., and Gallagher, M., Neurogenesis in a rat model of age-related cognitive decline, *Aging Cell*, 3, 227, 2004.

216. Goh, E.L. et al., Adult neural stem cells and repair of the adult central nervous system, *J. Hematother. Stem Cell Res.*, 12, 671, 2003.

217. Bernal, G.M. and Peterson, D.A., Neural stem cells as therapeutic agents for age-related bran repair, *Aging Cell*, 3, 345, 2004.

218. Emsley, J.G. et al., The repair of complex neuronal circuitry by transplanted and endogenous precursors, *NeuroRx*, 1, 452, 2004.

219. Lindvall, O., Kokaia, Z., and Martinez-Serrano, A., Stem cell therapy for human neurodegenerative disorders — how to make it work, *Nat. Med.*, 10 (Suppl), 542, 2004.

220. Lie, D.C. et al., Neurogenesis in the adult brain: new strategies for central nervous system diseases, *Annu. Rev. Pharmacol. Toxicol.*, 44, 399, 2004.

221. Goldman, S., Stem and progenitor cell-based therapy of the human central nervous system, *Nat. Biotechnol.*, 23, 862, 2005.

222. Mitchell, B.D. et al., Constitutive and induced neurogenesis in the adult mammalian brain: manipulation of endogenous precursors toward CNS repair, *Dev. Neurosci.*, 26, 101, 2004.

223. Kronenberg, G. et al., Physical exercise prevents age-related decline in precursor cell activity in the mouse dentate gyrus, *Neurobiol. Aging*, 27, 1505, 2006.

7 Expression Profile Analysis of Brain Aging

Stephen D. Ginsberg

CONTENTS

I. OVERVIEW

Modern molecular and cellular approaches to neuroscience have enabled the initiation of high throughput analysis of aging processes that occur within the central nervous system (CNS). To evaluate molecular events associated with aging in animal models and human postmortem tissues, microarray studies and other downstream genetic analyses are performed at the regional and cellular levels to characterize transcriptional patterns, or mosaics, that may provide clues into some of the mechanism(s) that drive senescence. This chapter reviews experimental and analytical issues associated with high throughput genomic analyses in the aging brain within the context of current datasets using several different aging paradigms. An overriding goal is to apply functional genomics- and proteomics-based approaches to aging research, in an effort to develop useful biomarkers of specific aging processes for eventual pharmacotherapeutic development and disease prevention.

II. INTRODUCTORY REMARKS

The molecular and cellular basis of the aging process is not well understood, particularly in humans, as the scientific community has yet to develop a reliable and predictive set of biomarkers that can be utilized to quantitate specific aspects of senescence within discrete regions and/or cell populations. The longevity of a given species depends on several parameters, including frailty (intrinsic vulnerability to death) and senescence (rate of change in frailty over time) [1, 2]. Actuarial rates and survival curves are not particularly useful for predicting aging rates in the brains of mammals. A general consensus is that using surrogate molecular and cellular markers to evaluate senescence throughout the lifespan of animal models is a plausible approach to gain greater insight into mechanisms that underlie aging in humans, with the hope of developing rational pharmacotherapeutic interventions to avoid the scourge of progressive late-onset neurodegenerative disorders and related phenomena that occur in the aging brain. It is unlikely that a single gene is responsible for aging. Rather, a complex pattern of genes probably influences a wide variety of critical parameters, including cellular defense, disease resistance, and generalized homeostasis. While an exact mosaic of gene products responsible for aging remains unknown, current research is beginning to identify candidate markers from a wide variety of transcript classes. Another obstacle using animal models in aging research has been the divergence of uniform genetic backgrounds in model systems, which has led to variable complexity in phenotypic expression. Moreover, from an experimental perspective, there still remains a relative lack of effective means to measure small, but potentially significant, changes in gene expression [3].

III. METHODOLOGICAL CONSIDERATIONS

A. OBTAINING RNA

Conventional molecular biology methods enable researchers to evaluate gene expression levels across a plethora of normative situations, experimental paradigms, and disease states. These methods include Southern analysis, Northern analysis, polymerase-chain reaction (PCR), ribonuclease (RNase) protection assay, and *in situ* hybridization, among others. These well-documented approaches typically quantitate the abundance of individual transcripts one (or a few) at a time. Recent developments in high throughput genomic-based technologies enable the assessment of hundreds to thousands of genes simultaneously in a coordinated fashion. Not surprisingly, the potential to understand physiological processes and disease pathogenesis has expanded exponentially with these applications. Microarray analysis has emerged as an important and effective tool to assess transcript levels in a myriad of systems and paradigms. A drawback to high throughput technologies is the need for significant amounts of high-quality input sources of RNA for acceptable levels of sensitivity and reproducibility.

1.   Preservation of mRNA

Sources of input RNA for RNA amplification can originate from a variety of *in vivo* and *in vitro* sources, including fresh, frozen, and fixed tissues. When employing mRNA as a starting material, it cannot be emphasized enough the importance of the preservation of RNA integrity in tissues and cells that will be used for extraction. RNA species are particularly sensitive to degradation by RNase. RNases are quite stable and retain their activity over a broad pH range [4]. Thus, RNase-free precautions should be taken prior to and during all RNA amplification procedures.

At present, no consensus protocol exists for optimal methods to fix brain tissues for use with microarray platforms. Successful microarray mining has been performed using tissue samples from animal models and human brains fixed in both crosslinking fixatives, such as 10% neutral-buffered formalin and 4% paraformaldehyde, as well as precipitating fixatives, such as 70% ethanol buffered with 150 mM sodium chloride [5–8]. Many variables, including antemortem characteristics, agonal state, duration of fixation, and length of storage, are also critical parameters for RNA preservation [9–11]. A useful and relatively expedient method for assessing RNA quality in tissue sections prior to performing expression profiling studies is the use of acridine orange (AO) histofluorescence. AO is a fluorescent dye that intercalates selectively into nucleic acids [12, 13]. AO that intercalates into RNA emits an orange-red fluorescence, whereas AO that intercalates into DNA emits a yellowish-green fluorescence. AO histofluorescence detects the presence of RNA species in neurons within human and animal model brains [14–16]. In addition, AO histofluorescence detects the sequestration of RNA species within senile plaques (SPs) and neurons that bear neurofibrillary tangles (NFTs) in Alzheimer's disease (AD) and other neurodegenerative disorders [17, 18] (Figure 7.1). However, individual RNA species (e.g., rRNA, tRNA, and mRNA) cannot be delineated by AO histofluorescence. Rather, this method serves as a basic diagnostic to ensure the likelihood that a specific brain tissue section has abundant RNA prior to performing expensive functional genomics studies [6]. A more definitive assessment of RNA quality and quantity can be obtained through bioanalysis. A bioanalyzer, such as the 2100 Bioanalyzer from Agilent Technologies, employs capillary gel electrophoresis to assay RNA quality and abundance [19–22]. In this manner, a readout in the form of an electropherogram or gel-based format provides a high-sensitivity means of RNA assessment prior to initiating PCR- or microarray-based studies.

2.   Regional Analysis

Regional analysis is an important strategy for identification of transcripts that are enriched in an organ, lamina, or nuclei that differ from adjacent or connected regions, but by definition contains an admixture of different cell types that comprise the region. Regions of brain (or other organs and tissues) can be readily dissected from fresh and frozen tissues and/or paraffin-embedded tissue sections [21, 23]. RNA is

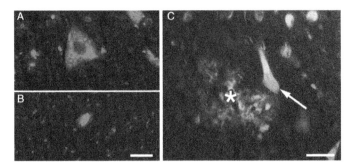

FIGURE 7.1 (SEE COLOR INSERT FOLLOWING PAGE 204) RNA sequestration to neurons and pathological lesions in late-onset progressive neurodegenerative disorders as evaluated by AO histofluorescence. (A) AO-positive motor neuron displaying robust cytoplasmic RNA species in the cervical spinal cord of a normal control subject. (B) Pyknotic motor neuron within the cervical spinal cord of an amyotrophic lateral sclerosis (ALS) patient. Note the intense accumulation of AO-positive RNA species within the degenerating neuron. (Scale bar A–B: 25 μm.) (C) Double-label epifluorescent image illustrating RNA sequestration to an SP (asterisk) and NFT (arrow) within the CA1 hippocampal region of an AD patient. The tissue section was double-stained with thioflavine-S to visualize neuropathological hallmarks and AO to visualize cytoplasmic RNA species. (Scale bar: 50 μm.)

then harvested from the desired tissue source using chemical extraction or magnetic extraction, and used for downstream genetic analyses including microarray and real-time quantitative (qPCR) based methods. An advantage of regional analyses is that RNA is abundant and differences between regions can be discerned readily without complex and relatively expensive RNA amplification methods. An obvious disadvantage of regional dissection is a lack of single-cell resolution, as epithelial cells, neurons, nonneuronal cells, vascular elements, and other intermingled cell types will contribute to the RNA being assessed.

3.   Single-Cell Analysis

Single-cell and single-population cell analysis enable the expression profile analysis of individual cell types. For example, neurons can be identified by selective expression of phenotypic markers in the case of cholinergic basal forebrain neurons [15] and midbrain dopaminergic neurons [24, 25]. Neurons that currently do not possess a signature phenotype can be identified using a variety of histochemical preparations such as cresyl violet for downstream genetic applications [21, 26, 27]. Microdissection is a strategy to acquire individual cells or populations of homogeneous cells to enable expression profiling using microarray platforms or by PCR-based technologies. Provided that procedures are performed on well-prepared tissue sections and RNase-free conditions are employed, both immunocytochemical and histochemical procedures can be utilized to identify specific cell(s) of interest. Two procedures for excising cells from tissue sections are single-cell microaspiration and laser capture microdissection (LCM). Single-cell microaspiration enables acquisition of an individual cell (or cells) using an inverted microscope connected to a micromanipulator and a vacuum source to dissect away the cells of interest from the surrounding tissues. An advantage of this technique is the high cellular and subcellular (including neurites, dendrites, and/or axons) level of resolution for aspiration of single elements [26, 28–30]. Disadvantages include experimenter error and a significant time requirement to perform microaspiration, especially if multiple cells are being acquired from different brain tissue sections. The advent of high throughput microaspiration systems has enabled rapid accession of single cells and populations for downstream molecular and cellular analyses. Notably, LCM is a method for acquiring cells from a myriad of tissue sources using histological and immunocytochemical methods. Positive extraction (an LCM method used by the PixCell from Arcturus) entails pulsing an infrared laser source over cells of interest onto a thermoplastic film that is embedded in the cap of a microfuge tube [31–33]. Raising the thermoplastic cap separates targeted cells, now attached to the film, from surrounding undisturbed tissue. Negative extraction (an LCM method utilized by P.A.L.M. Microlaser Technologies) employs a near-infrared laser source to cut around the cells of interest within a tissue section, and the microdissected material is catapulted into a microfuge tube [34]. Both positive and negative extraction methods allow captured cells to be examined microscopically to confirm their identity. This quality control step ensures the validity of the results obtained from downstream analysis. Single cells, as well as dozens to hundreds of cells, can be collected by LCM instrumentation, and DNA, protein, and RNA extraction methods can be performed on microdissected cells [34–37]. However, LCM use is most noted for RNA extraction and subsequent application to microarray platforms or qPCR [6, 31, 32].

B.   PCR and RNA Amplification

Amplification of genetic signals can be performed at both DNA and RNA levels, and the final amplified products are either DNA or RNA. A common method for DNA amplification is PCR [38]. Starting materials for PCR reactions can originate from genomic DNA or complementary DNA (cDNA) reverse-transcribed from RNA (e.g., RT-PCR). PCR is an effective method to amplify a DNA template. However, PCR is an exponential, nonlinear amplification, and variation can occur within individual mRNA species of different molecular mass and basepair composition. PCR-based methods tend to amplify abundant genes over rare genes and may distort quantitative relationships among gene populations [39]. Furthermore, amplified PCR products may not be proportional to the abundance of the starting material, potentially skewing relative gene expression level comparisons.

qPCR can quantitate amplicon product formation during each cycle of amplification and has eliminated many concerns that plague conventional PCR methods. Other advantages of real-time qPCR include high throughput capabilities, the ability to simultaneously multiplex reactions, enhanced sensitivity, reduced inter-assay variation, and lack of post-PCR manipulations. Various dye chemistries are currently being exploited in qPCR systems, including hydrolysis probes, molecular beacons, and double-stranded (ds) DNA binding dyes [40]. A prime example of a hydrolysis probe is the TaqMan assay. In this method, *Taq* polymerase enzyme cleaves a specific TaqMan probe during the extension phase of the PCR. The probe is dual-labeled with a reporter dye and a quenching dye at two separate ends; and as long as the probe is intact (in its free form), fluorescence emission of the reporter dye is absorbed by the quenching dye via fluorescence resonance energy transfer (FRET) [41, 42]. An increase in reporter fluorescence emission occurs when separation of the reporter and quencher dyes takes place during nuclease degradation in the PCR reaction [43]. This process occurs in every cycle of PCR and does not interfere with the exponential accumulation of the amplified product. Another methodology for qPCR-based detection involves the use of molecular beacons. Molecular beacons are probes that form a stem-loop structure from a single-stranded DNA molecule [44, 45]. They are particularly useful for identifying point mutations, as targets that differ by only a single nucleotide can be delineated. DNA binding dyes such as SYBR green incorporate selectively into ds DNA. SYBR green emits undetectable fluorescence levels when it is in its free form. Upon binding to ds DNA, a robust fluorescent signal is emitted [46]. An advantage of using ds DNA binding dye chemistry is that this method can be implemented to assay practically any target sequence with virtually any set of primers, making this application quite flexible and considerably less expensive than probe-based dye chemistries [47]. However, assay sensitivity can be diminished using a ds DNA binding dye system due to the increased risk of amplifying nonspecific PCR products. Careful primer set design and rigorous assay optimization can alleviate the majority of these nonspecific issues associated with ds DNA binding dyes.

In contrast to PCR-based technologies, RNA amplification-based procedures increase RNA in a linear fashion by amplifying the initial cDNA template sequence [23, 48, 49]. Resultant amplified products are representative of the original mRNA expression levels. RNA amplification is achieved through *in vitro* transcription (IVT). IVT is a process of RNA synthesis facilitated by an RNA polymerase under the direction of a DNA template coupled to a bacteriophage transcription promoter sequence. RNA polymerases typically used for IVT include T7, T3, and SP6 polymerase, named for the bacteriophage from which they were cloned. These three enzymes are single-subunit RNA polymerases that can transcribe genes without requiring additional proteins [50].

RNA amplification is a useful methodology because it can preserve quantitative relationships of classes of transcripts even when limited starting material is available. In addition to the linear amplification of small amounts of input RNA, RNA amplification procedures can increase the sensitivity of expression profiling paradigms on microarray platforms although abundant starting material is available [51, 52]. A method of linear amplification is amplified antisense RNA (aRNA) amplification [29, 30, 39]. aRNA is a T7 RNA polymerase-based amplification procedure using an IVT methodology that enables quantitation of the relative abundance of gene expression levels. Each round of aRNA results in an approximate thousand-fold amplification from the original amount of each polyadenylated mRNA in the sample [30, 53]. Two rounds of RNA amplification are usually required to generate sufficient quantities of aRNA for microarray studies. Although aRNA is a complicated procedure, this method has generated very interesting datasets utilizing a wide variety of input tissue sources and array platforms [28, 29, 54–59]. Additional experimental strategies have been developed by independent laboratories to improve RNA amplification methods for greater applicability and reproducibility [60–64]. A novel RNA amplification procedure has been developed in our laboratory that employs a method of terminal continuation (TC) [19–21, 23] (Figure 7.2). Two primers are used in the TC RNA amplification procedure, and one round of amplification is typically sufficient for downstream genetic analyses, including microarray-based studies [19, 23]. Results indicate that the threshold of detection of genes with low hybridization signal intensity is also greatly increased when using TC RNA amplification, as many genes that are at the limit of detection using conventional aRNA can be readily observed with the TC method [19, 20]. Furthermore, TC RNA transcription can be driven using a bacteriophage promoter sequence (e.g., T7, T3, or SP6) attached to either the 3'- or 5'-region of the oligonucleotide primers. Therefore, transcript orientation can be in an antisense orientation (similar to conventional aRNA methods) when the bacteriophage promoter sequence is placed on the 3' poly d(T) primer or in a sense orientation when the promoter sequence is attached to the 5' TC primer [19] (Figure 7.2), depending on the design of the experimental paradigm.

C.   HIGH THROUGHPUT STRATEGIES

Recent advances in high throughput cloning procedures have led to sequencing of the human genome and the genome of several other species. There is renewed interest in quantitative assessment of tissue-specific genes and proteins for discovery science. Although knowledge of the genetic sequence alone does not give *a priori* insight into the aging process, expression profiling technologies have created new avenues for aging research in animal models as well as human tissues through the use of both biopsy and postmortem samples. The development of reproducible microarrays has enabled high throughput analysis of hundreds to thousands of genes simultaneously. Synthesis of array platforms entails adhering cDNAs or expressed sequence-tagged cDNAs (ESTs) to solid supports such as glass slides, plastic slides, or nylon membranes [65, 66]. Oligonucleotide arrays are synthesized using photolithographic methods similar to computer chip production [67] that allow modified basepair sequences to adhere to array media [68]. Relatively long oligonucleotide features (>50-mer) are now routinely synthesized by robotic and ink-jet printing processes, making oligonucleotide arrays more sensitive and reproducible for the end user [65]. Array experiments essentially entail accessing mRNA from control and experimental paradigms and then generating fluorescent, biotin, or radioactive labeled probes that are hybridized to the desired array platform. Fluorescent hybridization signal intensity is measured with a laser scanner, and radioactive hybridization signal intensity is quantified using a phosphor imager, respectively. Gene expression data collected using array platforms do not usually allow absolute quantitation of mRNA levels, such as transcript copy number, but do generate an expression profile of the relative changes in mRNA levels [6, 48, 69]. Relative changes in individual mRNAs are often analyzed by univariate statistics for individual comparisons, with differential expression greater than approximately twofold accepted conventionally as relevant for further examination [69–71]. Complex multivariate statistics are often employed to cluster microarray data, due to the enormous volume of data generated from a single probe [72, 73]. A key aspect of microarray analysis is the ability to analyze many variables simultaneously without the luxury of having many independent

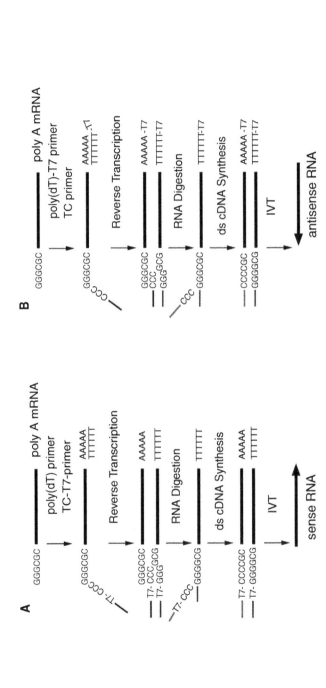

FIGURE 7.2 Outline of the TC RNA amplification methodology. (A) A poly d(T) primer and a TC primer (containing a bacteriophage promoter sequence for sense orientation) are added to the mRNA population to be amplified. First strand synthesis occurs as an mRNA-cDNA hybrid is formed after reverse transcription and terminal continuation of the oligonucleotide primers. Following RNase H digestion to remove the original mRNA template strand, second strand synthesis is performed using *Taq* polymerase. The resultant double-stranded product is utilized as the template for IVT, yielding high-fidelity, linear RNA amplification of sense orientation. (B) Schematic similar to (A), illustrating the TC RNA amplification procedure amplifying RNA in the antisense orientation. In this method, the bacteriophage promoter sequence is attached to the poly d(T) primer, not the TC primer. (*Source:* Adapted from Che and Ginsberg [19]. With permission.)

observations or replicates for each variable. Differentially expressed genes can be clustered into functional protein categories for multivariate coordinate gene expression analyses. Computational analysis is critical for optimal use of microarrays. Additionally, access to relational databases is ideal [74], especially when evaluating hundreds to thousands of ESTs or oligonucleotides that may be linked to genes and protein products of known function. Further, it is highly desirable to supplement microarray and qPCR data with measurements of protein expression by immunob lotting-, immunocytochemical-, ELISA-, or proteomic-based techniques. In terms of protein assessments, single-cell resolution can be attained in tissue sections using immunocytochemical methods. However, immunoblotting and proteomic-based procedures at present cannot (at least *in vivo*) be performed on single cells and must rely on larger tissue homogenate preparations with admixed cell types. One potentially exciting advance is that LCM is being utilized to collect homogeneous populations of cells for downstream antibody-based protein chips as well as mass spectroscopy analysis [6, 75].

IV. EXPRESSION PROFILING IN AGING BRAIN

A. OVERVIEW

Expression profiling studies of aged brain are derivatives of conventional aging paradigms whereby genomic and proteomic expression differences are characterized between young, adult, and senescent tissues [76, 77]. Although aging research within this context was initially descriptive in nature, viable expression profiling paradigms have enabled the formation of testable hypotheses based on the cellular and molecular sequelae of senescence [3, 78, 79]. A broad range of applications within age-related paradigms has been implemented, including the study of genetic factors, epigenetic and/or environmental alterations, oxidative stress, inflammation, and development of neurodegenerative pathology as evaluated by the use of postmortem human brain tissues and animal models of neurodegeneration (e.g., knockout, transgenic, and mutant phenotype) for expression profiling.

B. GENETIC STUDIES IN AGING BRAIN

The study of aging was one of the original areas tackled by geneticists, as researchers attempted to assess why longevity in humans appears to be a heritable trait. A preponderance of studies concludes that a large proportion variation in the human lifespan can be attributed to genetic variation [80–82], although specific age-related genes remain at large. Moreover, individual model organisms display significant variance in lifespan, despite the fact that these subjects possess a common genotype and reside in nearly identical environmental conditions [83]. Specific genes contributing to the genetic variation of senescence remain difficult to identify. One approach is to use association studies to compare and contrast aging pedigrees. Association studies typically use population-based genetic screening methods to compare the prevalence of genetic markers between extremely senescent individuals and randomly chosen individuals [84]. Potential markers are then identified by linkage disequilibrium, the non-random inheritance of alleles located in close proximity to each other in the genome. An increased prevalence of a genetic marker in senescent individuals would indicate that the marker may either be a causal genetic variant or located in close proximity to a causal variant [85]. Polymorphisms are analyzed for potential interactions or relationships with specific phenotypes, such as longevity. In this manner, the rate or frequency of a given polymorphism is evaluated in aged subjects as compared to random controls. These studies are arduous due to numerous polymorphisms that can exist within any given candidate gene. Furthermore, differentiating a causal gene from a susceptibility gene can be extremely difficult.

Another successful method to delineate potential causal/susceptibility genes is linkage analysis using a genome-scan approach. A current strategy is to employ markers termed "microsatellite markers" comprised of polymorphisms that likely represent random genetic variations [84]. Microsatellite maps have been generated that span the entire genome [86], and several studies have used linkage-based approaches to find candidate genes in age-related paradigms, including AD and Parkinson's disease (PD) [87–89]. Genome-wide linkage studies of aging cohorts have also been performed for macular degeneration of the eye [90–92]. Comparative studies across phyla have also been utilized to identify genetic changes associated with the aging process [93, 94]. Moreover, employing animal models to study senescence avoids some of the aforementioned confounds of evaluating genes associated with aging in humans.

C.   CALORIC RESTRICTION

There are many theories on aging, and one of the most widely accepted is the gradual age-related accumulation of irreparable and irreversible cellular and molecular damage. One environmental manipulation that can alter the aging process is caloric restriction (CR). For example, the lifespan of rodents can be increased by approximately 50% when CR is initiated in young adulthood and maintained throughout life [95]. CR also decreases the incidence of systemic age-related diseases, including cancer, cardiovascular disease, and diabetes in a variety of animal models [96, 97], making dietary restriction a plausible and relatively inexpensive preventive therapy to consider for aging human populations. CR also has profound behavioral and attentional effects [98]. Moreover, CR in rodents increases neurogenesis in the dentate gyrus [95, 99] and partially attenuates the effects of ischemia [100, 101] and of 1-methyl-4-phenyl-1,2,3,6-tetrahydropyridine (MPTP) poisoning within substantia nigra dopaminergic neurons [95, 102]. Thus, CR is an ideal paradigm for utilizing expression profiling methods to evaluate simultaneously many targets that may be relevant to senescence. Although in its infancy, compelling transcription mosaics following aging and CR in brain have been reported [94, 96, 103–106]. Although a review of systemic CR studies in age-related paradigms is beyond the scope of this chapter, pronounced effects of CR in tissues other than brain are worth noting, as genes responsible for metabolic and biosynthetic processes are downregulated in gastrocnemius muscle and heart [106, 107], whereas xenobiotic metabolism, cell cycle, and DNA replication transcripts are downregulated in the liver of aged mice [108]. Moreover, decreases in expression levels of genes associated with transcriptional regulation, transport, and signal transduction have been reported in the aging mouse submandibular gland [109]. In a provocative meta-analysis, datasets containing altered genes following CR were analyzed from 15 microarray papers using RNA extracted from flies, mice, monkeys, pigs, rats, and yeast [110]. Interestingly, the results displayed no single common gene altered by CR among different species, although relevant classes of transcripts that were consistently regulated across phyla included metabolic, stress related, immune response, and transcription activation related genes [110]. In brain, microarray analysis following aging has demonstrated alterations in several classes of transcripts, notably upregulation of genes involved in immune or inflammatory responses [103, 106]. Importantly, age-related upregulation of immune response and inflammatory related genes is attenuated significantly in both the cerebral cortex and cerebellum by CR [77, 103]. Taken together, results of microarray evaluations following aging and CR in the brain suggest an increase in immune and inflammatory responses that are at least partially attenuated by CR. Although mechanisms underlying the effects of CR remain unknown, potential mediators include the retardation of oxidative stress/lipid peroxidation, and increased production of neurotrophic factors such as brain-derived neurotrophic factor. Both effectors are plausible, as CR has been well documented to increase neurotrophic output and reduce reactive oxygen species (ROS) in several dietary restriction paradigms [105, 111].

1.   Oxidative Stress

Production of ROS, reactive nitrogen species (RNS), lipid peroxidation, and generalized increases in oxidative damage has been well-studied in age-related paradigms [105, 112, 113]. Furthermore, aging appears to involve a decreased transcriptional commitment to active intracellular and intercellular movement of ions, nutrients, and transmitters [93], with a concomitant increase in susceptibility to oxidative damage and metabolic deficits [114, 115]. Several microarray studies have identified differential regulation of markers of oxidative damage during the aging process. For example, Lu et al. [116] performed an Affymetrix oligonucleotide array analysis on an aging cohort of 30 subjects (age range 26 to 106 years) and discovered that expression profiles were most consistent for subjects less than 40, with another relatively homogeneous expression profile occurring in subjects older than approximately 70 [116]. In contrast, subjects between the ages of 40 and 70 had the most variability [116], indicating that the rate of change in expression levels likely occurs throughout middle age. This raises the distinct possibility that individual humans have divergent molecular and cellular rates of senescence as they progress from young adulthood through middle age and old age. These authors demonstrated upregulation of many genes related to oxidative damage and observed differential regulation of genes associated with DNA repair [116]. In accordance with these findings, the group also performed assays of promoter regions of several genes, and provide clear evidence of oxidative DNA damage during senescence [116], consistent with observations from independent research groups indicating that DNA damage is a prominent feature of aging and neurodegenerative disorders such as AD and motor neuron disease [115, 117, 118]. Moreover, RNA species appear to be vulnerable to oxidation in AD, and abnormal processing of proteins has been observed from oxidized mRNAs expressed *in vitro* [119]. Pronounced regulation of transcripts related to oxidative stress has also been observed in several aging paradigms in animal models [103, 120–122], enabling mechanistic evaluations and future studies of individual transcripts relevant to downstream neurodegenerative processes.

2.   Inflammation

Increases in several inflammatory responses are well documented during the aging process, and involve neuronal and nonneuronal (e.g., astrocytes, microglia, vascular elements, and epithelial cells) cells within the CNS [123–125]. For example, SPs, the extracellular amyloid deposits composed of Abeta peptides and other proteins that are prevalent throughout aged brain as well as in neurodegenerative disorders such as AD and Down's syndrome, are surrounded by astrocytes and infiltrated by microglial cells [17, 126, 127]. Inflammatory responses have been documented in virtually all age-related paradigms, ranging from normal senescence to neurodegenerative disorders such as AD, PD, ischemia, motor neuron disease, and multiple sclerosis [25, 117, 123, 128–130]. The prevalence of the inflammatory changes, however, is tempered by the question as to whether the inflammatory response is a primary event or a secondary response based upon primary neurodegenerative cell death, or injury-based stimuli [131–133]. In terms of microarray analysis of age-related studies, upregulation of genes linked to immune and/or inflammatory responses have been consistently observed across platforms and paradigms. For example, in one study of aging in mouse cortex, approximately 20% of the upregulated genes found in the entire study belonged to the inflammatory response/immune cascade class of transcripts [104]. These data suggest that the aging brain is associated with a state of heightened immune reactivity. The cause(s) of the observed amplified immune response remains unknown, although several lines of evidence point toward age-related increases in oxidative stress, DNA damage, and the accumulation of misfolded proteins as being primary factors [94, 116, 134]. Microarray studies that have demonstrated an upregulation of inflammatory-related markers include evaluations of postmortem tissues in AD hippocampus and cortex [128, 135, 136], spinal motor neurons in amyotrophic lateral sclerosis (ALS) [137, 138], cerebral cortex in Creutzfeldt-Jakob disease (CJD) [139], temporal cortex in epilepsy [140], multiple sclerosis lesions [130, 141], and substantia nigra in PD [25]. Upregulation of inflammatory markers has also been observed in a myriad of studies using animal models of aging, age-related disorders, and injury, including senescence in rat hippocampus [120], a mouse model of ALS [142], a mouse model of cerebral amyloidosis [143], a mouse model of experimental autoimmune encephalomyelitis (EAE) [130], MPTP poisoning [144], dentate gyrus following perforant path transection [145], dentate gyrus granule cells following trimethyltin hydroxide exposure [146], a rat model of ischemia [147], retroviral infection [148–150], and traumatic brain injury [151, 152]. Inflammatory expression profiling studies have also been performed on astrocytes *in vivo* [153–155], cultured astrocytes [155, 156], and cultured microglia [157, 158] to generate molecular fingerprints for these glial cell types relevant toward understanding inflammatory responses in the brain.

D. **NEURODEGENERATIVE PATHOLOGY WITHIN THE HIPPOCAMPUS**

The hippocampus is a prime target for expression profiling studies due to its central involvement in learning and memory and failure in a variety of neurodegenerative disorders, such as AD and ischemia. Indeed, microarray analysis has been utilized in the hippocampus for a variety of downstream genetic analyses in animal models, including regional hippocampal studies of alcohol consumption [159], aging [120], amyloid overexpression [143, 160], antidepressant administration [161], axotomy [145], epilepsy [162, 163], hippocampal cytoarchitecture [164, 165], hypergravity [166], hypoxia/ischemia [167, 168], learning and memory [169, 170], nerve agent exposure [171], and traumatic brain injury [172], among others. Regional analysis of hippocampal gene expression has also been performed on postmortem human brain tissues, including studies assessing AD [128, 135, 136, 173] and epilepsy [140, 162, 174].

Although the majority of microarray studies utilize regional dissections of brain as input sources of RNA, our laboratory has focused on utilizing single cells and homogeneous populations of neurons (termed "population cell analysis") within the hippocampal formation of human postmortem tissues and animal models as input sources via microaspiration techniques such as LCM coupled with RNA amplification (i.e., TC RNA amplification) to evaluate several neurodegenerative paradigms [14, 21, 26, 175]. As one example, the pathogenesis of NFTs in AD and related disorders is poorly understood, and is being studied using a variety of histopathological and biochemical methods [123, 176]. Our hypothesis that alterations in the expression of specific mRNAs may reflect mechanisms underlying the formation of NFTs and their consequences in affected neurons is being evaluated using microaspiration coupled with RNA amplification and hybridization to high-density and custom-designed cDNA arrays within CA1 pyramidal neurons [26, 57]. Relative to normal CA1 neurons, those harboring NFTs in AD brains displayed significant reductions in several classes of mRNAs known to encode proteins implicated in AD neuropathology, including protein phosphatases/kinases, cytoskeletal elements, synaptic-related markers, and receptor subunits such as glutamate receptors and dopamine (DA) receptors [26, 57] (Figure 7.3). Moreover, total hybridization signal intensity is downregulated in single AD NFT-bearing neurons compared to normal CA1 neurons by approximately 30%, consistent with evaluations of total polyadenylated mRNA expression in AD [177, 178]. Furthermore, a two- to fourfold decrease in the expression of the mRNAs for DA receptors DRD1-DRD5 (NCBI Unigene annotation for D1–D5 receptors) and the DA transporter (DAT) is observed in NFT-bearing neurons in AD versus non-tangle bearing neurons in control brains [26, 57] (Figure 7.3). These findings are consistent with neuropharmacological data showing decreased DRD2 receptor binding in the AD hippocampus [179, 180], and they underscore the advantages of single cell/population cell mRNA assessments because antibodies and neuropharmacological ligand-based studies have not been able to discriminate unequivocally between DA receptor subtypes.

In addition, age-related decline in DA receptor levels is observed in regional brain studies of animal models and human postmortem tissues [181, 182]. We performed single-cell RNA amplification combined with custom-designed cDNA array analysis to evaluate the effects of aging on DRD1–DRD5 DA receptor mRNA expression levels in hippocampal CA1 pyramidal neurons and entorhinal cortex layer II stellate cells from a cohort of normal control postmortem human brains aged 19 to 95 years [58]. Results indicate a significant age-related decline for all five DA receptor mRNAs in CA1 pyramidal neurons [26, 58]. Downregulation of DA receptor subtypes appears to be relatively selective, as no age-related decrement in other mRNAs is observed in CA1 pyramidal neurons, including the cytoskeletal elements beta-actin, three-repeat tau (3Rtau), and four-repeat tau (4Rtau) [58]. In contrast, no significant changes in DA receptor subtype expression are observed in entorhinal cortex stellate cells across the same cohort [26, 58]. Alterations in hippocampal DA function impact cognitive and mnemonic functions, and disruption in the functional integrity of hippocampal DA neurotransmission correlates with the pathophysiology of neurodegenerative disorders, including AD and neuropsychiatric disorders such as schizophrenia [183, 184]. Deficits in dopaminergic neurotransmission may also contribute to the cognitive decline associated with normal aging in humans and animal models [185–187]. In summary, senescence may be a factor responsible for cell-type-specific downregulation of DA receptor gene expression in a circuit crucial for learning and memory. Our single-cell studies extend and confirm previous observations at the regional/binding site level to include cell-type-specific localization of multiple classes of transcripts (e.g., DA receptors) simultaneously, which is relevant

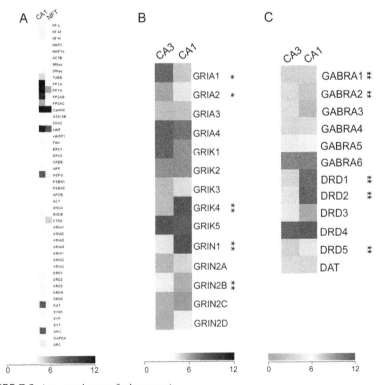

FIGURE 7.3 (see caption on facing page)

for understanding mechanisms that underlie pathological changes in neurodegenerative and neuropsychiatric disorders.

Despite the fact that the low molecular weight microtubule-associated protein tau is the principal component of NFTs found in select neuronal populations in AD [188, 189], no tau mutations have been described. However, pathogenic mutations in the tau gene cause frontotemporal dementia (FTD) [190], supporting the concept that post-transcriptional alterations in tau gene expression may play a role in the

FIGURE 7.3 (SEE COLOR INSERT FOLLOWING PAGE 204) Dendrograms illustrating relative expression levels of representative transcripts for several single-cell expression profile paradigms. (A) A comparison of expression profiles from normal control CA1 pyramidal neurons and NFT-bearing CA1 neurons in AD. (B) Color-coded matrix plots illustrating relative expression levels for individual glutamate receptor transcripts in CA1 and CA3 neurons. Single asterisk indicates a significant increase in expression of AMPA receptors GRIA1 and GRIA2 in CA3 neurons as compared to CA1 neurons. Double asterisks denote significant increases in relative expression levels in CA1 pyramidal neurons as compared to CA3 pyramidal neurons for kainate receptor KA1 (GRIK4) and NMDA receptors NMDAR1 (GRIN1) and NMDAR2B (GRIN2B). (C) Dendrogram and histogram depicting individual GABA A receptor and dopamine receptor mRNA expression levels in CA1 and CA3 pyramidal neurons microaspirated from human hippocampus. Color matrix plot illustrates expression levels for six GABA A receptors, five dopamine receptors, and the dopamine transporter in CA1 and CA3 pyramidal neurons. Double asterisk indicates genes that have significantly greater relative expression levels in CA1 neurons as compared to CA3 neurons including GABA A receptors (GABRA1, GABRA2), and the D1, D2, and D5 dopamine receptors (DRD1, DRD2, and DRD5).

Key: 3Rtau, three-repeat tau; 4Rtau, four-repeat tau; ACT, alpha-1-antichymotrypsin precursor; ACTB, beta-actin; APOE, apolipoprotein E; APP, amyloid-beta precursor protein; arc, activity regulated cytoskeletal-associated protein; CAMKII, calcium/calmodulin-dependent protein kinase II, alpha; CDK2, cyclin-dependent kinase 2; cdk5, cyclin-dependent kinase 5; cdk5R1, cyclin-dependent kinase 5, regulatory subunit 1 (p35); c-fos, cellular oncogene fos; c-jun, jun oncogene; CREB, cAMP responsive element binding protein; CTSD, cathepsin D; DAT, dopamine transporter; DRD1, dopamine receptor D1; DRD2, dopamine receptor D2; DRD3, dopamine receptor D3; DRD4, dopamine receptor D4; DRD5, dopamine receptor D5; ERK1, extracellular signal-regulated kinase 1 (p44); ERK2, extracellular signal-regulated kinase (p42); FAK, focal adhesion kinase; GABRA1, GABA A receptor, alpha 1; GABRA2, GABA A receptor, alpha 2; GABRA3, GABA A receptor, alpha 3; GABRA4, GABA A receptor, alpha 4; GABRA5, GABA A receptor, alpha 5; GABRA6, GABA A receptor, alpha 6; GAPDH, glyceraldehyde-3-phosphate dehydrogenase; GRIA1, AMPA1; GRIA2, AMPA2; GRIA3, AMPA3; GRIA4, AMPA4; GRIK1, kainate 1(GluR5); GRIK2, kainate 2(GluR6), GRIK3, kainate 3(GluR7); GRIN1, N-methyl D-aspartate 1(NMDAR1); GRIN2A, NMDAR2A; GRIN2B, NMDAR2B; GRIN2C, NMDAR2C; GRIN2D, NMDAR2D; GRX, glutaredoxin; GSK-3B, glycogen synthase kinase-3 beta; HSPG, heparan sulfate proteoglycan; MAP1b, microtubule-associated protein 1b; MAP2, microtubule-associated protein 2; NF-H, neurofilament heavy subunit; NF-L, neurofilament light subunit; NF-M, neurofilament medium subunit; PP1A, protein phosphatase 1 catalytic subunit, alpha isoform; PP1G, protein phosphatase 1, catalytic subunit, gamma isoform; PP2AB, protein phosphatase 2, regulatory subunit A, beta isoform; PP2AC, protein phosphatase 2, catalytic subunit, alpha isoform; PSEN1, presenilin 1; PSEN2, presenilin 2; SNCA, alpha synuclein; SNCB, beta synuclein; SYN1, synapsin 1; SYP, synaptophysin; SYT, synaptotagmin; TUBB, beta-tubulin.

pathogenesis of tauopathy, including AD. Although mechanism(s) underlying the tauopathic process(es) remain unknown, it is possible that neuronal tau mRNA expression levels are altered during the progression of AD. Interestingly, tau gene expression level differences have not been reported either at the regional [191–194] or single cell level [57, 58] at any stage during the development of AD. However, there are indications of fluctuation in both 3Rtau and 4Rtau mRNA levels [191, 194, 195]. These observations are perplexing, given the pronounced alteration in tau protein levels and phosphorylation states in AD. Our laboratory has performed single-cell gene expression profiling coupled with custom-designed cDNA array analysis to evaluate tau expression and other cytoskeletal elements within individual neuronal populations in patients with no cognitive impairment (NCI), mild cognitive impairment (MCI), and AD [196]. Results reveal a shift in the ratio of 3Rtau to 4Rtau mRNAs within individual human cholinergic basal forebrain (CBF) neurons within nucleus basalis (NB) and CA1 hippocampal neurons during the progression of AD, but not during normal aging. Specifically, single-cell results indicate that tau transcript expression and other cytoskeletal elements — including beta-tubulin, microtubule-associated proteins MAP1b and MAP2, and the low, medium, and high neurofilament subunits levels — did not differ significantly across the cohort. However, when the ratios of 3Rtau/4Rtau were calculated, a significant difference in the proportion of 3Rtau/4Rtau mRNA was found in MCI and AD relative to NCI [196]. The shift is due to a decrease in 3Rtau as opposed to an increase in 4Rtau levels. Remarkably, this shift in the 3Rtau/4Rtau ratio was present in both MCI and AD, suggesting that this dysregulation impacts neuronal function and marks a transition from normal cognition to prodromal AD. A shift in 3Rtau to 4Rtau may precipitate a cascade of events in the selective vulnerability of neurons, ultimately leading to frank NFT formation in tauopathies, including AD. Studies on additional transcripts, including the neuropeptide galanin and galanin receptors GALR1, GALR2, and GALR3, also did not display expression level differences within individual CBF neurons in NCI, MCI, and AD [197]. In contrast, ongoing studies of individual CBF neurons have demonstrated differential regulation in AD and MCI vs. NCI in other relevant transcript classes, including high-affinity nerve growth factor trk receptors, synaptic-related markers, and glutamate receptors [15, 26], providing an interesting comparator to the 3Rtau/4Rtau results. While the functional significance of a shift in the 3Rtau/4Rtau ratio remains unknown, several lines of evidence indicate that 3Rtau and 4Rtau likely play different roles in select neurons [198, 199], and consequently may be differentially dysregulated during the pathogenesis of various neurodegenerative diseases. These data suggest a subtle, yet pervasive change in gene dosage of 3Rtau and 4Rtau within vulnerable neurons in MCI and AD, which does not occur during normal aging. In summary, shifts in the ratio of tau genes may be a fundamental mechanism whereby normal tau expression is dysregulated, leading to NFT formation.

E.   CONCLUDING REMARKS

Because the mechanisms underlying the aging process are likely to be quite complex, there is a high probability that expression profiles within the CNS will reveal a hierarchy of mosaics at the regional, laminar, nuclear, and cellular levels. There is currently no widely accepted biomarker for aging. A goal of modern molecular neuroscience is to develop reliable molecular fingerprints for age-related research similar to the translational design of cancer-related paradigms [3, 200, 201]. Aging is likely a polygenic phenomenon, and microarray analysis can help to identify transcripts contributing to longer life and define genes contributing positively or adversely to the aging process. The application of microarray technology has generated significant interest across several disciplines and spans a multiplicity of biological systems. However, the brain remains a difficult organ to study, in part due to the regional and cellular heterogeneity of brain regions and cell types [6, 21]. Thus, a combination of single cell/population cell analysis is a highly desirable paradigm whereby expression profiles of single populations of neuronal and nonneuronal subtypes can be analyzed and compared under normal and pathological conditions [15, 26, 153, 154, 175]. The transcript profile in a homogeneous population of neurons may be more informative than patterns derived from whole brain or regional tissue homogenates [6], as each neuronal subtype is likely to have a unique molecular signature in normative and diseased states. The next level of understanding of cellular and molecular mechanisms underlying the neurobiology of aging, and of associated pathophysiology of late-onset progressive neurodegenerative disorders such as AD, ALS, and PD, lies in the ability to combine these aforementioned technologies with appropriate models to recapitulate the structure and connectivity of these systems *in vivo* and *in vitro*. As our ability to refine expression profiling paradigms increases, the development of pharmacotherapeutic agents and delivery systems that are more effective, as well as selective or potentially specific for individual cell types, becomes more realistic. An important caveat for microarray studies and functional genomics evaluations as a whole is that changes in mRNA levels may not always result in concomitant and/or coincident alterations in respective protein levels. Notwithstanding this issue, mosaics that are generated using expression profiling methods in age-related studies are an exciting and important contributor to the current repertoire of tools available to understand the complex mechanisms that underlie cellular and molecular programs of senescence.

ACKNOWLEDGMENTS

I would like to acknowledge support from grants AG10688, AG14449, AG17617, NS43939, NS48447, and the Alzheimer's Association. I thank Drs. Shaoli Che, Scott E. Counts, Scott E. Hemby, and Elliott J. Mufson for their long-term collaborative efforts on these projects. I thank Dr. Melissa J. Alldred for critical review of the manuscript. I acknowledge the efforts of Ms. Irina Elarova, Ms. Shaona Fang, and

Ms. Krisztina M. Kovacs for their expert technical assistance. I am also grateful to the families of the patients studied here who made this research possible.

REFERENCES

1. De Magalhaes, J.P., From cells to ageing: a review of models and mechanisms of cellular senescence and their impact on human ageing, *Exp. Cell Res.*, 300, 1, 2004.
2. McElwee, J.J., Addressing the age-old question of old age, *Genome Biol.*, 5, 337, 2004.
3. Galvin, J.E. and Ginsberg, S.D., Expression profiling in the aging brain: a perspective, *Ageing Res. Rev.*, 4, 529, 2005.
4. Blumberg, D.D., Creating a ribonuclease-free environment, *Methods Enzymol.*, 152, 20, 1987.
5. Coombs, N.J., Gough, A.C., and Primrose, J.N., Optimisation of DNA and RNA extraction from archival formalin-fixed tissue, *Nucleic Acids Res.*, 27, e12, 1999.
6. Ginsberg, S.D. et al., Cell and tissue microdissection in combination with genomic and proteomic applications, in *Neuroanatomical Tract Tracing 3: Molecules-Neurons-Systems*, Zaborszky, L., Wouterlood, F., and Lanciego, J.L., Eds., Springer/Kluwer/Plenum, New York, 2006, pp. 109–141.
7. Goldsworthy, S.M. et al., Effects of fixation on RNA extraction and amplification from laser capture microdissected tissue, *Mol. Carcinog.*, 25, 86, 1999.
8. Su, J.M. et al., Comparison of ethanol versus formalin fixation on preservation of histology and RNA in laser capture microdissected brain tissues, *Brain Pathol.*, 14, 175, 2004.
9. Bahn, S. et al., Gene expression profiling in the post-mortem human brain — no cause for dismay, *J. Chem. Neuroanat.*, 22, 79, 2001.
10. Leonard, S. et al., Biological stability of mRNA isolated from human postmortem brain collections, *Biol. Psychiatry*, 33, 456, 1993.
11. Van Deerlin, V.M.D., Ginsberg, S.D., Lee, V.M.-Y., and Trojanowski, J.Q., The use of fixed human post mortem brain tissue to study mRNA expression in neurodegenerative diseases: applications of microdissection and mRNA amplification, in *Microarrays for the Neurosciences: An Essential Guide*, Geschwind, D.H. and Gregg, J.P. , Eds., MIT Press, Boston, 2002, pp. 201 235.
12. Mikel, U.V. and Becker Jr., R.L., A comparative study of quantitative stains for DNA in image cytometry, *Analyt. Quant. Cytol. Histol.*, 13, 253, 1991.
13. von Bertalanffy, L. and Bickis, I., Identification of cytoplasmic basophilia (ribonucleic acid) by fluorescence microscopy, *J. Histochem. Cytochem.*, 4, 481, 1956.
14. Ginsberg, S.D. and Che, S., RNA amplification in brain tissues, *Neurochem. Res.*, 27, 981, 2002.
15. Mufson, E.J., Counts, S.E., and Ginsberg, S.D., Single cell gene expression profiles of nucleus basalis cholinergic neurons in Alzheimer's disease, *Neurochem. Res.*, 27, 1035, 2002.
16. Topaloglu, H. and Sarnat, H.B., Acridine orange-RNA fluorescence maturing neurons in the perinatal rat brain, *Anat. Rec.*, 224, 88, 1989.
17. Ginsberg, S.D., Crino, P.B., Lee, V.M.-Y., Eberwine, J.H., and Trojanowski, J.Q., Sequestration of RNA in Alzheimer's disease neurofibrillary tangles and senile plaques, *Ann. Neurol.*, 41, 200, 1997.

18. Ginsberg, S.D., Galvin, J.E. , Chiu, T.-S., Lee, V.M.-Y., Masliah, E., and Trojanowski, J.Q., RNA sequestration to pathological lesions of neurodegenerative disorders, *Acta Neuropathol.*, 96, 487, 1998.

19. Che, S. and Ginsberg, S.D., Amplification of transcripts using terminal continuation, *Lab. Invest.*, 84, 131, 2004.

20. Che, S. and Ginsberg, S.D., RNA amplification methodologies, in *Trends in RNA Research*, McNamara, P.A., Ed., Hauppage, NY, Nova Science Publishing, pp. 277–301, 2000.

21. Ginsberg, S.D. and Che, S., Combined histochemical staining, RNA amplification, regional, and single cell analysis within the hippocampus, *Lab. Invest.*, 84, 952, 2004.

22. Miller, C.L., Diglisic, S., Leister, F., Webster, M., and Yolken, R.H., Evaluating RNA status for RT-PCR in extracts of postmortem human brain tissue, *BioTechniques*, 36, 628, 2004.

23. Ginsberg, S.D., RNA amplification strategies for small sample populations, *Methods*, 37, 229, 2005.

24. Fasulo, W.H. and Hemby, S.E., Time-dependent changes in gene expression profiles of midbrain dopamine neurons following haloperidol administration, *J. Neurochem.*, 87, 205, 2003.

25. Grunblatt, E. et al., Gene expression profiling of Parkinsonian substantia nigra pars compacta; alterations in ubiquitin-proteasome, heat shock protein, iron and oxidative stress regulated proteins, cell adhesion/cellular matrix and vesicle trafficking genes, *J. Neural. Transm.*, 111, 1543, 2004.

26. Ginsberg, S.D. et al., Single cell gene expression analysis: implications for neurodegenerative and neuropsychiatric disorders, *Neurochem. Res.*, 29, 1054, 2004.

27. Vincent, V.A. et al., Analysis of neuronal gene expression with laser capture microdissection, *J. Neurosci. Res.*, 69, 578, 2002.

28. Crino, P.B. et al., Presence and phosphorylation of transcription factors in dendrites, *Proc. Natl. Acad. Sci. U.S.A.*, 95, 2313, 1998.

29. Eberwine, J. et al., Analysis of subcellularly localized mRNAs using *in situ* hybridization, mRNA amplification, and expression profiling, *Neurochem. Res.*, 27, 1065, 2002.

30. Kacharmina, J.E., Crino, P.B., and Eberwine, J., Preparation of cDNA from single cells and subcellular regions, *Methods Enzymol.*, 303, 3, 1999.

31. Bonner, R.F. et al., Laser capture microdissection: molecular analysis of tissue, *Science*, 278, 1481, 1997.

32. Emmert-Buck, M. et al., Laser capture microdissection, *Science*, 274, 998, 1996.

33. Mikulowska-Mennis, A. et al., High-quality RNA from cells isolated by laser capture microdissection, *BioTechniques*, 33, 176, 2002.

34. Niyaz, Y. et al., Noncontact laser microdissection and pressure catapulting: sample preparation for genomic, transcriptomic, and proteomic analysis, *Methods Mol. Med.*, 114, 1, 2005.

35. Craven, R.A. et al., Laser capture microdissection and two-dimensional polyacrylamide gel electrophoresis: evaluation of tissue preparation and sample limitations, *Am. J. Pathol.*, 160, 815, 2002.

36. Ehrig, T. et al., Quantitative amplification of genomic DNA from histological tissue sections after staining with nuclear dyes and laser capture microdissection, *J. Mol. Diagn.*, 3, 22, 2001.

37. Simone, N.L. et al., Sensitive immunoassay of tissue cell proteins procured by laser capture microdissection, *Am. J. Pathol.*, 156, 445, 2000.

38. Mullis, K.B., The unusual origin of the polymerase chain reaction, *Sci. Am.*, 262, 56, 1990.
39. Phillips, J. and Eberwine, J.H., Antisense RNA amplification: a linear amplification method for analyzing the mRNA population from single living cells, *Methods Enzymol. Suppl.*, 10, 283, 1996.
40. Bustin, S.A., Quantification of mRNA using real-time reverse transcription PCR (RT-PCR): trends and problems, *J. Mol. Endocrinol.*, 29, 23, 2002.
41. Giulietti, A. et al., An overview of real-time quantitative PCR: applications to quantify cytokine gene expression, *Methods*, 25, 386, 2001.
42. Shintani-Ishida, K., Zhu, B.L., and Maeda, H., TaqMan fluorogenic detection system to analyze gene transcription in autopsy material, *Methods Mol. Biol.*, 291, 415, 2005.
43. Cardullo, R.A. et al., Detection of nucleic acid hybridization by nonradiative fluorescence resonance energy transfer, *Proc. Natl. Acad. Sci. U.S.A.*, 85, 8790, 1988.
44. Bonnet, G. et al., Thermodynamic basis of the enhanced specificity of structured DNA probes, *Proc. Natl. Acad. Sci. U.S.A.*, 96, 6171, 1999.
45. Tan, L. et al., Molecular beacons for bioanalytical applications, *Analyst*, 130, 1002, 2005.
46. Kricka, L.J., Stains, labels and detection strategies for nucleic acids assays, *Ann. Clin. Biochem.*, 39, 114, 2002.
47. Providenti, M.A. et al., The copy-number of plasmids and other genetic elements can be determined by SYBR-Green-based quantitative real-time PCR, *J. Microbiol. Methods*, 7, 7, 2005.
48. Eberwine, J. et al., mRNA expression analysis of tissue sections and single cells, *J. Neurosci.*, 21, 8310, 2001.
49. Eberwine, J. et al., Analysis of gene expression in single live neurons, *Proc. Natl. Acad. Sci. U.S.A.*, 89, 3010, 1992.
50. Steitz, T.A., The structural basis of the transition from initiation to elongation phases of transcription, as well as translocation and strand separation, by T7 RNA polymerase, *Curr. Opin. Struct. Biol.*, 14, 4, 2004.
51. Feldman, A.L. et al., Advantages of mRNA amplification for microarray analysis, *BioTechniques*, 33, 906, 2002.
52. Polacek, D.C. et al., Fidelity and enhanced sensitivity of differential transcription profiles following linear amplification of nanogram amounts of endothelial mRNA, *Physiol. Genomics*, 13, 147, 2003.
53. Eberwine, J., Crino, P., and Dichter, M., Single-cell mRNA amplification: implications for basic and clinical neuroscience, *The Neuroscientist*, 1, 200, 1995.
54. Chow, N. et al., Expression profiles of multiple genes in single neurons of Alzheimer's disease, *Proc. Natl. Acad. Sci. U.S.A.*, 95, 9620, 1998.
55. Ghasemzadeh, M.B. et al., Multiplicity of glutamate receptor subunits in single striatal neurons: an RNA amplification study, *Mol. Pharmacol.*, 49, 852, 1996.
56. Ginsberg, S.D. et al, Predominance of neuronal mRNAs in individual Alzheimer's disease senile plaques, *Ann. Neurol.*, 45, 174, 1999.
57. Ginsberg, S.D. et al., Expression profile of transcripts in Alzheimer's disease tangle-bearing CA1 neurons, *Ann. Neurol.*, 48, 77, 2000.
58. Hemby, S.E., Trojanowski, J.Q., and Ginsberg, S.D., Neuron-specific age-related decreases in dopamine receptor subtype mRNAs, *J. Comp. Neurol.*, 456, 176, 2003.
59. Madison, R.D. and Robinson, G.A., lRNA internal standards quantify sensitivity and amplification efficiency of mammalian gene expression profiling, *BioTechniques*, 25, 504, 1998.

60. Dafforn, A. et al., Linear mRNA amplification from as little as 5 ng total RNA for global gene expression analysis, *BioTechniques*, 37, 854, 2004.

61. Iscove, N.N. et al., Representation is faithfully preserved in global cDNA amplified exponentially from sub-picogram quantities of mRNA, *Nat. Biotechnol.*, 20, 940, 2002.

62. Schneider, J. et al., Systematic analysis of T7 RNA polymerase based *in vitro* linear RNA amplification for use in microarray experiments, *BMC Genomics*, 5, 29, 2004.

63. Wang, E. et al., High-fidelity mRNA amplification for gene profiling, *Nat. Biotechnol.*, 18, 457, 2000.

64. Xiang, C.C. et al., A new strategy to amplify degraded RNA from small tissue samples for microarray studies, *Nucleic Acids Res.*, 31, E53, 2003.

65. Auburn, R.P. et al., Robotic spotting of cDNA and oligonucleotide microarrays, *Trends Biotechnol.*, 23, 374, 2005.

66. Brown, P.O. and Botstein, D., Exploring the new world of the genome with DNA microarrays, *Nat. Genet.*, 21(Suppl.), 33, 1999.

67. Fodor, S.P. et al., Light-directed, spatially addressable parallel chemical synthesis, *Science*, 251, 767, 1991.

68. Lockhart, D.J. and Barlow, C., Expressing what's on your mind: DNA arrays and the brain, *Nat. Rev. Neurosci.*, 2, 63, 2001.

69. Galvin, J.E. and Ginsberg, S.D., Expression profiling and pharmacotherapeutic development in the central nervous system, *Alzheimer Dis. Assoc. Disord.*, 18, 264, 2004.

70. Colantuoni, C. et al., High throughput analysis of gene expression in the human brain, *J. Neurosci. Res.*, 59, 1, 2000.

71. Taib, Z., Statistical analysis of oligonucleotide microarray data, *C. R. Biol.*, 327, 175, 2004.

72. Aittokallio, T. et al., Computational strategies for analyzing data in gene expression microarray experiments, *J. Bioinform. Comput. Biol.*, 1, 541, 2003.

73. Klur, S., Toy, K., et al., Evaluation of procedures for amplification of small-size samples for hybridization on microarrays, *Genomics*, 83, 508, 2004.

74. Chesler, E.J. et al., Genetic correlates of gene expression in recombinant inbred strains: a relational model system to explore neurobehavioral phenotypes, *Neuroinformatics*, 1, 343, 2003.

75. Krieg, R.C. et al., Proteomic analysis of human bladder tissue using SELDI approach following microdissection techniques, *Methods Mol. Biol.*, 293, 255, 2005.

76. Kim, S.I. et al., Neuroproteomics: expression profiling of the brain's proteomes in health and disease, *Neurochem. Res.*, 29, 1317, 2004.

77. Park, S.K. and Prolla, T.A., Lessons learned from gene expression profile studies of aging and caloric restriction, *Ageing Res. Rev.*, 4, 55, 2005.

78. Lund, P.K. et al., Transcriptional mechanisms of hippocampal aging, *Exp. Gerontol.*, 39, 1613, 2004.

79. Selkoe, D.J., Aging, amyloid, and Alzheimer's disease: a perspective in honor of Carl Cotman, *Neurochem. Res.*, 28, 1705, 2003.

80. Gudmundsson, H. et al., Inheritance of human longevity in Iceland, *Eur. J. Hum. Genet.*, 8, 743, 2000.

81. Longo, V.D. and Finch, C.E., Evolutionary medicine: from dwarf model systems to healthy centenarians? *Science*, 299, 1342, 2003.

82. Slagboom, P.E. et al., Genetics of human aging. The search for genes contributing to human longevity and diseases of the old, *Ann. N.Y. Acad. Sci.*, 908, 50, 2000.

83. Kirkwood, T.B. et al., What accounts for the wide variation in life span of genetically identical organisms reared in a constant environment? *Mech. Ageing Dev.*, 126, 439, 2005.
84. Hauser, E.R. and Pericak-Vance, M.A., Genetic analysis for common complex disease, *Am. Heart J.*, 140, S36, 2000.
85. Cordell, H.J. and Clayton, D.G., Genetic association studies, *Lancet*, 366, 1121, 2005.
86. Bently, D.R. and Dunham, I., Mapping human chromosomes, *Curr. Opin. Genet. Dev.*, 5, 328, 1995.
87. Olson, J.M., Goddard, K.A., and Dudek, D.M., A second locus for very-late-onset Alzheimer disease: a genome scan reveals linkage to 20p and epistasis between 20p and the amyloid precursor protein region, *Am. J. Hum. Genet.*, 71, 54, 2002.
88. Pericak-Vance, M.A. et al., Identification of novel genes in late-onset Alzheimer's disease, *Exp Gerontol.*, 35, 1343, 2000.
89. Scott, W.K. et al., Complete genomic screen in Parkinson disease: evidence for multiple genes, *J. Am. Med. Assoc.*, 286, 2239, 2001.
90. Abecasis, G.R. et al., Age-related macular degeneration: a high-resolution genome scan for susceptibility loci in a population enriched for late-stage disease, *Am. J. Hum. Genet.*, 74, 482, 2004.
91. Majewski, J. et al., Age-related macular degeneration--a genome scan in extended families, *Am. J. Hum. Genet.*, 73, 540, 2003.
92. Seddon, J.M. et al., A genomewide scan for age-related macular degeneration provides evidence for linkage to several chromosomal regions, *Am. J. Hum. Genet.*, 73, 780, 2003.
93. McCarroll, S.A. et al., Comparing genomic expression patterns across species identifies shared transcriptional profile in aging, *Nat. Genet.*, 36, 197, 2004.
94. Prolla, T.A., Multiple roads to the aging phenotype: insights from the molecular dissection of progerias through DNA microarray analysis, *Mech. Ageing Dev.*, 126, 461, 2005.
95. Mattson, M.P. et al., Prophylactic activation of neuroprotective stress response pathways by dietary and behavioral manipulations, *NeuroRx*, 1, 111, 2004.
96. Mattison, J.A. et al., Age-related decline in caloric intake and motivation for food in rhesus monkeys, *Neurobiol. Aging*, 26, 1117, 2005.
97. Spindler, S.R., Rapid and reversible induction of the longevity, anticancer and genomic effects of caloric restriction, *Mech. Ageing Dev.*, 126, 960, 2005
98. Overton, J.M. and Williams, T.D., Behavioral and physiologic responses to caloric restriction in mice, *Physiol. Behav.*, 81, 749, 2004.
99. Bondolfi, L. et al., Impact of age and caloric restriction on neurogenesis in the dentate gyrus of C57BL/6 mice, *Neurobiol. Aging*, 25, 333, 2004.
100. Mattson, M.P. and Wan, R., Beneficial effects of intermittent fasting and caloric restriction on the cardiovascular and cerebrovascular systems, *J. Nutr. Biochem.*, 16, 129, 2005.
101. Shinmura, K., Tamaki, K., and Bolli, R., Short-term caloric restriction improves ischemic tolerance independent of opening of ATP-sensitive K+ channels in both young and aged hearts, *J. Mol. Cell. Cardiol.*, 39, 285, 2005.
102. Duan, W. and Mattson, M.P., Dietary restriction and 2-deoxyglucose administration improve behavioral outcome and reduce degeneration of dopaminergic neurons in models of Parkinson's disease, *J. Neurosci. Res.*, 57, 195, 1999.
103. Lee, C.K., Weindruch, R., and Prolla, T.A., Gene-expression profile of the ageing brain in mice, *Nat. Genet.*, 25, 294, 2000.

104. Prolla, T.A., DNA microarray analysis of the aging brain, *Chem. Senses*, 27, 299, 2002.

105. Sohal, R.S. and Weindruch, R., Oxidative stress, caloric restriction, and aging, *Science*, 273, 59, 1996.

106. Weindruch, R. et al., Microarray profiling of gene expression in aging and its alteration by caloric restriction in mice, *J. Nutr.*, 131, 918S, 2001.

107. Edwards, M.G. et al., Impairment of the transcriptional responses to oxidative stress in the heart of aged C57BL/6 mice, *Ann. N.Y. Acad. Sci.*, 1019, 85, 2004.

108. Cao, S.X. et al., Genomic profiling of short- and long-term caloric restriction effects in the liver of aging mice, *Proc. Natl. Acad. Sci. U.S.A.*, 98, 10630, 2001.

109. Hiratsuka, K. et al., Microarray analysis of gene expression changes in aging in mouse submandibular gland, *J. Dent. Res.*, 81, 679, 2002.

110. Han, E.S. and Hickey, M., Microarray evaluation of dietary restriction, *J. Nutr.*, 135, 1343, 2005.

111. Maswood, N. et al., Caloric restriction increases neurotrophic factor levels and attenuates neurochemical and behavioral deficits in a primate model of Parkinson's disease, *Proc. Natl. Acad. Sci. U.S.A.*, 101, 18171, 2004.

112. Barja, G., Free radicals and aging, *Trends Neurosci.*, 27, 595, 2004.

113. Serrano, F. and Klann, E., Reactive oxygen species and synaptic plasticity in the aging hippocampus, *Ageing Res. Rev.*, 3, 431, 2004.

114. Suji, G. and Sivakami, S., Glucose, glycation and aging, *Biogerontology*, 5, 365. 2004.

115. Vijg, J. and Suh, Y., Genetics of longevity and aging, *Annu. Rev. Med.*, 56, 193, 2005.

116. Lu, T. et al., Gene regulation and DNA damage in the ageing human brain, *Nature*, 429, 883, 2004.

117. Liu, Z. and Martin, L.J., Motor neurons rapidly accumulate DNA single-strand breaks after *in vitro* exposure to nitric oxide and peroxynitrite and *in vivo* axotomy, *J. Comp. Neurol.*, 432, 35, 2001.

118. Smith, M.A. et al., Radical AGEing in Alzheimer's disease, *Trends Neurosci.*, 18, 172, 1995.

119. Shan, X., Tashiro, H., and Lin, C.L., The identification and characterization of oxidized RNAs in Alzheimer's disease, *J. Neurosci.*, 23, 4913, 2003.

120. Blalock, E.M. et al., Gene microarrays in hippocampal aging: statistical profiling identifies novel processes correlated with cognitive impairment, *J. Neurosci.*, 23, 3807, 2003.

121. Kim, S.N. et al., Age-dependent changes of gene expression in the *Drosophila* head, *Neurobiol. Aging*, 26, 1083, 2005.

122. McMurray, M.A. and Gottschling, D.E., Aging and genetic instability in yeast, *Curr. Opin. Microbiol.*, 7, 673, 2004.

123. Ginsberg, S.D. et al., Molecular pathology of Alzheimer's disease and related disorders, in *Cerebral Cortex, Vol. 14. Neurodegenerative and Age-related Changes in Structure and Function of Cerebral Cortex*, Peters A. and Morrison J.H., Eds., Kluwer Academic/Plenum, New York, 1999, pp. 603–653.

124. Licastro, F. and Chiappelli, M., Brain immune responses cognitive decline and dementia: relationship with phenotype expression and genetic background, *Mech. Ageing Dev.*, 124, 539, 2003.

125. McGeer, P.L. and McGeer, E.G., Mechanisms of cell death in Alzheimer disease — immunopathology, *J. Neural Transm. Suppl.*, 54, 159, 1998.

126. Itagaki, S. et al., Relationship of microglia and astrocytes to amyloid deposits of Alzheimer disease, *J. Neuroimmunol.*, 24, 173, 1989.

127. McGeer, P.L. et al., Reactive microglia in patients with senile dementia of the Alzheimer type are positive for the histocompatibility glycoprotein HLA-DR, *Neurosci. Lett.*, 79, 195, 1987.

128. Blalock, E.M. et al., Incipient Alzheimer's disease: microarray correlation analyses reveal major transcriptional and tumor suppressor responses, *Proc. Natl. Acad. Sci. U.S.A.*, 101, 2173, 2004.

129. Lippoldt, A., Reichel, A., and Moenning, U., Progress in the identification of stroke-related genes: emerging new possibilities to develop concepts in stroke therapy, *CNS Drugs*, 19, 821, 2005.

130. Lock, C. et al., Gene-microarray analysis of multiple sclerosis lesions yields new targets validated in autoimmune encephalomyelitis, *Nat. Med.*, 8, 500, 2002.

131. Danton, G.H. and Dietrich, W.D., Inflammatory mechanisms after ischemia and stroke, *J. Neuropathol. Exp. Neurol.*, 62, 127, 2003.

132. McGeer, P.L. and McGeer, E.G., Innate immunity, local inflammation, and degenerative disease, *Sci. Aging Knowledge Environ.*, 2002(29), re3, 2002.

133. Wersinger, C. and Sidhu, A., Inflammation and Parkinson's disease, *Curr. Drug Targets Inflamm. Allergy*, 1, 221, 2002.

134. Gems, D. and McElwee, J.J., Ageing: microarraying mortality, *Nature*, 424, 259, 2003.

135. Loring, J.F. et al., A gene expression profile of Alzheimer's disease, *DNA Cell. Biol.*, 20, 683, 2001.

136. Lukiw, W.J., Gene expression profiling in fetal, aged, and Alzheimer hippocampus: a continuum of stress-related signaling, *Neurochem. Res.*, 29, 1287, 2004.

137. Jiang, Y.M. et al., Gene expression profile of spinal motor neurons in sporadic amyotrophic lateral sclerosis, *Ann. Neurol.*, 57, 236, 2005.

138. Malaspina, A., Kaushik, N., and de Belleroche, J., Differential expression of 14 genes in amyotrophic lateral sclerosis spinal cord detected using gridded cDNA arrays, *J. Neurochem.*, 77, 132, 2001.

139. Xiang, W. et al., Cerebral gene expression profiles in sporadic Creutzfeldt-Jakob disease, *Ann. Neurol.*, 58, 242, 2005.

140. Lukasiuk, K. and Pitkänen, A., Large-scale analysis of gene expression in epilepsy research: is synthesis already possible? *Neurochem. Res.*, 29, 1164, 2004.

141. Mycko, M.P. et al., cDNA microarray analysis in multiple sclerosis lesions: detection of genes associated with disease activity, *Brain*, 126, 1048, 2003.

142. Yoshihara, T. et al., Differential expression of inflammation- and apoptosis-related genes in spinal cords of a mutant SOD1 transgenic mouse model of familial amyotrophic lateral sclerosis, *J. Neurochem.*, 80, 158, 2002.

143. Dickey, C.A. et al., Selectively reduced expression of synaptic plasticity-related genes in amyloid precursor protein + presenilin-1 transgenic mice, *J. Neurosci.*, 23, 5219, 2003.

144. Grunblatt, E. et al., Gene expression analysis in N-methyl-4-phenyl-1,2,3,6-tetrahydropyridine mice model of Parkinson's disease using cDNA microarray: effect of R-apomorphine, *J. Neurochem.*, 78, 1, 2001.

145. Ginsberg, S.D., Glutamatergic neurotransmission expression profiling in the mouse hippocampus after perforant-path transection, *Am. J. Geriatr. Psychiatry*, 13, 1052, 2005.

146. Lefebvre d'Hellencourt, C. and Harry, G.J., Molecular profiles of mRNA levels in laser capture microdissected murine hippocampal regions differentially responsive to TMT-induced cell death, *J. Neurochem.*, 93, 206, 2005.

147. Schmidt-Kastner, R. et al., DNA microarray analysis of cortical gene expression during early recirculation after focal brain ischemia in rat, *Brain Res. Mol. Brain Res.*, 108, 81, 2002.

148. Gebicke-Haerter, P.J., Microarrays and expression profiling in microglia research and in inflammatory brain disorders, *J. Neurosci. Res.*, 81, 327, 2005.

149. Labrada, L. et al., Age-dependent resistance to lethal alphavirus encephalitis in mice: analysis of gene expression in the central nervous system and identification of a novel interferon-inducible protective gene, mouse ISG12, *J. Virol.*, 76, 11688, 2002.

150. Roberts, E.S. et al., Induction of pathogenic sets of genes in macrophages and neurons in NeuroAIDS, *Am. J. Pathol.*, 162, 2041, 2003.

151. Matzilevich, D.A. et al., High-density microarray analysis of hippocampal gene expression following experimental brain injury, *J. Neurosci. Res.*, 67, 646, 2002.

152. O'Dell, D.M. et al., Traumatic brain injury alters the molecular fingerprint of TUNEL-positive cortical neurons *in vivo*: a single-cell analysis, *J. Neurosci.*, 20, 4821, 2000.

153. Burbach, G.J. et al., Laser microdissection reveals regional and cellular differences in GFAP mRNA upregulation following brain injury, axonal denervation, and amyloid plaque deposition, *Glia*, 48, 76, 2004.

154. Burbach, G.J. et al., Laser microdissection of immunolabeled astrocytes allows quantification of astrocytic gene expression, *J. Neurosci. Methods*, 138, 141, 2004.

155. Nakagawa, T. and Schwartz, J.P., Gene expression patterns in *in vivo* normal adult astrocytes compared with cultured neonatal and normal adult astrocytes, *Neurochem. Int.*, 45, 203, 2004.

156. Kim, S.Y. et al., Microarray analysis of changes in cellular gene expression induced by productive infection of primary human astrocytes: implications for HAD, *J. Neuroimmunol.*, 157, 17, 2004.

157. Baker, C.A. and Manuelidis, L., Unique inflammatory RNA profiles of microglia in Creutzfeldt-Jakob disease, *Proc. Natl. Acad. Sci. U.S.A.*, 100, 675, 2003.

158. Paglinawan, R. et al., TGFbeta directs gene expression of activated microglia to an anti-inflammatory phenotype strongly focusing on chemokine genes and cell migratory genes, *Glia*, 44, 219, 2003.

159. Saito, M. et al., Microarray analysis of gene expression in rat hippocampus after chronic ethanol treatment, *Neurochem. Res.*, 27, 1221, 2002.

160. Reddy, P.H. et al., Gene expression profiles of transcripts in amyloid precursor protein transgenic mice: up-regulation of mitochondrial metabolism and apoptotic genes is an early cellular change in Alzheimer's disease, *Hum. Mol. Genet.*, 13, 1225, 2004.

161. Drigues, N. et al., cDNA gene expression profile of rat hippocampus after chronic treatment with antidepressant drugs, *J. Neural Transm.*, 110, 1413, 2002.

162. Becker, A.J. et al., Correlated stage- and subfield-associated hippocampal gene expression patterns in experimental and human temporal lobe epilepsy, *Eur. J. Neurosci.*, 18, 2792, 2003.

163. Newton, S.S. et al., Gene profile of electroconvulsive seizures: induction of neurotrophic and angiogenic factors, *J. Neurosci.*, 23, 10841, 2003.

164. Lein, E.S., Zhao, X., and Gage, F.H., Defining a molecular atlas of the hippocampus using DNA microarrays and high-throughput in situ hybridization, *J. Neurosci.*, 24, 3879, 2004.

165. Zhao, X. et al., Transcriptional profiling reveals strict boundaries between hippocampal subregions, *J. Comp. Neurol.*, 441, 187, 2001.

166. Del Signore, A. et al., Hippocampal gene expression is modulated by hypergravity, *Eur. J. Neurosci.*, 19, 667, 2004.

167. Gilbert, R.W. et al., DNA microarray analysis of hippocampal gene expression measured twelve hours after hypoxia-ischemia in the mouse, *J. Cereb. Blood Flow Metab.*, 23, 1195, 2003.

168. Qiu, J. et al., Effects of NF-kappaB oligonucleotide "decoys" on gene expression in P7 rat hippocampus after hypoxia/ischemia, *J. Neurosci. Res.*, 77, 108, 2004.

169. Cavallaro, S., D'Agata, V., and Alkon, D.L., Programs of gene expression during the laying down of memory formation as revealed by DNA microarrays, *Neurochem. Res.*, 27, 1201, 2002.

170. Cavallaro, S. et al., Gene expression profiles during long-term memory consolidation, *Eur. J. Neurosci.*, 13, 1809, 2001.

171. Blanton, J.L. et al., Global changes in the expression patterns of RNA isolated from the hippocampus and cortex of VX exposed mice, *J. Biochem. Mol. Toxicol.*, 18, 115, 2004.

172. Marciano, P.G. et al., Expression profiling following traumatic brain injury: a review, *Neurochem. Res.*, 27, 1147, 2002.

173. Colangelo, V. et al., Gene expression profiling of 12633 genes in Alzheimer hippocampal CA1: transcription and neurotrophic factor down-regulation and up-regulation of apoptotic and pro-inflammatory signaling, *J. Neurosci. Res.*, 70, 462, 2002.

174. Becker, A.J., Wiestler, O.D., and Blumcke, I., Functional genomics in experimental and human temporal lobe epilepsy: powerful new tools to identify molecular disease mechanisms of hippocampal damage, *Prog. Brain Res.*, 135, 161, 2002.

175. Ginsberg, S.D. and Che, S., Expression profile analysis within the human hippocampus: comparison of CA1 and CA3 pyramidal neurons, *J. Comp. Neurol.*, 487, 107, 2005.

176. Trojanowski, J.Q. and Lee, V.M., The Alzheimer's brain: finding out what's broken tells us how to fix it, *Am. J. Pathol.*, 167, 1183, 2005.

177. Griffin, W.S. et al., Polyadenylated messenger RNA in paired helical filament-immunoreactive neurons in Alzheimer disease, *Alz. Dis. Assoc. Dis.*, 4, 69, 1990.

178. Harrison, P.J., et al., Regional and neuronal reductions of polyadenylated messenger RNA in Alzheimer's disease, *Psychol. Med.*, 21, 855, 1991.

179. Joyce, J.N. et al., Dopamine D2 receptors in the hippocampus and amygdala in Alzheimer's disease, *Neurosci. Lett.*, 154, 171, 1993.

180. Ryoo, H.L. and Joyce, J.N., Loss of dopamine D2 receptors varies along the rostro-caudal axis of the hippocampal complex in Alzheimer's disease, *J. Comp. Neurol.*, 348, 94, 1994.

181. Emborg, M.E. et al., Age-related declines in nigral neuronal function correlate with motor impairments in rhesus monkeys, *J. Comp. Neurol.*, 401, 253, 1998.

182. Ma, S.Y. et al., Dopamine transporter-immunoreactive neurons decrease with age in the human substantia nigra, *J. Comp. Neurol.*, 409, 25, 1999.

183. Gsell, W., Jungkunz, G., and Riederer, P., Functional neurochemistry of Alzheimer's disease, *Curr. Pharm. Des.*, 10, 265, 2004.

184. Jann, M.W., Implications for atypical antipsychotics in the treatment of schizophrenia: neurocognition effects and a neuroprotective hypothesis, *Pharmacotherapy*, 24, 1759, 2004.

185. Amenta, F. et al., Age-related changes of dopamine receptors in the rat hippocampus: a light microscope autoradiography study, *Mech. Ageing. Dev.*, 122, 2071, 2001.

186. Rinne, J.O., Lonnberg, P., and Marjamaki, P., Age-dependent decline in human brain dopamine D1 and D2 receptors, *Brain Res.*, 508, 349, 1990.

187. Volkow, N.D. et al., Dopamine transporters decrease with age, *J. Nucl. Med.*, 37, 554, 1996.

188. Kosik, K.S., Joachim, C.L., and Selkoe, D.J., Microtubule-associated protein tau is a major antigenic component of paired helical filaments in Alzheimer's disease, *Proc. Natl. Acad. Sci. U.S.A.*, 83, 4044, 1986.

189. Lee, V.M.-Y. et al., A68: a major subunit of paired helical filaments and derivatized forms of normal tau, *Science*, 251, 675, 1991.

190. Goedert, M. and Jakes, R., Mutations causing neurodegenerative tauopathies, *Biochim. Biophys. Acta*, 1739, 240, 2005.

191. Boutajangout, A. et al., Expression of tau mRNA and soluble tau isoforms in affected and non-affected brain areas in Alzheimer's disease, *FEBS Lett.*, 576, 183, 2004.

192. Chambers, C.B. et al., Overexpression of four-repeat tau mRNA isoforms in progressive supranuclear palsy but not in Alzheimer's disease, *Ann. Neurol.*, 46, 325, 1999.

193. Goedert, M. et al., Cloning and sequencing of the cDNA encoding an isoform of microtubule-associated protein tau containing four tandem repeats: differential expression of tau protein mRNAs in human brain, *EMBO J.*, 8, 393, 1989.

194. Hyman, B.T., Augustinack, J.C., and Ingelsson, M., Transcriptional and conformational changes of the tau molecule in Alzheimer's disease, *Biochim. Biophys. Acta*, 1739, 150, 2005.

195. Yasojima, K., McGeer, E.G., and McGeer, P.L., Tangled areas of Alzheimer brain have upregulated levels of exon 10 containing tau mRNA, *Brain Res.*, 831, 301, 1999.

196. Ginsberg, S.D. et al., Shift in the ratio of 3-repeat tau and 4-repeat tau mRNAs in individual cholinergic basal forebrain neurons in mild cognitive impairment and Alzheimer's disease, *J. Neurochem.*, 96, 1401, 2006.

197. Counts, S.E. et al., Galanin fiber hypertrophy within the cholinergic nucleus basalis during the progression of Alzheimer's disease, *Dement. Geriatr. Cogn. Disord.*, 21, 205, 2006.

198. King, M.E. et al., Differential assembly of human tau isoforms in the presence of arachidonic acid, *J. Neurochem.*, 74, 1749, 2000.

199. Levy, S.F. et al., Three- and four-repeat tau regulate the dynamic instability of two distinct microtubule subpopulations in qualitatively different manners. Implications for neurodegeneration, *J. Biol. Chem.*, 280, 13520, 2005.

200. McClain, K.L. et al., Expression profiling using human tissues in combination with RNA amplification and microarray analysis: assessment of Langerhans cell histiocytosis, *Amino Acids*, 28, 279, 2005.

201. Melov, S. and Hubbard, A., Microarrays as a tool to investigate the biology of aging: a retrospective and a look to the future, *Sci. Aging. Knowledge Environ.*, 2004, re7, 2004.

Section III

Assessing Functional Changes in
the Aging Nervous System

8 Subtle Alterations in Glutamatergic Synapses Underlie the Aging-Related Decline in Hippocampal Function

Lei Shi, *Michelle Adams,* *and Judy K. Brunso-Bechtold*

CONTENTS

I.   INTRODUCTION

Aging-related cognitive decline has enormous, tangible costs to national and family health care. The intangible costs are equally detrimental and include decreased

---

* Authors made equal contributions.

quality of life as well as diminished ability to function in and contribute to society. Earlier studies have documented increased difficulties for the elderly on a variety of mental tasks. For example, neuropsychological assessment revealed that after the age of 60, people often have impairments in certain types of memory, particularly recall of recent events (i.e., episodic memory) [1]. A progressive decrease in cognitive ability with advancing age has been well documented not only in humans, but also in rodent models. A clear understanding of the neural changes that accompany aging-related cognitive declines in animal models will aid in the development of strategies to prevent, and therapies to ameliorate, the progression of cognitive decline in the elderly. Although the definition of cognitive function can be broad, including learning and memory, attention, mood, motivation, and planning, the present discussion concentrates on the changes in the cognitive ability most closely associated with the hippocampus. The anatomical, physiological, and biochemical changes in the hippocampus that may contribute to those cognitive abilities also are evaluated.

In this chapter, we will first provide the behavioral evidence characterizing the aging-related decline in performance on hippocampus-dependent tasks in rodent models. We will then consider the aging-related anatomical, physiological, and biochemical changes that occur in the whole hippocampus, as well as in hippocampal subregions. Taken together, the available data suggest that subtle changes in synaptic composition and function, rather than a significant loss of neurons or synapses, are the critical underlying factors for aging-related cognitive decline. The potential for factors such as insulin-like growth factor 1, estrogen, or caloric restriction to impact those aging-related synaptic changes also are considered.

II. BEHAVIORAL CHARACTERIZATION OF AGING-RELATED COGNITIVE DECLINE

A wide variety of behavioral tests have been used to evaluate cognitive changes across the lifespan in rodents, including tests that specifically depend on the hippocampus, such as the radial arm maze [2, 3], the T-mazes [4, 5], and the Morris water maze (MWM) [6, 7]. Of these tests, the most commonly used is the MWM procedure [8]. In this test, a platform is submerged in a circular tank filled with opacified water, and the animal is placed in the water at different starting points. In training trials, spatial learning is assessed as the rat learns to find the hidden platform using spatial cues placed around the perimeter of the tank. Spatial reference memory is assessed in probe trials during which the platform is made unavailable in order to demonstrate whether the rat remembers the location of the platform. Results from the MWM test provide an estimation of spatial learning as well as spatial reference memory and have been correlated with neurobiological markers. Significant impairment on both the training and the probe of MWM has been reported consistently in aged rodents [6, 9–11]. As animals age, they demonstrate an increasingly broad variation in MWM performance. Specifically, some aged animals perform in the same range as young animals, whereas others demonstrate significant impairment [12, 13].

Importantly, the MWM test of spatial learning and reference memory has been shown to depend on the integrity of the hippocampus. In particular, the impairment in MWM performance seen in old rats are quite similar to those seen in young animals with hippocampal lesions [14–16]. MWM performance is a sensitive correlate of hippocampal change in old animals [12, 13, 17], and the hippocampus has been shown to play a dominant role in the acquisition and retrieval of spatial information, as well as in the consolidation and storage of memory [14].

III. MAINTENANCE OF HIPPOCAMPUS NEURONS IN THE AGING BRAIN

The hippocampus or hippocampal formation contains four distinct regions: (1) the dentate gyrus (DG), (2) the hippocampus proper, (3) the subiculum, and (4) the entorhinal cortex (Figure 8.1) [18]. The hippocampus proper includes the CA1, CA2, and CA3 subregions; CA2 and CA3 generally are considered together and unless specified, in the present chapter CA3 will refer to both subregions. Each region of the hippocampus (HC) is comprised of a three-layered cortex. For example, the DG consists of three layers: (1) the molecular layer, containing the outer, middle, and inner molecular sub-layers (OML, MML, IML, respectively; Figure 8.1C); (2) the granule cell layer (asterisk, Figure 8.1C); and (3) the hilus (Figure 8.1C), also referred to as the polymorphic layer [18]. The principal projection neurons of the DG are the granule cells, which are small cells with elliptical somata. They are organized compactly and form an inferior and superior blade in the rat DG. The apical dendrites of the granule cells have a characteristic cone-shaped tree of spiny dendrites with all of the branches directed toward the superficial portion of the molecular layer (Figure 8.1B). The most distal tips of the dendritic tree end just at the hippocampal fissure. In CA1 and CA3, the pyramidal cell layers contain the projection neurons (asterisks, Figure 8.1, D and E). In CA3, the layers dorsomedial to the pyramidal cells contain the apical dendrites of these neurons (Figure 8.1B) and are divided into stratum lucidum, adjacent to the pyramidal cell layer; stratum radiatum; and the most distal sub-layer, stratum lacunosum-moleculare (SL, SR, SL-M, respectively; Figure 8.1D). The layer ventrolateral to the pyramidal cell layer is stratum oriens (SO, Figure 8.1D). In CA1, stratum oriens is dorsal to the pyramidal cell layer (SO, Figure 8.1E) and ventral to the pyramidal cell layer are two sublayers, the proximal stratum radiatum and the distal stratum lacunosum-moleculare (SR, SL-M, respectively; Figure 8.1E). The subregions of the hippocampus are interconnected by largely unidirectional input in a pathway referred to as the trisynaptic pathway (summarized in Figure 8.1B). The flow of information into the hippocampal formation begins with projections from layers II and III of entorhinal cortex to the outer and middle molecular layers of the dentate gyrus; granule cells of the dentate gyrus project to stratum lucidum moleculare of CA3 via the mossy fibers; CA3 pyramidal cells project to stratum radiatum of CA1 via Schaffer collateral input; finally, CA1 pyramidal cells project back to the entorhinal cortex. In addition, there are projections from the entorhinal cortex directly to CA3 and CA1, as well as an intrinsic projection within CA3 to the stratum radiatum.

Early reports proposed that, similar to neurodegenerative diseases such as Alzheimer's [19], aging-related cognitive impairment was associated with a loss of total

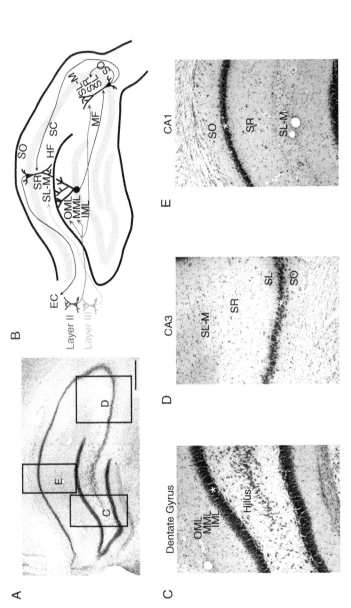

FIGURE 8.1 (SEE COLOR INSERT FOLLOWING PAGE 204) Illustrations depicting the rat hippocampus: (A) a low power photomicrograph showing the hippocampal regions dentate gyrus (C), CA3 (D), and CA1 (E); (B) schematic illustration of the hippocampal circuitry demonstrating the trisynaptic pathway; and (C, D, E) high-power images of hippocampal regions enclosed by the boxes in A. Abbreviations: EC, entorhinal cortex; HF, hippocampal fissure; OML, outer molecular layer; MML, middle molecular layer; IML, inner molecular layer; SL-M, stratum lacunosum moleculare; SR, stratum radiatum; SL, stratum lucidum. * Indicates pyramidal cell layers. (Scale bars: (A) 300 μm and (C–E) 150 μm.)

neurons across the lifespan [20, 21]. However, recent studies using unbiased stereo-logical quantification techniques have shown that the total number of neurons in the granular cell layer of DG as well as the pyramidal cell layers in CA1 and CA3 of hippocampus are maintained throughout life [22–25]. Notably, even in a population of old rats with a wide range of spatial learning abilities, there was no aging-related loss of neurons in the hippocampus [23]. These studies indicate that the aging-related decline in spatial learning and memory is not associated with an overall loss of hippocampal neurons. Such stability of neuron number suggests that the functional impairments in the aging brain are likely to be due to changes in connectivity of existing neurons at structural, physiological, and/or molecular levels.

IV. MAINTENANCE OF ULTRASTRUCTURALLY IDENTIFIED SYNAPSES IN THE AGING HIPPOCAMPUS

One possible anatomical substrate for aging-related learning and memory impairment is a compromise in the synaptic connections within the hippocampus. Synapses are highly labile structures and are responsive to microenvironmental changes in the brain, resulting in a continual refinement of neuronal circuitry [26, 27]. Such synaptic plas-ticity is essential for information storage and for experience-dependent learning and memory, as well as for other phenomena associated with cognition [28, 29]. It is likely that the learning and memory impairment in old animals is associated with synaptic changes in the hippocampus. As the fundamental element of neuronal connectivity, synapses are essential for brain function including information processing and trans-mission [30, 31]. A synapse is composed of a presynaptic component that includes an axon with a presynaptic terminal containing vesicles of neurotransmitter and a postsyn-aptic element, such as a dendritic spine, a dendrite, or cell soma, with a postsynaptic density (PSD) containing an aggregation of neurotransmitter receptors and signaling proteins (Figure 8.2) [32]. In the hippocampus, most synapses are located on dendritic spines that protrude from the dendritic shaft [30, 33].

Although many different techniques have been used to quantify aging synapses, quantification of ultrastructurally identified synapses provides the most accurate estimate. Early studies quantifying synapses in the hippocampus employed non-stereological methods that are inherently biased [34]. More recent studies have used unbiased stereological methods (see Chapter 4) to quantify synapses in individual hippocampal subregions during aging. In DG, a decrease of ultrastructurally defined, axospinous synapses in the middle and inner molecular layers was reported in old (28 months) compared to young (5 months) Fischer-344 rats [35]. Another recent study evaluating ultrastructurally identified synapses in the middle molecular layer of the DG of young (10 months), middle aged (18 months), and old (29 months) Fischer-344 × Brown Norway (F344 × BN) rats [36] found no change across the lifespan, suggesting that after 10 months of age, synapses in the DG of F344 × BN rats have stabilized. A similar stereological study also demonstrated a maintenance of synapses at young (4 months), middle aged (18 months), and old (29 months) F344 × BN rats in the stratum lucidum of hippocampal CA3 [37]. Finally, in CA1,

aged-impaired, and aged-unimpaired, as defined by MWM performance. Semiquantitative Western blot analysis revealed similar levels of the presynaptic markers synaptophysin, synaptotagmin, and SNAP-25 among the three groups, indicating an absence of association of hippocampal levels of these presynaptic proteins with either age or cognitive impairment. In another study, Smith et al. [60] used confocal laser microscopy to quantify synaptophysin immunoreactivity in different layers of hippocampal subregions of behaviorally characterized young and aged Long-Evans rats. The results suggested that the intensity of synaptophysin immunoreactivity, averaged across the whole hippocampus did not differ among the young, aged impaired, or aged unimpaired groups. Interestingly, however, the synaptophysin immunoreactivity was significantly lower in stratum lacunosum moleculare of CA3 in aged rats with spatial learning deficits compared to the other two groups. Moreover, there also was a significant correlation between the MWM performance of aged rats and the intensity of synaptophysin immunoreactivity in the outer molecular and middle molecular layers of DG, as well as in the stratum lacunosum moleculare of CA3. Utilizing synaptophysin immunoreactivity as a marker to quantify presynaptic boutons at the light microscopic level of C57BL/6 mice, stereological quantification did not reveal any differences on this measure among young, middle-aged, and old animals in either DG, CA3, or CA1 [25]. Thus, aging-related spatial learning impairments occur in the absence of marked, widely distributed changes in hippocampal presynaptic markers, although limited changes do occur in specific layers of hippocampal subregions.

B.   POSTSYNAPTIC NMDA AND AMPA RECEPTOR SUBUNITS

Nearly all presynaptic terminals that contact dendritic spines release the excitatory neurotransmitter glutamate, and receptors for glutamate are integral components of the postsynaptic membrane. The postsynaptic membrane of a typical hippocampal spine contains at least two distinct types of glutamate receptors: (1) AMPA and (2) NMDA receptors [32, 61]. These receptors are the primary mediators of excitatory synaptic transmission in the central nervous system [62] and are required for hippocampal synaptic plasticity, as well as for spatial learning and memory [63–65]. Moreover, NMDA and AMPA receptors have been implicated in the structural changes associated with synaptic plasticity, including synapse formation, maintenance, and remodeling [43, 44, 66].

The majority of functional NMDA receptors are hetero-oligomers composed of NR1 and different NR2 subunits, including NR2A and NR2B [67–70]. NR1 is the organizing subunit that is essential for NMDA receptor formation and function. Therefore, NR1 is an obligatory subunit for normal functioning NMDA receptors, in combination with NR2 subunits. In the hippocampus, heteromeric NMDA receptors composed of NR1 with NR2A or NR2B subunits demonstrate significantly higher efficacy than homomeric receptors composed of NR1 alone [67–69]. NMDA receptor activation depends on glutamate binding (with glycine as a co-agonist) and membrane depolarization to remove the Mg^{2+} ion blocking the channel pore [71, 72]. The requirement of two separate events to open NMDA receptors enables them to function as "molecular coincidence detectors" and makes them uniquely suitable for mediating Hebbian plasticity [73–75]. Moreover, it has been established that activation of NMDA receptors is critical for the induction and maintenance of synaptic plasticity in the hippocampus [76–78].

AMPA receptors are composed of GluR1–4 subunits. In this class of glutamate receptors, GluR2 is the organizing subunit that is critical for AMPA receptor assembly and expression [79]. GluR2 also renders AMPA receptors more resistant to excitotoxicity in response to biological challenge by decreasing Ca^{2+} permeability [79–82]. The GluR1 subunit is essential for the formation of heteromeric AMPA receptors, which demonstrate higher conductance capacity compared to homomeric receptors formed by GluR2 alone [80–82]. In contrast with the relatively slow kinetics of the NMDA receptors, AMPA receptor activation accounts for fast postsynaptic responses [83, 84]. Compelling electrophysiological evidence indicates that the number of postsynaptic AMPA receptors is a major determinant of synaptic efficacy [85–87].

Recent studies have reported an aging-related loss of subunits of the NMDA and AMPA types of glutamate receptors in the hippocampus as well as a decline in glutamate-mediated excitatory transmission [70, 88–91]. The loss and/or diminished function of NMDA and AMPA receptors can contribute not only to impaired synaptic transmission, but also to ultrastructural changes that occur in the PSD of synapses in the aging hippocampus. Previous studies have addressed the issue of aging-related changes in hippocampal levels of NMDA and AMPA receptors in different animal models, ages, and regions, using a variety of technical approaches [92–94]. NMDA receptor binding in subdissected hippocampus of Sprague-Dawley rats revealed an overall decrease in NMDA receptors between very young (3 months) and old animals (25 to 29 months) in CA1 and CA3, but not in DG [95]. In whole hippocampus, NMDA subunits NR1 [89, 90, 96], NR2A [97], and NR2B [88, 89, 96, 97], as well as the AMPA subunits GluR1 and GluR2 [88, 89, 96, 97], have been reported to decline with age. Moreover, recent studies using Western blot analysis of subdissected hippocampal subregions indicate a decline in NMDA and AMPA subunits across the lifespan in CA1 and CA3, and to a lesser degree in DG (black bars, Figure 8.3) [36, 39, 98]. Interestingly, by including a middle-aged group (18 months) as well as a young (10 months) and an old group (28 months), these studies were able to reveal that all of the aging-related subunit declines, except for the AMPA subunit GluR2 in CA3, occurred not between middle and old age, but between young and middle age (Figure 8.3).

Based on the functional significance of glutamate receptor subunits, it is likely that declines in NMDA and AMPA receptor subunits are associated with impaired synaptic plasticity. For example, as both NMDA and AMPA receptor subunits are essential for LTP induction and maintenance [86, 88, 99, 100], the aging-related loss and/or functional impairment of glutamate receptors can contribute to the LTP deficits in the brains of aged animals [14, 101–105]. Declines in NMDA and AMPA receptors each induce cellular changes. Specifically, the aging-related decrease of functional NMDA receptors in rats has been shown to lead to impaired synaptic transmission and LTP induction, and thus to compromised synaptic plasticity [76, 78, 88, 89, 96, 97]. As AMPA receptors mediate most of the fast excitatory synaptic transmission and their number is the major determinant of synaptic efficacy [85], an aging-related loss of these receptors is also associated with impaired synaptic transmission and compromised synaptic plasticity [106]. Moreover, a diminished expression of AMPA

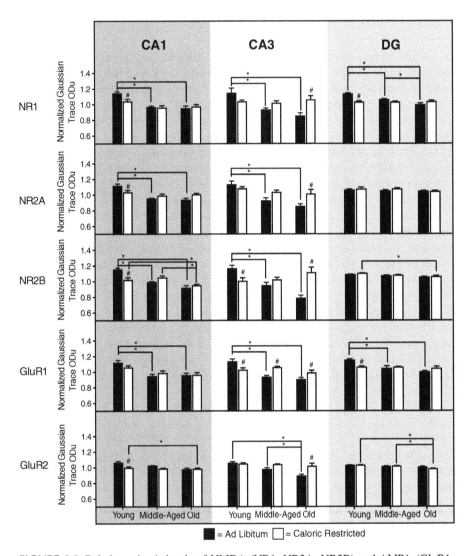

FIGURE 8.3 Relative subunit levels of NMDA (NR1, NR2A, NR2B) and AMPA (GluR1, GluR2) subtypes of glutamate receptors in CA1, CA3, and DG (dentate gyrus) of young (10 months), middle-aged young (18 months), and old young (28 months) F344 × BN rats that were fed *ad libitum* (AL, black bars) or caloric restricted (CR, white bars) beginning at 4 months of age. *p < 0.05 for indicated comparisons; #p < 0.05 compared to age-matched AL.

receptors in both perforated and nonperforated synapses may have a deleterious effect on cognitive function, even when the synapse number is constant [38]. Without AMPA receptors, glutamatergic synapses in hippocampus are functionally silent. Thus, a loss of AMPA receptors may transform functional synapses into silent ones during aging and contribute to aging-related cognitive impairment [48, 49].

The hippocampal levels of NMDA/AMPA receptors also have been correlated directly with cognitive performance, particularly on spatial learning and memory tasks [88, 107]. For example, experimental reduction of NMDA or AMPA receptors or of their specific subunits using transgenic rodent models has resulted in deficits in spatial learning and memory [63, 64, 78, 88, 108–110]. Similarly, spatial learning and memory were impaired by administration of NMDA receptor antagonists [111–113]. Moreover, in aged animals with impaired MWM performance, both decreased levels of NMDA and AMPA receptor subunits and impaired synaptic transmission via those receptors have been reported [88, 89, 91, 96, 97]. Finally, even in the absence of a global aging-related decrease in hippocampal glutamate receptors, glutamate receptor subunits levels are correlated with cognitive performance. For example, although neither Western blot analysis nor confocal immunocytochemistry revealed an overall or region-specific difference in hippocampal NR1 levels between young and aged animals [107], individual spatial learning performance correlated with NR1 immunofluorescence levels in hippocampal CA3 neurons. These findings suggest that dendritic NR1 is generally preserved in the hippocampus of aged rats but the levels of this receptor subunit in selective elements of hippocampal circuitry are linked to spatial learning.

VII. FACTORS THAT CONTRIBUTE TO AGING-RELATED CHANGES IN HIPPOCAMPAL SYNAPSES: POTENTIAL THERAPEUTIC STRATEGIES

Although synaptic changes such as those described in this chapter may contribute to aging-associated learning and memory impairment, the mechanisms underlying these changes have not been characterized fully. Nevertheless, microenvironmental changes in the aging brain may be key elements in the functional decline that occurs across the lifespan. In particular, evidence suggests that insulin-like growth factor-1 (IGF-1), estrogen, and calorie restriction are microenvironmental factors that may have significant impacts on the structure and/or function of synapses in senescent animals.

A. INSULIN-LIKE GROWTH FACTOR-1 (IGF-1)

IGF-1 is a growth factor that can influence a broad range of physiological processes in the brain (see Chapter 12). Importantly, brain levels of IGF-1 have been associated with spatial learning and memory performance on the MWM [11, 97]. IGF-1 has been shown to support diverse aspects of synaptic function, including nerve regeneration and synaptogenesis at the neuromuscular junction and in the DG of hippocampus [114–118]. In addition, IGF-1 exerts trophic effects on both the pre- and postsynaptic compartments. Presynaptically, the extent of axonal sprouting in rat DG correlates with the level of IGF-1 expression [119]. Postsynaptically, IGF-1 stimulates dendritic branching of cortical neurons in organotypic slice culture [120]. Moreover, it is essential for the maintenance of dendritic length and complexity as well as the density of dendritic spines on pyramidal cells in frontoparietal cortex [121]. These findings suggest that IGF-1 exerts a significant influence on the formation and maintenance of neuronal connectivity in the rodent central nervous system.

Serum and brain levels of IGF-1 [122], as well as brain levels of the type 1 IGF receptor [123], have been reported to decline in the aging brain. Moreover, aged rodents

(AL) live 20 to 40% longer than AL animals [152–154]. Not only does CR extend lifespan, but it also retards aging by delaying the onset of various diseases as well as by attenuating spatial learning and memory deficits [153, 155, 156]. For example, the aging-related impairment on MWM performance in old F344 × BN rats was ameliorated by CR [157]. Similarly, life-long CR ameliorated the aging-related impairment of spatial learning and memory in C57B1/6 mice [158]. Aging-related changes in synaptic plasticity and neurotransmitter systems can be ameliorated by CR as well. Specifically, CR prevents the deficit in LTP induction in the hippocampus of old F-344 rats and may do so by ameliorating the compromise of NMDA-mediated transmission in the aging brain [158–160].

Recent studies in our laboratory suggested that aging-related declines in subunits of hippocampal NMDA and AMPA receptors in F344 × BN rats do not occur in rats on a CR diet. As described previously and illustrated in Figure 8.3, in both CA1 and CA3, levels of most NMDA and AMPA subunits decrease significantly between young and middle age and remain stable thereafter in AL rats. In contrast, subunit levels are significantly lower in young CR compared to young AL rats, and those lower levels are maintained across the lifespan in CR rats. In CA3, the levels of most receptor subunits are significantly higher in old CR compared to old AL rats. Importantly, this difference is not due to *elevated* subunit levels in old CR rats, but rather to significantly *reduced* subunit levels in old AL rats. In DG, only NR1 and GluR1 subunits decrease with age in AL rats. Nevertheless, as in CA1 and CA3, those subunits are significantly lower in young CR compared to young AL rats and remain stable at middle and old age. Accordingly, CR changes the progressive pattern of aging-related declines in NMDA and AMPA receptor subunits and induces a metabolic stability for these glutamate receptor subunits. Importantly, in both AL and CR rats, ultrastructurally identified synapses in CA1 and DG were stable across the lifespan. Thus, despite some regional and subunit variations, NMDA and AMPA receptor subunit levels in AL and CR animals across the lifespan reveal three overall trends that are more evident in CA1 and CA3 than in DG. First, there is an aging-related decline in NMDA and AMPA receptor subunit levels in AL rats. Second, subunit levels are lower in young CR than in young AL rats. Third, subunit levels of most NMDA and AMPA receptor subunits are the same in young, middle-aged, and old CR rats.

The available evidence suggests that the capacity of an organism to maintain steady state is a prime determinant of longevity. Senescence-related loss of function is due to impairment of a homeostatic state and CR enhances longevity by increasing metabolic stability [161]. Evidence suggests that metabolic stability is a better predictor of longevity than metabolic rate, and an organism's ability to maintain stable levels of free radicals may be more important than how fast it produces them [162, 163]. CR delays deleterious consequences of aging by inducing a stable state of biological parameters that normally demonstrate aging-related declines [164, 165]. Moreover, in the presence of continued CR, a stable state in those parameters is maintained across the lifespan [161, 164]. Thus, it may be that changes in critical biological parameters result in functional decline in the aging brain, and CR may eliminate such changes by inducing a stable state in those parameters.

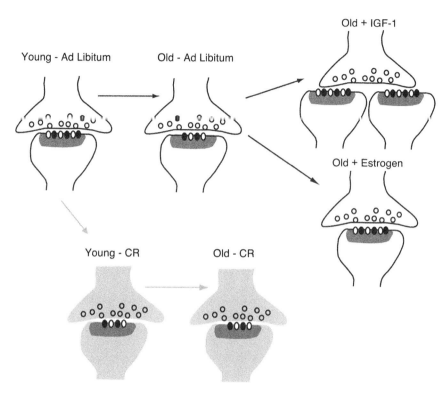

FIGURE 8.4 A schematic diagram illustrating age-related changes in excitatory synapses and the effects of IGF-1, estrogen, and caloric restriction on these synapses. Aging is associated with a decrease in synaptic glutamate receptors. Both IGF-1 and estrogen increase glutamate receptor subunit levels and IGF-1 also increases the number of multiple spine bouton synapses. Caloric restriction decreases glutamate receptor subunit levels in young animals, but then maintains those levels across the lifespan. Note the black and white ovals represent AMPA and NMDA glutamate receptor subunits, the open circles represent synaptic vesicles, and the dark gray zone represents the postsynaptic density.

VIII. SUMMARY

Aging-related cognitive impairment is reflected in performance deficits on hippocampal-dependent tasks such as the MWM test of spatial learning and memory. Although changes in hippocampal synapses are likely to underlie this cognitive impairment, there is little, if any, aging-related loss of synapses. Consequently, it appears that overall synapse loss is not a determining factor for this aging-related impairment of cognitive performance. In contrast, subtle synaptic changes, including loss of glutamate receptors in hippocampal subregions, occur across the lifespan (Young-*Ad Libitum* → Old-*Ad Libitum*; Figure 8.4) and these subtle changes may well contribute to aging-related cognitive impairment. Significantly, several manipulations that have been associated with amelioration of aging-related cognitive impairment also modify the aging-related changes that occur in the numerically stable population of hippocampal synapses. For example, IGF-1 can increase the number of MSB synapses (Old + IGF-1; Figure 8.4) and estrogen can increase the number of NR1 subunits in the PSD (Old + Estrogen; Figure 8.4). NMDA and AMPA subunit levels in young CR rats are lower than in young AL rats; however, in CR rats, those subunit levels of glutamate receptors do not change between young and old age (Young-CR → Old-CR; Figure 8.4). In summary, future studies of hormonal and metabolic interventions that can impact subtle, but functionally integral aspects of synapses may provide clues to potential therapeutic strategies for the amelioration of cognitive decline in the elderly.

REFERENCES

1. Shimamura, A.P., Neuropsychological perspectives on memory and cognitive decline in normal human aging., *Sem. Neurosci.*, 6, 387, 1994.
2. Detoledo-Morrell, L., Geinisman, Y., and Morrell, F., Age-dependent alterations in hippocampal synaptic plasticity: relation to memory disorders, *Neurobiol. Aging*, 9, 581, 1988.
3. Ingram, D.K., London, E.D., and Goodrick, C.L., Age and neurochemical correlates of radial maze performance in rats, *Neurobiol. Aging*, 2, 41, 1981.
4. Liu, P. et al., Hippocampal nitric oxide synthase and arginase and age-associated behavioral deficits, *Hippocampus*, 15, 642, 2005.
5. Ordy, J.M. et al., An animal model of human-type memory loss based on aging, lesion, forebrain ischemia, and drug studies with the rat, *Neurobiol. Aging*, 9, 667, 1988.
6. Gage, F.H. et al., Experimental approaches to age-related cognitive impairments, *Neurobiol. Aging*, 9, 645, 1988.
7. Engstrom, D.A. et al., Increased responsiveness of hippocampal pyramidal neurons to nicotine in aged, learning-impaired rats, *Neurobiol. Aging*, 14, 259, 1993.
8. Morris, R., Developments of a water-maze procedure for studying spatial learning in the rat, *J. Neurosci. Meth.*, 11, 47, 1984.
9. Barnes, C.A. et al., Acetyl-1-carnitine. 2. Effects on learning and memory performance of aged rats in simple and complex mazes, *Neurobiol. Aging*, 11, 499, 1990.
10. Gallagher, M., Burwell, R., and Burchinal, M., Severity of spatial learning impairment in aging: development of a learning index for performance in the Morris water maze, *Behav. Neurosci.*, 107, 618, 1993.
11. Markowska, A.L., Mooney, M., and Sonntag, W.E., Insulin-like growth factor-1 ameliorates age-related behavioral deficits, *Neuroscience*, 87, 559, 1998.
12. Zhang, H.Y. et al., Muscarinic receptor-mediated GTP-Eu binding in the hippocampus and prefrontal cortex is correlated with spatial memory impairment in aged rats, *Neurobiol. Aging*, in press, 2007.
13. Nicholson, D.A. et al., Reduction in size of perforated postsynaptic densities in hippocampal axospinous synapses and age-related spatial learning impairments, *J. Neurosci.*, 24, 7648, 2004.
14. D'Hooge, R. and De Deyn, P.P., Applications of the Morris water maze in the study of learning and memory, *Brain Res. Brain Res. Rev.*, 36, 60, 2001.
15. Moser, E., Moser, M.B., and Andersen, P., Spatial learning impairment parallels the magnitude of dorsal hippocampal lesions, but is hardly present following ventral lesions, *J. Neurosci.*, 13, 3916, 1993.

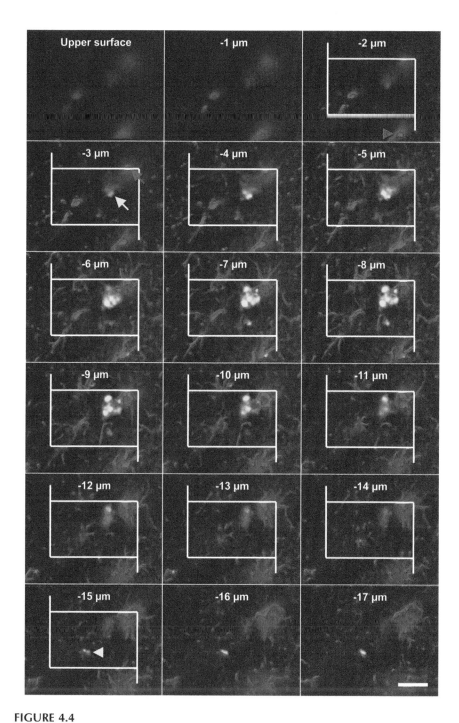

FIGURE 4.4

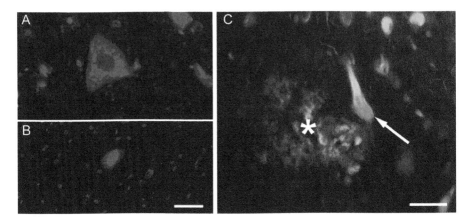

FIGURE 7.1

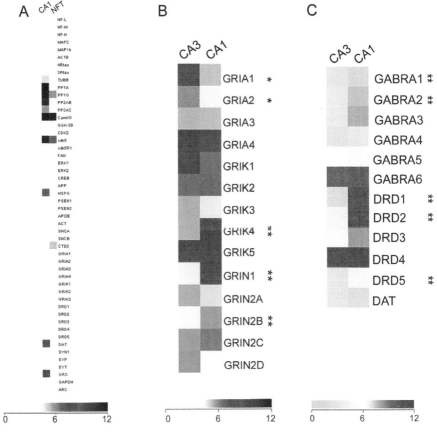

FIGURE 7.3

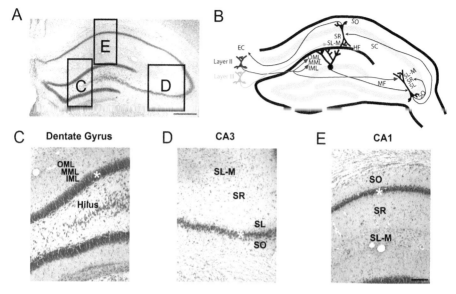

FIGURE 8.1

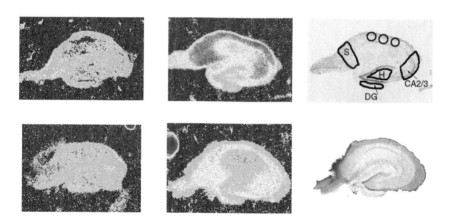

FIGURE 9.6

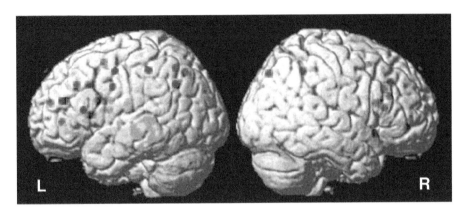

FIGURE 11.2

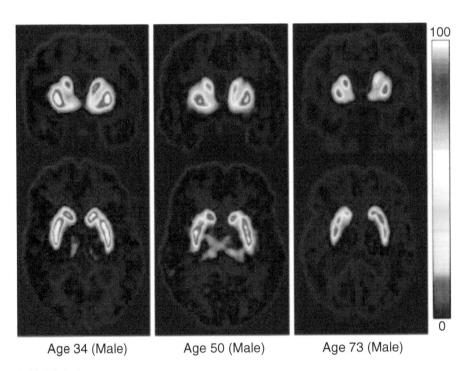

| Age 34 (Male) | Age 50 (Male) | Age 73 (Male) |

FIGURE 11.3

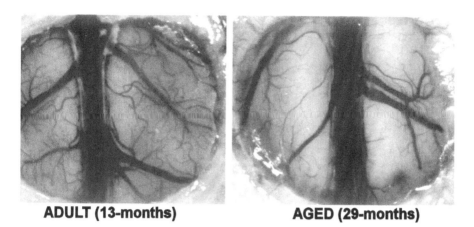

ADULT (13-months) **AGED (29-months)**

FIGURE 12.1

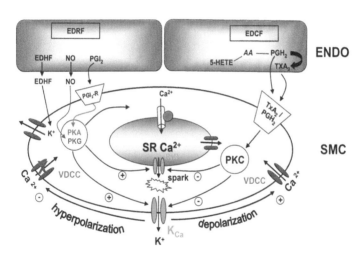

FIGURE 12.3

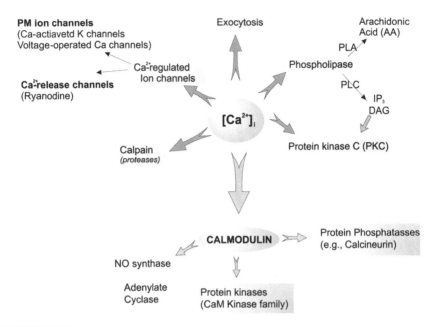

FIGURE 14.1

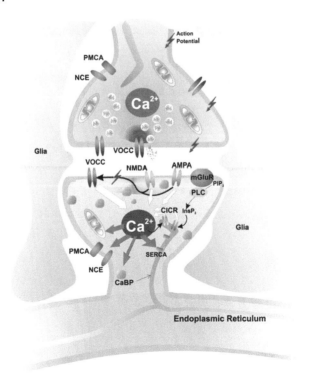

FIGURE 14.2

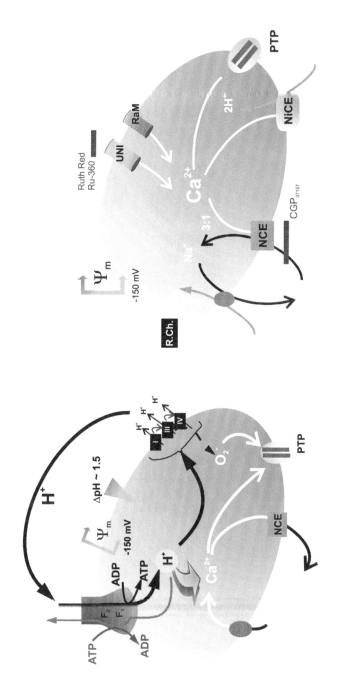

FIGURE 14.3

Control   Blueberry   Spinach   Spirulina

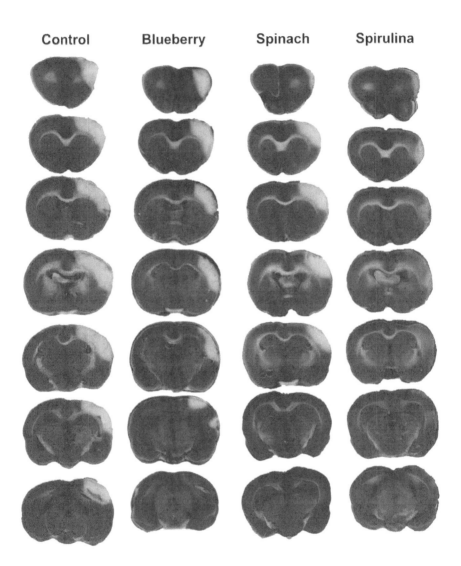

FIGURE 15.3

16. Morris, R.G. et al., Ibotenate lesions of hippocampus and/or subiculum: dissociating components of allocentric spatial learning, *Eur. J. Neurosci.*, 2, 1016, 1990.

17. Tombaugh, G.C., Rowe, W.B., and Rose, G.M., The slow afterhyperpolarization in hippocampal CA1 neurons covaries with spatial learning ability in aged Fisher 344 rats, *J. Neurosci.*, 25, 2609, 2005.

18. Johnston, D. and Amaral, D., Hippocampus, in *The Synaptic Organization of the Brain*, 5th ed., Shepherd, G., Ed., Oxford, 2004, chap. 11.

19. Morrison, J.H. and Hof, P.R., Life and death of neurons in the aging brain, *Science*, 278, 412, 1997.

20. Henderson, G., Tomlinson, B.E., and Gibson, P.H., Cell counts in human cerebral cortex in normal adults throughout life using an image analysing computer, *J. Neurol. Sci.*, 46, 113, 1980.

21. Devaney, K.O. and Johnson, H.A., Neuron loss in the aging visual cortex of man, *J. Gerontol.*, 35, 836, 1980.

22. West, M.J., Slomianka, L., and Gundersen, H.J., Unbiased stereological estimation of the total number of neurons in thesubdivisions of the rat hippocampus using the optical fractionator, *Anat. Rec.*, 231, 482, 1991.

23. Rapp, P.R. and Gallagher, M., Preserved neuron number in the hippocampus of aged rats with spatial learning deficits, *Proc. Natl. Acad. Sci. U.S.A.*, 93, 9926, 1996.

24. Rasmussen, T. et al., Memory impaired aged rats: no loss of principal hippocampal and subicular neurons, *Neurobiol. Aging*, 17, 143, 1996.

25. Calhoun, M.E. et al., Hippocampal neuron and synaptophysin-positive bouton number in aging C57BL/6 mice, *Neurobiol. Aging*, 19, 599, 1998.

26. Causing, C.G. et al., Synaptic innervation density is regulated by neuron-derived BDNF, *Neuron*, 18, 257, 1997.

27. Adams, B. et al., Nerve growth factor accelerates seizure development, enhances mossy fiber sprouting, and attenuates seizure-induced decreases in neuronal density in the kindling model of epilepsy, *J. Neurosci.*, 17, 5288, 1997.

28. Burke, S.N. and Barnes, C.A., Neural plasticity in the ageing brain, *Nat. Rev. Neurosci.*, 7, 30, 2006.

29. Martin, S.J., Grimwood, P.D., and Morris, R.G., Synaptic plasticity and memory: an evaluation of the hypothesis, *Annu. Rev. Neurosci.*, 23, 649, 2000.

30. Sorra, K.E. and Harris, K.M., Overview on the structure, composition, function, development, and plasticity of hippocampal dendritic spines, *Hippocampus*, 10, 501, 2000.

31. Harris, K.M., Structure, development, and plasticity of dendritic spines, *Curr. Opin. Neurobiol.*, 9, 343, 1999.

32. Kennedy, M.B., Signal-processing machines at the postsynaptic density, *Science*, 290, 750, 2000.

33. Matus, A., Brinkhaus, H., and Wagner, U., Actin dynamics in dendritic spines: a form of regulated plasticity at excitatory synapses, *Hippocampus*, 10, 555, 2000.

34. Geinisman, Y. et al., Hippocampal markers of age-related memory dysfunction: behavioral, electrophysiological and morphological perspectives, *Prog. Neurobiol.*, 45, 223, 1995.

35. Geinisman, Y. et al., Age-related loss of axospinous synapses formed by two afferent systems in the rat dentate gyrus as revealed by the unbiased stereological dissector technique, *Hippocampus*, 2, 437, 1992.

36. Linville, C. et al., Synapse number is unchanged across lifespan in calorically restricted Fisher 344 × Brown Norway rats, *Soc. Neurosci. Abst.*, 35, 848.14, 2005.

37. Poe, B.H. et al., Effects of age and insulin-like growth factor-1 on neuron and synapse numbers in area CA3 of hippocampus, *Neuroscience*, 107, 231, 2001.
38. Geinisman, Y. et al., Aging, spatial learning, and total synapse number in the rat CA1 stratum radiatum, *Neurobiol. Aging*, 25, 407, 2004.
39. Shi, L. et al., Effects of caloric restriction (CR) or NMDA/AMPA receptors and multiple spine bouton (MSB) synapses in hippocampal CAI across lifespan, *Amer. Aging Assoc. Abst.*, 34, 44, 2005.
40. Geinisman, Y., Structural synaptic modifications associated with hippocampal LTP and behavioral learning, *Cereb. Cortex*, 10, 952, 2000.
41. Buchs, P.A. and Muller, D., Induction of long-term potentiation is associated with major ultrastructural changes of activated synapses, *Proc. Natl. Acad. Sci. U.S.A.*, 93, 8040, 1996.
42. Toni, N. et al., Remodeling of synaptic membranes after induction of long-term potentiation, *J. Neurosci.*, 21, 6245, 2001.
43. Hering, H. and Sheng, M., Dendritic spines: structure, dynamics and regulation, *Nat. Rev. Neurosci.*, 2, 880, 2001.
44. Luscher, C. et al., Synaptic plasticity and dynamic modulation of the postsynaptic membrane, *Nat. Neurosci.*, 3, 545, 2000.
45. Ziff, E.B., Enlightening the postsynaptic density, *Neuron*, 19, 1163, 1997.
46. Baude, A. et al., High-resolution immunogold localization of AMPA type glutamate receptor subunits at synaptic and non-synaptic sites in rat hippocampus, *Neuroscience*, 69, 1031, 1995.
47. Desmond, N.L. and Weinberg, R.J., Enhanced expression of AMPA receptor protein at perforated axospinous synapses, *Neuroreport*, 9, 857, 1998.
48. Ganeshina, O. et al., Synapses with a segmented, completely partitioned postsynaptic density express more AMPA receptors than other axospinous synaptic junctions, *Neuroscience*, 125, 615, 2004.
49. Ganeshina, O. et al., Differences in the expression of AMPA and NMDA receptors between axospinous perforated and nonperforated synapses are related to the configuration and size of postsynaptic densities, *J. Comp Neurol.*, 468, 86, 2004.
50. Geinisman, Y. et al., Associative learning elicits the formation of multiple-synapse boutons, *J. Neurosci.*, 21, 5568, 2001.
51. Nikonenko, I. et al., Activity-induced changes of spine morphology, *Hippocampus*, 12, 585, 2002.
52. Jones, T.A. et al., Induction of multiple synapses by experience in the visual cortex of adult rats, *Neurobiol. Learn. Mem.*, 68, 13, 1997.
53. Toni, N. et al., LTP promotes formation of multiple spine synapses between a single axon terminal and a dendrite, *Nature*, 402, 421, 1999.
54. Jones, T.A., Multiple synapse formation in the motor cortex opposite unilateral sensorimotor cortex lesions in adult rats, *J. Comp Neurol.*, 414, 57, 1999.
55. Sorra, K.E., Fiala, J.C., and Harris, K.M., Critical assessment of the involvement of perforations, spinules, and spine branching in hippocampal synapse formation, *J. Comp Neurol.*, 398, 225, 1998.
56. Neuhoff, H., Roeper, J., and Schweizer, M., Activity-dependent formation of perforated synapses in cultured hippocampal neurons, *Eur. J. Neurosci.*, 11, 4241, 1999.
57. Jones, T.A. et al., Motor skills training enhances lesion-induced structural plasticity in the motor cortex of adult rats, *J. Neurosci.*, 19, 10153, 1999.
58. Shi, L. et al., Differential effects of aging and insulin-like growth factor-1 on synapses in CA1 of rat hippocampus, *Cereb. Cortex*, 15, 571, 2005.

59. Nicolle, M.M., Gallagher, M., and McKinney, M., No loss of synaptic proteins in the hippocampus of aged, behaviorally impaired rats, *Neurobiol. Aging*, 20, 343, 1999.

60. Smith, T.D. et al., Circuit-specific alterations in hippocampal synaptophysin immunoreactivity predict spatial learning impairment in aged rats, *J. Neurosci.*, 20, 6587, 2000.

61. Takumi, Y. et al., Different modes of expression of AMPA and NMDA receptors in hippocampal synapses, *Nat. Neurosci.*, 2, 618, 1999.

62. Hollmann, M. and Heinemann, S., Cloned glutamate receptors, *Annu. Rev. Neurosci.*, 17, 31, 1994.

63. McHugh, T.J. et al., Impaired hippocampal representation of space in CA1-specific NMDAR1 knockout mice, *Cell*, 87, 1339, 1996.

64. Nakazawa, K. et al., Requirement for hippocampal CA3 NMDA receptors in associative memory recall, *Science*, 297, 211, 2002.

65. Lee, H.K. et al., Phosphorylation of the AMPA receptor GluR1 subunit is required for synaptic plasticity and retention of spatial memory, *Cell*, 112, 631, 2003.

66. Fischer, M. et al., Glutamate receptors regulate actin-based plasticity in dendritic spines, *Nat. Neurosci.*, 3, 887, 2000.

67. Monyer, H. et al., Heteromeric NMDA receptors: molecular and functional distinction of subtypes, *Science*, 256, 1217, 1992.

68. Kutsuwada, T. et al., Molecular diversity of the NMDA receptor channel, *Nature*, 358, 36, 1992.

69. Meguro, H. et al., Functional characterization of a heteromeric NMDA receptor channel expressed from cloned cDNAs, *Nature*, 357, 70, 1992.

70. Barria, A. and Malinow, R., Subunit-specific NMDA receptor trafficking to synapses, *Neuron*, 35, 345, 2002.

71. Riedel, G., Platt, B., and Micheau, J., Glutamate receptor function in learning and memory, *Behav. Brain Res.*, 140, 1, 2003.

72. MacDonald, J.F. and Nowak, L.M., Mechanisms of blockade of excitatory amino acid receptor channels, *Trends Pharmacol. Sci.*, 11, 167, 1990.

73. Collingridge, G.L. and Singer, W., Excitatory amino acid receptors and synaptic plasticity, *Trends Pharmacol. Sci.*, 11, 290, 1990.

74. Zador, A., Koch, C., and Brown, T.H., Biophysical model of a Hebbian synapse, *Proc. Natl. Acad. Sci. U.S.A.*, 87, 6718, 1990.

75. Schiller, J., Schiller, Y., and Clapham, D.E., NMDA receptors amplify calcium influx into dendritic spines during associative pre- and postsynaptic activation, *Nat. Neurosci.*, 1, 114, 1998.

76. Potier, B. et al., NMDA receptor activation in the aged rat hippocampus, *Exp. Gerontol.*, 35, 1185, 2000.

77. Malenka, R.C. and Nicoll, R.A., NMDA-receptor-dependent synaptic plasticity: multiple forms and mechanisms, *Trends Neurosci.*, 16, 521, 1993.

78. Tsien, J.Z., Huerta, P.T., and Tonegawa, S., The essential role of hippocampal CA1 NMDA receptor-dependent synaptic plasticity in spatial memory, *Cell*, 87, 1327, 1996.

79. Sans, N. et al., Aberrant formation of glutamate receptor complexes in hippocampal neurons of mice lacking the GluR2 AMPA receptor subunit, *J. Neurosci.*, 23, 9367, 2003.

80. Boulter, J. et al., Molecular cloning and functional expression of glutamate receptor subunit genes, *Science*, 249, 1033, 1990.

81. Nakanishi, N., Shneider, N.A., and Axel, R., A family of glutamate receptor genes: evidence for the formation of heteromultimeric receptors with distinct channel properties, *Neuron*, 5, 569, 1990.

82. Verdoorn, T.A. et al., Structural determinants of ion flow through recombinant glutamate receptor channels, *Science*, 252, 1715, 1991.

83. Spruston, N., Jonas, P., and Sakmann, B., Dendritic glutamate receptor channels in rat hippocampal CA3 and CA1 pyramidal neurons, *J. Physiol*, 482(Pt 2), 325, 1995.

84. Umemiya, M., Senda, M., and Murphy, T.H., Behaviour of NMDA and AMPA receptor-mediated miniature EPSCs at rat cortical neuron synapses identified by calcium imaging, *J. Physiol*, 521(Pt. 1), 113, 1999.

85. Malenka, R.C. and Nicoll, R.A., Long-term potentiation—a decade of progress? *Science*, 285, 1870, 1999.

86. Malinow, R. and Malenka, R.C., AMPA receptor trafficking and synaptic plasticity, *Annu. Rev. Neurosci.*, 25, 103, 2002.

87. Luscher, C. et al., Role of AMPA receptor cycling in synaptic transmission and plasticity, *Neuron*, 24, 649, 1999.

88. Clayton, D.A. et al., A hippocampal NR2B deficit can mimic age-related changes in long-term potentiation and spatial learning in the Fischer 344 rat, *J. Neurosci.*, 22, 3628, 2002.

89. Clayton, D.A. and Browning, M.D., Deficits in the expression of the NR2B subunit in the hippocampus of aged Fisher 344 rats, *Neurobiol. Aging*, 22, 165, 2001.

90. Magnusson, K.R., Nelson, S.E., and Young, A.B., Age-related changes in the protein expression of subunits of the NMDA receptor, *Brain Res. Mol. Brain Res.*, 99, 40, 2002.

91. Newcomer, J.W. and Krystal, J.H., NMDA receptor regulation of memory and behavior in humans, *Hippocampus*, 11, 529, 2001.

92. Tamaru, M. et al., Age-related decreases of the N-methyl-D-aspartate receptor complex in the rat cerebral cortex and hippocampus, *Brain Res.*, 542, 83, 1991.

93. Wenk, G.L. et al., Loss of NMDA, but not GABA-A, binding in the brains of aged rats and monkeys, *Neurobiol. Aging*, 12, 93, 1991.

94. Magnusson, K.R. and Cotman, C.W., Age-related changes in excitatory amino acid receptors in two mouse strains, *Neurobiol. Aging*, 14, 197, 1993.

95. Wenk, G.L. and Barnes, C.A., Regional changes in the hippocampal density of AMPA and NMDA receptors across the lifespan of the rat, *Brain Res.*, 885, 1, 2000.

96. Mesches, M.H. et al., Sulindac improves memory and increases NMDA receptor subunits in aged Fischer 344 rats, *Neurobiol. Aging*, 25, 315, 2004.

97. Sonntag, W.E. et al., Age and insulin-like growth factor-1 modulate N-methyl-D-aspartate receptor subtype expression in rats, *Brain Res. Bull.*, 51, 331, 2000.

98. Adams M.M. et al., Effect of caloric restriction and age on synaptic proteins in hippocampal CA3, *Soc. Neurosci. Abst.*, 35, 731.13, 2005.

99. Grosshans, D.R. et al., Analysis of glutamate receptor surface expression in acute hippocampal slices, *Sci. STKE.*, 2002, L8, 2002.

100. Hayashi, Y. et al., Driving AMPA receptors into synapses by LTP and CaMKII: requirement for GluR1 and PDZ domain interaction, *Science*, 287, 2262, 2000.

101. Bach, M.E. et al., Age-related defects in spatial memory are correlated with defects in the late phase of hippocampal long-term potentiation *in vitro* and are attenuated by drugs that enhance the cAMP signaling pathway, *Proc. Natl. Acad. Sci. U.S.A.*, 96, 5280, 1999.

102. Rosenzweig, E.S. et al., Role of temporal summation in age-related long-term potentiation-induction deficits, *Hippocampus*, 7, 549, 1997.

103. Tombaugh, G.C. et al., Theta-frequency synaptic potentiation in CA1 in vitro distinguishes cognitively impaired from unimpaired aged Fischer 344 rats, *J. Neurosci.*, 22, 9932, 2002.

104. Oh, M.M. et al., Watermaze learning enhances excitability of CA1 pyramidal neurons, *J. Neurophysiol.*, 90, 2171, 2003.

105. Liao, D., Hessler, N.A., and Malinow, R., Activation of postsynaptically silent synapses during pairing-induced LTP in CA1 region of hippocampal slice, *Nature*, 375, 400, 1995.

106. Broutman, G. and Baudry, M., Involvement of the secretory pathway for AMPA receptors in NMDA-induced potentiation in hippocampus, *J. Neurosci.*, 21, 27, 2001.

107. Adams, M.M. et al., Hippocampal dependent learning ability correlates with N-methyl-D-aspartate (NMDA) receptor levels in CA3 neurons of young and aged rats, *J. Comp. Neurol.*, 432, 230, 2001.

108. Filliat, P. et al., Behavioral effects of NBQX, a competitive antagonist of the AMPA receptors, *Pharmacol. Biochem. Behav.*, 59, 1087, 1998.

109. Lee, I. and Kesner, R.P., Differential contribution of NMDA receptors in hippocampal subregions to spatial working memory, *Nat. Neurosci.*, 5, 162, 2002.

110. Yan, J. et al., Place-cell impairment in glutamate receptor 2 mutant mice, *J. Neurosci.*, 22, RC204, 2002.

111. Davis, S., Butcher, S.P., and Morris, R.G., The NMDA receptor antagonist D-2-amino-5-phosphonopentanoate (D-AP5) impairs spatial learning and LTP in vivo at intracerebral concentrations comparable to those that block LTP *in vitro*, *J. Neurosci.*, 12, 21, 1992.

112. Butelman, E.R., A novel NMDA antagonist, MK-801, impairs performance in a hippocampal-dependent spatial learning task, *Pharmacol. Biochem. Behav.*, 34, 13, 1989.

113. Morris, R.G. et al., Selective impairment of learning and blockade of long-term potentiation by an N-methyl-D-aspartate receptor antagonist, AP5, *Nature*, 319, 774, 1986.

114. Fernandez, A.M. et al., Neuroprotective actions of peripherally administered insulin-like growth factor I in the injured olivo-cerebellar pathway, *Eur. J. Neurosci.*, 11, 2019, 1999.

115. Gehrmann, J. et al., Expression of insulin-like growth factor-I and related peptides during motoneuron regeneration, *Exp. Neurol.*, 128, 202, 1994.

116. Ishii, D.N., Glazner, G.W., and Pu, S.F., Role of insulin-like growth factors in peripheral nerve regeneration, *Pharmacol. Ther.*, 62, 125, 1994.

117. Recio-Pinto, E., Rechler, M.M., and Ishii, D.N., Effects of insulin, insulin-like growth factor-II, and nerve growth factor on neurite formation and survival in cultured sympathetic and sensory neurons, *J. Neurosci.*, 6, 1211, 1986.

118. O'Kusky, J.R., Ye, P., and D'Ercole, A.J., Insulin-like growth factor-I promotes neurogenesis and synaptogenesis in the hippocampal dentate gyrus during postnatal development, *J. Neurosci.*, 20, 8435, 2000.

119. Woods, A.G. et al., Deafferentation-induced increases in hippocampal insulin-like growth factor-1 messenger RNA expression are severely attenuated in middle aged and aged rats, *Neuroscience*, 83, 663, 1998.

120. Niblock, M.M., Brunso-Bechtold, J.K., and Riddle, D.R., Insulin-like growth factor I stimulates dendritic growth in primary somatosensory cortex, *J. Neurosci.*, 20, 4165, 2000.

121. Cheng, C.M. et al., Insulin-like growth factor 1 is essential for normal dendritic growth, *J. Neurosci. Res.*, 73, 1, 2003.

122. Carter, C.S., Ramsey, M.M., and Sonntag, W.E., A critical analysis of the role of growth hormone and IGF-1 in aging and lifespan, *Trends Genet.*, 18, 295, 2002.

123. Sonntag, W.E. et al., Alterations in insulin-like growth factor-1 gene and protein expression and type 1 insulin-like growth factor receptors in the brains of ageing rats, *Neuroscience*, 88, 269, 1999.

124. Xu, X. and Sonntag, W.E., Growth hormone-induced nuclear translocation of Stat-3 decreases with age: modulation by caloric restriction, *Am. J. Physiol*, 271, E903, 1996.

125. Zhang, F.X., Rubin, R., and Rooney, T.A., N-Methyl-D-aspartate inhibits apoptosis through activation of phosphatidylinositol 3-kinase in cerebellar granule neurons. A role for insulin receptor substrate-1 in the neurotrophic action of n-methyl-D-aspartate and its inhibition by ethanol, *J. Biol. Chem.*, 273, 26596, 1998.

126. Barria, A., Derkach, V., and Soderling, T., Identification of the Ca2+/calmodulin-dependent protein kinase II regulatory phosphorylation site in the alpha-amino-3-hydroxyl-5-methyl-4-isoxazole-propionate-type glutamate receptor, *J. Biol. Chem.*, 272, 32727, 1997.

127. Mammen, A.L. et al., Phosphorylation of the alpha-amino-3-hydroxy-5-methylisoxazole4-propionic acid receptor GluR1 subunit by calcium/calmodulin-dependent kinase II, *J. Biol. Chem.*, 272, 32528, 1997.

128. Sherwin, B.B., Estrogen effects on cognition in menopausal women, *Neurology*, 48, S21, 1997.

129. Roberts, J.A. et al., Reproductive senescence predicts cognitive decline in aged female monkeys, *Neuroreport*, 8, 2047, 1997.

130. Berry, B., McMahan, R., and Gallagher, M., Spatial learning and memory at defined points of the estrous cycle: effects on performance of a hippocampal-dependent task, *Behav. Neurosci.*, 111, 267, 1997.

131. Stackman, R.W. et al., Stability of spatial working memory across the estrous cycle of Long-Evans rats, *Neurobiol. Learn. Mem.*, 67, 167, 1997.

132. Warren, S.G. and Juraska, J.M., Spatial and nonspatial learning across the rat estrous cycle, *Behav. Neurosci.*, 111, 259, 1997.

133. Frick, K.M. et al., Reference memory, anxiety and estrous cyclicity in C57BL/6NIA mice are affected by age and sex, *Neuroscience*, 95, 293, 2000.

134. Packard, M.G. and Teather, L.A., Intra-hippocampal estradiol infusion enhances memory in ovariectomized rats, *Neuroreport*, 8, 3009, 1997.

135. Gould, E. et al., Gonadal steroids regulate dendritic spine density in hippocampal pyramidal cells in adulthood, *J. Neurosci.*, 10, 1286, 1990.

136. Woolley, C.S., Estrogen-mediated structural and functional synaptic plasticity in the female rat hippocampus, *Horm. Behav.*, 34, 140, 1998.

137. Woolley, C.S., Wenzel, H.J., and Schwartzkroin, P.A., Estradiol increases the frequency of multiple synapse boutons in the hippocampal CA1 region of the adult female rat, *J. Comp Neurol.*, 373, 108, 1996.

138. Woolley, C.S. et al., Naturally occurring fluctuation in dendritic spine density on adult hippocampal pyramidal neurons, *J. Neurosci.*, 10, 4035, 1990.

139. Woolley, C.S. and McEwen, B.S., Estradiol mediates fluctuation in hippocampal synapse density during the estrous cycle in the adult rat, *J. Neurosci.*, 12, 2549, 1992.

140. Woolley, C.S. and McEwen, B.S., Roles of estradiol and progesterone in regulation of hippocampal dendritic spine density during the estrous cycle in the rat, *J. Comp Neurol.*, 336, 293, 1993.

141. Woolley, C.S. and McEwen, B.S., Estradiol regulates hippocampal dendritic spine density via an N-methyl-D-aspartate receptor-dependent mechanism, *J. Neurosci.*, 14, 7680, 1994.

142. Murphy, D.D. and Segal, M., Regulation of dendritic spine density in cultured rat hippocampal neurons by steroid hormones, *J. Neurosci.*, 16, 4059, 1996.

143. Weiland, N.G., Estradiol selectively regulates agonist binding sites on the N-methyl-D-aspartate receptor complex in the CA1 region of the hippocampus, *Endocrinology*, 131, 662, 1992.

144. Gazzaley, A.H. et al., Differential regulation of NMDAR1 mRNA and protein by estradiol in the rat hippocampus, *J. Neurosci.*, 16, 6830, 1996.

145. Foy, M.R. et al., 17beta-estradiol enhances NMDA receptor-mediated EPSPs and long-term potentiation, *J. Neurophysiol.*, 81, 925, 1999.

146. Cordoba Montoya, D.A. and Carrer, H.F., Estrogen facilitates induction of long term potentiation in the hippocampus of awake rats, *Brain Res.*, 778, 430, 1997.

147. Warren, S.G. et al., LTP varies across the estrous cycle: enhanced synaptic plasticity in proestrus rats, *Brain Res.*, 703, 26, 1995.

148. Good, M., Day, M., and Muir, J.L., Cyclical changes in endogenous levels of oestrogen modulate the induction of LTD and LTP in the hippocampal CA1 region, *Eur. J. Neurosci.*, 11, 4476, 1999.

149. Frick, K.M., Fernandez, S.M., and Bulinski, S.C., Estrogen replacement improves spatial reference memory and increases hippocampal synaptophysin in aged female mice, *Neuroscience*, 115, 547, 2002.

150. Markham, J.A., Pych, J.C., and Juraska, J.M., Ovarian hormone replacement to aged ovariectomized female rats benefits acquisition of the morris water maze, *Horm. Behav.*, 42, 284, 2002.

151. Adams, M.M. et al., Estrogen modulates synaptic N-methyl-D-aspartate receptor subunit distribution in the aged hippocampus, *J. Comp Neurol.*, 474, 419, 2004.

152. Weindruch, R. et al., The retardation of aging in mice by dietary restriction: longevity, cancer, immunity and lifetime energy intake, *J. Nutr.*, 116, 641, 1986.

153. Sohal, R.S. and Weindruch, R., Oxidative stress, caloric restriction, and aging, *Science*, 273, 59, 1996.

154. Yu, B.P., Masoro, E.J., and McMahan, C.A., Nutritional influences on aging of Fischer 344 rats. I. Physical, metabolic, and longevity characteristics, *J. Gerontol.*, 40, 657, 1985.

155. Ingram, D.K. et al., Dietary restriction benefits learning and motor performance of aged mice, *J. Gerontol.*, 42, 78, 1987.

156. Stewart, J., Mitchell, J., and Kalant, N., The effects of life-long food restriction on spatial memory in young and aged Fischer 344 rats measured in the eight-arm radial and the Morris water mazes, *Neurobiol. Aging*, 10, 669, 1989.

157. Markowska, A.L. and Savonenko, A., Retardation of cognitive aging by life-long diet restriction: implications for genetic variance, *Neurobiol. Aging*, 23, 75, 2002.

158. Magnusson, K.R., Influence of diet restriction on NMDA receptor subunits and learning during aging, *Neurobiol. Aging*, 22, 613, 2001.

159. Eckles-Smith, K. et al., Caloric restriction prevents age-related deficits in LTP and in NMDA receptor expression, *Brain Res. Mol. Brain Res.*, 78, 154, 2000.

160. Okada, M. et al., How does prolonged caloric restriction ameliorate age-related impairment of long-term potentiation in the hippocampus? *Brain Res. Mol. Brain Res.*, 111, 175, 2003.

161. Demetrius, L., Caloric restriction, metabolic rate, and entropy, *J. Gerontol. A Biol. Sci. Med. Sci.*, 59, B902, 2004.

162. McCarter, R.J. and McGee, J.R., Transient reduction of metabolic rate by food restriction, *Am. J. Physiol.*, 257, E175, 1989.

163. Kirkwood, T.B. and Shanley, D.P., Food restriction, evolution and ageing, *Mech. Ageing Dev.*, 126, 1011, 2005.
164. Yu, B.P. and Chung, H.Y., Stress resistance by caloric restriction for longevity, *Ann. N.Y. Acad. Sci.*, 928, 39, 2001.
165. Koubova, J. and Guarente, L., How does calorie restriction work? *Genes Dev.*, 17, 313, 2003.

9 Assessment of Second Messenger Function in the Hippocampus of Aged Rats with Cognitive Impairment

Michelle M. Nicolle, Hai-Yan Zhang, and Jennifer L. Bizon

CONTENTS

I. INTRODUCTION

The hippocampus is an anatomical region that is critical for certain types of learning and memory that are vulnerable to the effects of normal aging. Early data indicated that these cognitive deficits could be attributed to age-related neuronal loss. However, in the mid-1990s, it was discovered that frank neural degeneration was not a consequence of the normal aging process. First observed in rodents, this finding has since been replicated in primates, including humans (reviewed in [1] and [2]). Given the fact that hippocampal neuronal number is relatively preserved, even at very advanced ages, dysfunctions associated with neuronal integrity (e.g., proper encoding, gene expression and cell signaling) have become an important avenues of exploration as causative factors of age-related mnemonic impairment [3–5]). Indeed, as this chapter discusses in detail, age-related deficits in signal transduction do occur and are presumed to reflect deficient transfer of information both within the hippocampal formation and between the hippocampus and other brain structures critical for proper cognitive function (e.g., [6–8]).

The animal model that we have used to investigate the behavioral relevance of age-related changes in signal transduction mechanisms is reliable and well-established [9, 10]. Briefly, hippocampal-dependent spatial memory is assessed in young and aged male Long-Evans rats in the Morris water maze. Using data from probe trials that are interpolated throughout our training protocol, an individual measure of spatial learning ability is derived for each rat (i.e., a "spatial learning index"). As shown in Figure 9.1, plotting individual young and aged rat spatial performance using the spatial learning index reveals that this measure reliably distinguishes two groups of aged rats: (1) those that learn on par with the young cohorts (i.e., aged-unimpaired rats) and (2) those that perform outside the range of young rats, demonstrating impairment on the task (i.e., aged-impaired rats) [9]. The variability in spatial learning performance observed in this population of aged rats both mimics that observed in humans and affords investigators the opportunity to not only compare neurobiological factors that change as a function of age but, also, to directly link such changes to a functional behavioral measure of hippocampal integrity. Among aged rats, the correlation between individual learning indices and neurobiological measures related to the efficacy of signal transduction mechanisms is the

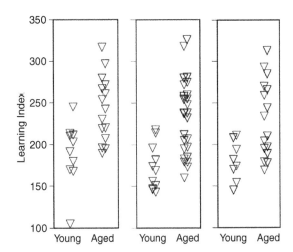

FIGURE 9.1 Individual Learning Index scores from three separate experiments. The data show that the behavioral phenotype of young (6 months old) and aged (25 to 27 months old) Long-Evans rats is measured in a reliable manner. (*Source:* From Nicolle [5]. With permission.)

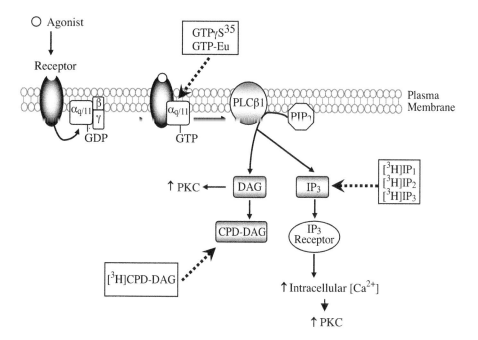

FIGURE 9.2 $G\alpha_{q/11}$-coupled phosphoinositide signaling cascade. When the receptor is activated by agonist, it will interact with a trimeric G protein, causing the $G\alpha_{q/11}$ to release a bound molecule of GDP and to replace it with a molecule of GTP. The signal is transduced to PLCβ1, which liberates DAG and IP_3 from PIP_2. Both DAG and IP_3 can affect PKC and intracellular calcium levels. Receptor/G protein coupling can be measured by either the GTPγ^{35}S or GTP-Eu binding assays. The production of IP_3 can be measured by the incorporation of [^{3}H]myo-inositol into [^{3}H]IP_1/IP_2/IP_3 and the production of DAG can be measured by the incorporation of [^{3}H]cytidine into [^{3}H]CDP-DAG.

primary methodology used in our studies. Although all data in this chapter are related to this one particular model, both the neurobiological and behavioral changes have been replicated in other strains of rodents and even primates. The approaches and techniques described here should be useful and applicable to other animal models of cognitive aging.

The acetylcholine muscarinic and metabotropic glutamate receptors that are coupled to phosphoinositide (PI) turnover are particularly relevant in the study of the aged hippocampus because they are located postsynaptically on the granule cells of the dentate gyrus and pyramidal cells of hippocampus proper [11]. Indeed, these are the same hippocampal neurons that are maintained in number, even at very advanced ages in subjects with severe memory impairment [12, 13].

The muscarinic M1, M3, and M5 receptor subtypes and the metabotropic glutamate receptor subtypes mGluR1 and mGluR5 are coupled to PI turnover via the G-protein α subunit q/11 ($G\alpha_{q/11}$). Figure 9.2 diagrams the intracellular events that follow stimulation of $G\alpha_{q/11}$-coupled receptors. In brief, $G\alpha_{q/11}$ activates phospholipase C-β1 (PLCβ1) [14–16], which in turn liberates inositol 1,4,5-trisphosphate (IP$_3$) and diacylglycerol (DAG) from phosphatidylinositol bisphosphate (PIP$_2$). IP$_3$

and DAG increase intracellular calcium and protein kinase C (PKC), two signaling molecules tightly linked to synaptic plasticity (reviewed in [17]).

The remainder of this chapter systematically presents data in the phosphoinositide cell signaling pathway using the combined approach of behavioral characterization described above and neurobiological assessments of different levels of intracellular signaling cascades with functional behavioral characterization that provides a measure of hippocampal integrity. Specifically, animals are initially behaviorally characterized to provide a measure of hippocampal function and, subsequently, the hippocampus and related structures are dissected and examined for changes in the machinery necessary for proper signaling within and between neurons. This approach allows us to determine whether age-related changes in cell signaling relate to, and perhaps contribute to, cognitive deficits that emerge in aging. First, we present data on the quantification of the protein "machinery" needed for signal transduction: determination of receptor and effector levels of various components of the signaling cascade. Second, we describe the quantification of the functional ability of this machinery to generate downstream signaling in the hippocampus of young and aged rats and its relevance to age-related cognitive decline.

II. QUANTIFICATION OF PROTEIN MACHINERY

As described above, there are proteins at all levels in the second messenger signaling cascade that work in concert to stimulate PI turnover. Importantly, if expression of any of these proteins was decreased in the aged brain, the result could significantly contribute to deficient neuronal communication and, ultimately, impaired learning and memory processes. Thus, the quantification of the availability of key proteins involved in the second messenger signal transduction cascade is an essential first step in investigating this signaling pathway as a causative factor in age-related cognitive decline. The critical machinery includes the G-protein receptor, G-protein subunits, and downstream enzymes and precursor molecules necessary for transduction. Neurotransmitter receptor and downstream effector levels can both be examined using Western blotting techniques in hippocampal tissue homogenates. Receptor binding can also be assayed in a more regionally specific manner using hippocampal slices.

A.   RECEPTOR BINDING

Receptor binding, measured in tissue homogenates or slices (using autoradiography), is a well-established pharmacological method that has several advantages, which are described below. First, the method accurately quantifies the density of neurotransmitter receptor binding sites using a radiolabeled standard scale. Second, such assays conducted in fresh-frozen tissue sections or homogenates require relatively little tissue, such that tissue from the same subjects used for receptor quantification also can be used for additional studies of receptor function (e.g., assessment of receptor-stimulated GTPγ^{35}S binding, discussed in Section IV of this chapter), providing several measurements related to cellular signaling in the same animal. Finally, because receptor binding autoradiography affords anatomical specificity, regional

TABLE 9.1
Regional [³H]PZ Binding in
Young and Aged Rats

Brain Region	Young n = 4	Aged n = 8
Dorsal Hippocampal Formation		
CA1	287 ± 17	303 ± 8
CA3	140 ± 6	153 ± 9
Dentate gyrus	285 ± 10	306 ± 7
Ventral Hippocampal Formation		
CA1	283 ± 13	303 ± 9
CA3	168 ± 14	187 ± 8
Dentate gyrus	151 ± 14	160 ± 23

Note: Binding site densities reflect mean ± SEM (fmol/mg tissue wet weight).

Source: Modified from Smith, T.D. et al., *Neurobiol. Aging,* 16, 161, 1995. With permission.

changes may be identified that could be missed in assays using tissue homogenate preparations.

An early study in young and aged behaviorally characterized Long-Evans rats quantified muscarinic M1 receptor binding using an autoradiographic approach. Data from that study and others indicated that aging does not affect the binding density of [³H]pirezipine, an M1 antagonist, in the hippocampus (Table 9.1) [18]. The preservation of M1 receptors in the aged hippocampus of Long-Evans rats was later confirmed by immunoprecipitation of M1 receptor subunits and also in membrane preparations (Figure 9.3). Each method reported similar results: a maintenance of M1 receptor levels across the lifespan. This result has been replicated by other laboratories in Long-Evans rats [19] and with a variety of techniques (e.g., Western blotting, which is described in detail below). All data to date have supported the conclusion that M1 receptor levels are not altered as a function of chronological age.

B. WESTERN BLOTTING

Western blotting was also used to analyze components of the PI turnover protein machinery that are downstream of the effector (e.g., $G\alpha_{q/11}$, phospholipase Cβ1 (PLC β1), protein kinase C (PKC)). This method has the advantage of using antibodies that are usually more specific to receptor subtypes than agonists. However, Western blot data are more difficult to quantify accurately compared to receptor autoradiography using isotopes. We therefore developed a rigorous Western blot technique that affords the standardization of large numbers of animals assayed, out of necessity, in separate gels.

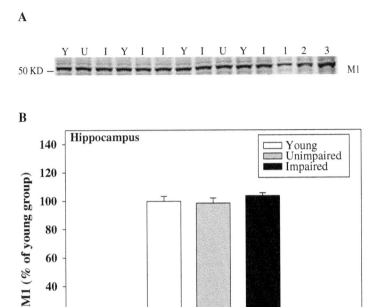

FIGURE 9.3 M1 Western blot data from the hippocampus of young and aged Long-Evans rats. Panel A shows representative Western blots for M1. The lanes numbered 1, 2, and 3 mark the standard curve, with lane 1 containing the lowest standard concentration. Y: 6 months old, U: 26 months old, aged unimpaired, I: 26 months old, aged impaired. Panel B shows the data plotted by behavioral group ± SE from three separate experiments. (*Source:* From Zhang et al. [26]. With permission.)

Such standardization is required as large numbers of animals are necessary to afford statistical power sufficient to link changes in protein level to spatial learning performance (a typical behavioral cohort for our experiments includes 24 rats: n — 8 young, n = 16 aged). Tissue homogenates from dissected hippocampus are normalized to equal protein concentrations across all animals in the study. The immunoreactivity for the protein of interest is then quantified by performing a Western blot on the tissue homogenate of total protein or in a preparation of membrane protein. Our stringent methodology includes constructing a standard curve of at least three protein concentrations that bracket the optical density of the samples (Figure 9.3 and Figure 9.4). Such a curve serves two purposes. First, it is included on both the right and the left side of the gel to provide an assessment of equal side-to-side transfer of protein from the gel to the blotting membrane. Second, it is important that the standard curve be linear to avoid saturation of the signal with high levels of immunoreactivity that could result in a ceiling effect, a particular problem when using chemiluminescent reagents to visualize the immunoreactivity. Many laboratories use actin immunoreactivity to verify equal protein loading of each sample but, because levels of actin could be altered in the aged brain, the use of a standard protein curve better alleviates this potential confound.

Although chemiluminescent detection of secondary antibodies is a common and effective method used to quantify immunoreactivity levels, near-infrared (IR) imaging has four- to eightfold greater sensitivity compared with the traditional chemiluminescent detection [20]. IR imaging possesses a 16- to 250-fold wider quantifiable linear range than traditional chemiluminescent detection. Moreover, by imaging at the infrared wavelengths, a cleaner background and higher signal-to-noise ratio can be achieved, as compared to the visible wavelength range used by other detection systems. Another advantage of IR imaging is that it can detect two different proteins at the same time in the same lane using two secondary antibodies that fluoresce at different wavelengths (e.g., red and green). This approach avoids problems associated with antibody stripping (e.g., inconsistent protein loss or confusion due to inadequate stripping). Although our lab uses the Odyssey Imaging system (LI-COR Biosciences, Lincoln, Nebraska), it should be noted other systems are also available that are sensitive to analysis of Western blots generated with near-infrared secondary antibody labels (e.g., Quantum (Qdot) Western Blotting Kits, QuantumDot Corporation, Hayward, California).

Chemiluminescent visualization was used for detection in our early studies designed to quantify protein immunoreactivity of $G\alpha_{q/11}$ and PLCβ1 from the hippocampus of spatially characterized young and aged Long-Evans rats [5]. Experimental samples fall within the linear range of the standard curve and quantification of the immunoreactivity intensity indicated that there was no loss of the $G\alpha_{q/11}$ protein with age, and expression of this protein did not correlate with spatial learning impairment. Importantly, however, $G\alpha_{q/11}$ activated PLCβ1 and, in contrast to the $G\alpha_{q/11}$ results, PLCβ1 immunoreactivity significantly decreased by 20% in the aged hippocampus [5]. This age-related decrease was not, however, correlated with spatial learning impairment among aged rats (R = −0.27, ns). These data strongly suggest that a different component of the signaling pathway (either instead or in addition to the changes in PLCβ1 levels) contributes to cognitive dysfunction in a subset of the aged rats.

As described above, PLCβ1 liberates IP_3 and DAG, which can increase PKC levels. Muscarinic receptor activation can increase the calcium-activated PKCγ isoform [21]. In addition, learning has been associated with the increase of PKCγ immunoreactivity in the hippocampus and also the translocation of PKCγ from the cytosol (soluble) to the membrane-bound (particulate) fraction [21, 22]. In aged Long-Evans rats, we have analyzed PKC levels (γ, α, $β_2$ isoforms) using Western blotting in soluble and particulate hippocampal protein fractions. Higher PKCγ levels, but not PKCα or $β_2$, in the soluble fraction were associated with greater memory impairment in the aged rats. These data suggest that lack of translocation of PKCγ to the particulate fraction could contribute to impaired hippocampal-dependent learning [23].

As levels and binding densities of key proteins in Long-Evans rats were unchanged or minimally affected by age, it suggested that dysfunction downstream of the agonist binding to the receptor contributes to dysfunctional cellular signaling and failed communication between neurons. The remainder of this chapter focuses on several functional assays that we have used to investigate muscarinic and metabotropic glutamate receptor function in the hippocampus in relation to age-related cognitive impairment. Each assay varies in the type of tissue required (fresh or fresh-frozen) and in the number of "molecular steps" from agonist activation to output measure. Together, however, an approach of using a variety of assays that are designed to systematically assess individual transmitter systems and second messenger signals has yielded a significant amount of data that demonstrates a contribution of blunted cellular signaling to age-related cognitive impairment. The methodology described below, applied to these and other signaling pathways in aging and other neurological conditions, should continue to elucidate neurobiological underpinnings of cognitive dysfunction.

III.　QUANTIFICATION OF RECEPTOR-MEDIATED SIGNALING

A.　RECEPTOR-MEDIATED PHOSPHOINOSITIDE TURNOVER

As shown in Figure 9.2, $G\alpha_{q/11}$-coupled receptors stimulate the generation of phosphoinositides (PI). In the PI turnover assay, tissue minces are prelabeled with a radioactive precursor to phosphoinositide, [^{3}H]myo-inositol. Agonist binding to the receptor stimulates the incorporation of the [^{3}H]myo-inositol into [^{3}H]IP-1. Lithium is included in the assay to allow for the accumulation of [^{3}H]IP-1. Without lithium, the radiolabeled polyphosphoinositides would be quickly degraded [24]. Agonist stimulation is calculated as the net value over basal (unstimulated) levels. The net stimulation is then examined using a curve-fitting program that fits the data to a sigmoidal dose response curve (we use GraphPad Prism, San Diego, California, for these analyses). Basic pharmacological assessment of individual dose response curves provides information regarding the basal metabolism, the concentration of the agonist that stimulates the half maximal effector response (EC$_{50}$) and maximal effector response (E_{MAX}). An example of the type of data obtained using this protocol, integrated with the assessment of cognitive function, is shown in Table 9.2 and Figure 9.4 [5]. An analysis of the data by chronological age demonstrates a stability of basic metabolism, measured by the basal cellular incorporation of [^{3}H]myo-inositol and the basal PI turnover activity (Table 9.2). Stimulation of PI turnover by the metabotropic glutamate receptor agonist 1S,3R ACPD in these same animals revealed no change in the Hill slope or the EC$_{50}$, but a significant decrease in the E_{MAX} in the aged group of about 50% compared to the young group. The functional implications of the age-related change in E_{MAX} are apparent when the data are analyzed based upon performance on the hippocampal-dependent spatial learning task in the Morris water maze. A simple regression between the E_{MAX} and the spatial learning index demonstrated a highly significant relationship between cognitive performance and the magnitude of PI turnover stimulated by agonist, such that the PI response was generally attenuated to a greater degree in aged rats with the greatest spatial learning impairments.

A strength, but also a limitation, of the PI turnover assay is the requirement for freshly dissected brain tissue. The benefit of fresh tissue is that it allows for a more

TABLE 9.2
Parameters of 1S,3R ACPD-stimulated PI turnover in young and aged rats ± SEM

	Young	Aged
Cell-associated radioactivity (dpm)	8421 ± 987	7808 ± 166
Basal [³H]IP1 release (dpm)	497 ± 33	446 ± 31
Log EC_{50}	−5.17 ± 0.10	−5.11 ± 0.08
Hill slope	1.20 ± 0.18	1.78 ± 0.36
1S,3R ACPD E_{MAX}[a,b]	562 ± 27	414 ± 24

[a] dpm with basal dpm subtracted.

[b] $p < 0.05$.

Source: From Nicolle et al., [5]. With permission.

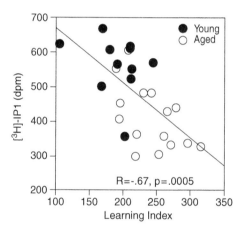

FIGURE 9.4 Maximal mGluR-mediated phosphoinositide turnover plotted as a function of spatial learning ability. Individual data points for young and aged rats are shown for the 1S,3R ACPD E_{MAX}. The solid line indicates the linear regression between PI turnover and learning index for young and aged animals grouped together. (*Source:* From Nicolle [5]. With permission.)

accurate representation of *in vivo* conditions compared to studies that use previously frozen tissue. For PI turnover, the only assay component that must be added exogenously is the radiolabeled precursor, [³H]myo-inositol. Assays using frozen tissue require the addition of other cellular components to mimic the *in vivo* conditions, such as PIP_2 or GDP. However, although this assay provides very valuable information, it is very difficult to run this assay on more than one animal's tissue sample at a time due to the magnitude of assay and the temporal considerations involved in using freshly dissected tissue. Therefore, the comparison of the data across subjects is suspect to inter-assay variability and special care must be taken to control from such confounds. We control for sample variability by including an [^{14}C]IP-1 standard in all the columns used for separation of the inositol phosphates. The experimentally generated inositol phosphates labeled with tritium ([^{3}H]) are in contrast to the known amount of [^{14}C]IP-1 added to each sample. When the samples are read in the liquid scintillation counter, the two different isotopic signals can be separated to allow for normalization of the experimentally generated inositol phosphates to the extraction of the standard [^{14}C]IP-1.

B.   RECEPTOR-MEDIATED GTP BINDING

Receptor-stimulated GTP binding directly measures the initial interaction between the receptor and its G-protein(s). It measures the agonist-stimulated exchange of GDP for GTP on the G-protein α-subunit using a non-hydrolysable GTP analogue, either the traditional radioactively labeled GTPγ^{35}S (guanosine-5′-O-(3-[^{35}S]thio)-triphosphate) or the fluorescently labeled GTP-Eu (europium) [25]. Normally, GTPases quickly remove the GTP to terminate the cellular signal. However, because the GTP is nonhydrolysable and remains bound to the activated G protein α subunit, it accumulates and provides a measure of the magnitude of receptor coupling. Both the GTPγ^{35}S and the GTP-Eu assays can be performed in previously frozen tissue homogenates.

As an alternative to the traditional GTPγ^{35}S binding assay, the GTP-Eu binding assay was developed with the consideration of moving the G-protein coupling assay to a nonradioactive format [25]. The GTP-Eu binding assay uses the nonhydrolysable lanthanide chelate europium instead of ^{35}S to label the GTP. Quantification of the europium label is based on the well-established quantification of lanthanide chelates using time-resolved fluorescence (TRF). The unique fluorescence properties of lanthanide chelates include their long lifetime, usually longer than several hundreds microseconds; compared to an organic fluorescence reagent's lifetime of several nanoseconds. Most importantly, they also have a large Stokes shift that reduces the nonspecific fluorescent signal and creates a high signal-to-noise ratio. Typically, the lanthanide chelate complexes are excited by UV absorption (340 nm for europium in particular), and emit light of wavelength longer than 500 nm (615 nm for europium in particular). Finally, the fluorescent peak profiles of lanthanide chelates are sharp, with half-widths of 10 to 20 nm.

In young and aged behaviorally characterized Long-Evans rats, we used muscarinic receptor-stimulated GTP-Eu binding to analyze an upstream component of the impaired receptor-mediated PI turnover [26]. Our results indicate that upstream to the age attenuation of PI turnover, there is a similar age-related decrease in muscarinic receptor-stimulated GTP-Eu binding in the hippocampus of aged rats. In addition, this change is most significant in the aged rats with learning impairment (Figure 9.5). This result suggests that the age-related deficit in receptor-mediated PI turnover occurs early in the signal transduction cascade at the interface between the receptor and the G-protein α subunit.

An advantage of the receptor-stimulated GTP binding assays, whether GTPγ^{35}S or GTP-Eu, is that inter-assay variability is reduced due to the processing of triplicate samples from each subject simultaneously, either in test tubes (GTPγ^{35}S) or in a

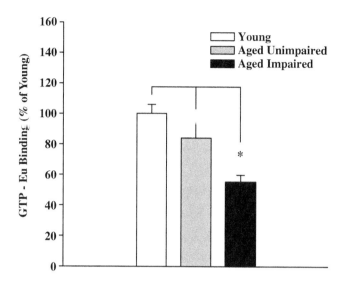

FIGURE 9.5 Oxotremorine-M-mediated GTP-Eu binding in the hippocampus of aged rats. Data were expressed as percentage of young group ± SE and plotted by behavioral group. The aged impaired rats had significantly less oxotremorine-M stimulated GTP-Eu binding than either the young or the aged, learning unimpaired groups. * p < 0.01. (*Source:* From Zhang et al. [26]. With permission.)

96-well plate (GTP-Eu). This methodology is in contrast to the limitation of running tissue from a single animal per assay, as when measuring PI turnover. Running all cohorts in a single assay decreases the variability across experiments and thus increases the reliability of the assay. A technical limitation of the receptor-stimulated GTP binding assays, however, is the availability of sub-type specific agonists that couple to the G-protein signaling system of interest. For example, the popular muscarinic agonist oxotremorine-M stimulates not only the $G\alpha_{q/11}$ PI-coupled receptors (M1, M3, and M5 subtypes) but also $G\alpha_{i/o}$ adenyl cyclase-coupled receptors (M2 and M4 subtypes). Therefore, if age-related changes in oxotremorine-M-mediated GTP binding occur in areas of the brain that contain both PI and adenyl cyclase-coupled muscarinic receptors, it is not possible to determine if deficiencies result from both muscarinic receptor subtypes or if, rather, one subtype is particularly vulnerable to the effects of age. Although the relative contribution of receptor subtypes to GTP binding may be determined using subtype specific antagonists, the results should still be interpreted cautiously.

Another technical consideration in GTP binding assays involves the specifics of the buffer composition across neurotransmitter systems. In our laboratory, we noted that the magnitude of the metabotropic glutamate receptor-stimulated response was much lower than the muscarinic receptor-stimulated response. After optimization of the ion composition of the buffers, however, we were able to obtain an optimal signal using the mGluR Type 1 agonist 3,5-dihydroxyphenylglycine (DHPG). The differences in the buffer compositions are shown in Table 9.3, and such considerations are important when examining a variety of transmitter systems.

TABLE 9.3
Ionic Concentrations in Buffer for Muscarinic (OXOTREMORINe-M) and Metabotropic Glutamate Receptor (DHPG) Agonists

Agonist	MgCl$_2$	GDP	NaCl	EGTA	EDTA
Oxotremorine-M	5 mM	10 μM	100 mM	0.2 mM	—
DHPG	10 mM	50 μM	100 mM	1 mM	1 mM

IV. FUNCTIONAL ASSAYS USING TISSUE SLICES FOR REGIONALLY SPECIFIC ANALYSES

The anatomical specificity that is absent in studies using tissue homogenates can be accomplished using film autoradiographic techniques. Film autoradiography has been used for imaging of receptor stimulation of the upstream GTPγ^{35}S incorporation and the more downstream incorporation of [^{3}H]cytidine into [^{3}H]CDP-DAG. In addition, the methods used for tissue preparation in the GTPγ^{35}S binding assay are amenable to traditional receptor binding; adjacent tissue sections can be analyzed for receptor binding using highly quantifiable, traditional radioligand autoradiography techniques to provide a measure of receptor level in the same animals.

A.   RECEPTOR-STIMULATED GTPγ^{35}S AUTORADIOGRAPHY

GTPγ^{35}S autoradiography is elegantly described in [27] and is only briefly described here. Like the homogenate assay, this assay provides a measure of the receptor-mediated activation of G-protein, with the added refinement of anatomical resolution. Slides from a large number of individual subjects can be prepared and frozen, and subsequently processed together to eliminate inter-assay variability. Comparable sets of sequential tissue sections can be analyzed for responses to several agonists or for receptor binding autoradiography. Additionally, adjacent sections can be histologically stained to assist in defining anatomical boundaries for anatomically specific analyses. Although we have not used this assay in our study of young and aged Long-Evans rats, it has been used to quantify the regional responses to drugs of addiction in rodents (e.g., [28, 29]) and is a direction of future research in cognitive aging.

The added anatomical specificity of GTPγ^{35}S autoradiography can be offset by the amount of time it takes to image and quantify the data. For example, examination of muscarinic receptor-stimulated GTPγ^{35}S binding in hippocampal homogenates from 24 rats will take approximately 1 week, taking into account membrane preparation, determination of membrane protein in a BCA assay, and the actual running of the receptor/GTPγ^{35}S binding assay. In contrast, an anatomical study will require about tenfold more time due to the sectioning of the tissue (~2 weeks), assay (~1 day), exposure to film (varies from days to weeks), then the careful imaging of anatomical regions and sub-regions and subsequent number crunching and data analysis. Nevertheless, these temporal considerations indeed may prove necessary and worthwhile to fully understand the underlying signaling deficiencies that contribute to age-related memory impairment. Notably, in our studies of behaviorally characterized young and aged rats (described in Section IV.A of this chapter), we discovered subregion-specific neurobiological changes that were not detected in studies using homogenate studies (compare [3] with [30]).

B.   Receptor-Stimulated [³H] CDP-DAG Autoradiography

To analyze the effectiveness of agonists to stimulate PI turnover further downstream from the G-protein while maintaining anatomical resolution, a method originally described by Hwang et al. [31] can be employed. This method takes advantage of an insoluble product of PI turnover cascade: the generation of membrane-bound cytidine diphosphate diacylglycerol (CDP-DAG). Using [³H]cytidine as a precursor and in the presence of Li⁺ (a reagent that inhibits the recycling of IP₃ and allows the accumulation of [³H]CDP-DAG [32]), the receptor-stimulated incorporation of [³H]cytidine into membrane-bound [³H]CDP-DAG can be visualized and quantified using traditional autoradiography techniques. An example of muscarinic receptor-mediated [³H]CDP-DAG in young and aged rats is shown in Figure 9.6.

In young and aged learning-impaired Long-Evans rats, anatomical visualization of muscarinic receptor-mediated PI turnover using [³H]CDP-DAG autoradiography revealed that basal PI turnover was decreased in the subiculum and the dentate gyrus but not in CA1 or CA3 [30]. Notably, these differences were only detected when using the more time-consuming, regionally specific autoradiographic approach

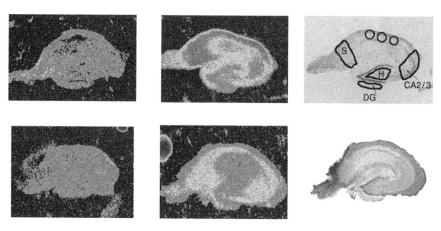

FIGURE 9.6 (SEE COLOR INSERT FOLLOWING PAGE 204) Representative autoradiograms and histologies from a young rat and an aged, learning-impaired rat. Left: basal [³H]CDP-DAG levels. Middle: increased incorporation of [³H]CDP-DAG after stimulation with 100 μM oxotremorine-M. Right: the oxotremorine-M section was subsequently stained with toluidine blue. Areas of quantification are indicated by outlines on the top right panel. S, subiculum; H, hilus; DG, dentate gyrus; CA2/3 and CA1, fields of the hippocampus. (*Source:* From Nicolle et al. [30]. With permission.)

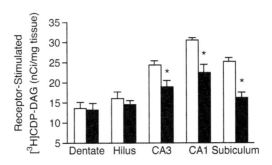

FIGURE 9.7 Muscarinic receptor-mediated [³H]CDP-DAG ± SEM in regions of the hippocampus in young and aged, learning-impaired rats. (*Source:* From Nicolle et al. [30]. With permission.)

(described in Section III.A in this chapter). Indeed, the specific agonist-stimulated response was also affected by age in a subregion-specific manner; aged learning impaired rats showed a significantly blunted response that was restricted to the subiculum (−36%), CA3 (−22%), and CA1 (−27%), whereas receptor-mediated signaling in the dentate gyrus and hilus was maintained (Figure 9.7). In summary, whereas assays using homogenates are a practical starting point in understanding changes in receptor level, binding, and signaling, negative data should be interpreted cautiously as regionally specific changes may be obscured when analyses are conducted on homogenates that contain a number of anatomically distinct regions.

Perhaps the most challenging aspect of [³H]CDP-DAG autoradiography is the sectioning of 15-μm sections from a 350-μm slab of dissected hippocampus. To stabilize the 350-μm slab, it can be horizontally placed flat on the bottom of a plastic embedding cup filled with Tissue Tek and then sliced using a cryostat. The first 15-μm sections from the outer edges of the slab should be disposed and not used for analysis due to the potential damage on the surface of the tissue slice.

There is some concern that freezing tissue prior to assay is detrimental to receptor/G-protein complexes. However, guanine nucleotides inhibit agonist binding in frozen tissue sections, providing evidence of maintained function of the receptor/G-protein complex [33]. In addition, in 1991, O'Neill et al. [34] demonstrated the presence of functional G-proteins and phospholipase C in frozen tissue. It has been noted by this lab and others, however, that the strength of the signal diminishes with longer tissue storage at low temperatures.

V. CONCLUSIONS

Studies in behaviorally characterized aged rat have demonstrated that decrements in muscarinic and metabotropic glutamate receptor function in the hippocampus are related to cognitive impairment. Alterations in signal transduction have been observed as far upstream as receptor/G-protein coupling and as far downstream as PI turnover, although the molecular machinery, measured by Western blotting and receptor autoradiography, remains intact. Receptor-mediated $G\alpha_{q/11}$ signaling ultimately influences intracellular calcium levels, via the IP_3 receptors on the endoplasmic reticulum or via protein kinase C and interaction with cell membrane calcium channels. Regulation of calcium signaling has far-reaching consequences, from modulation of synaptic plasticity to cellular toxicity. Our recent data indicating that age-related alterations in receptor signaling occur very early in the cascade at the level of the G-protein suggest that receptor/G-protein coupling is a mechanism to consider for repair and/or protection in the aged brain.

REFERENCES

1. Morrison, J.H. and Hof, P.R., Life and death of neurons in the aging brain, *Science*, 278, 412, 1997.
2. Erickson, C.A. and Barnes, C.A., The neurobiology of memory changes in normal aging, *Exp. Gerontol.*, 38, 61, 2003.
3. Chouinard, M.L. et al., Hippocampal muscarinic receptor function in spatial learning-impaired aged rats, *Neurobiol. Aging*, 16, 955, 1995.
4. Morrison, J.H. and Hof, P.R., Selective vulnerability of corticocortical and hippocampal circuits in aging and Alzheimer's disease, *Prog. Brain Res.*, 136, 467, 2002.
5. Nicolle, M.M. et al., Metabotropic glutamate receptor-mediated hippocampal phosphoinositide turnover is blunted in spatial learning impaired aged rats, *J. Neurosci.*, 19, 9604, 1999.
6. Gallagher, M. et al., Effects of aging on the hippocampal formation in a naturally occurring animal model of mild cognitive impairment, *Exp. Gerontol.*, 38, 71, 2003.
7. Tanila, H. et al., Brain aging: changes in the nature of information coding by the hippocampus, *J. Neurosci.*, 17, 5155, 1997.
8. Tanila, H. et al., Brain aging: impaired coding of novel environmental cues, *J. Neurosci.*, 17, 5167, 1997.
9. Gallagher, M., Burwell, R., and Burchinal, M., Severity of spatial learning impairment in aging: development of a learning index for performance in the Morris water maze, *Behav. Neurosci.*, 107, 618, 1993.
10. Rapp, P.R., Rosenberg, R.A., and Gallagher, M., An evaluation of spatial information processing in aged rats, *Behav. Neurosci.*, 101, 3, 1987.
11. Levey, A.I. et al., Expression of m1-m4 muscarinic acetylcholine receptor proteins in rat hippocampus and regulation by cholinergic innervation, *J. Neurosci.*, 15, 4077, 1995.
12. Rapp, P.R. and Gallagher, M., Preserved neuron number in the hippocampus of aged rats with spatial learning deficits, *Proc. Natl. Acad. Sci. U.S.A.*, 93, 9926, 1996.
13. Rasmussen, T. et al., Memory impaired aged rats: No loss of principle hippocampal and subicular neurons, *Neurobiol. Aging*, 17, 143, 1996.
14. Berstein, G. et al., Reconstitution of agonist-stimulated phosphatidylinositol 4,5-bisphosphate hydrolysis using purified m1 muscarinic receptor, $G_{q/11}$, and phospholipase C-β1, *J. Biol. Chem.*, 267, 8081, 1992.
15. Smrcka, A.V. et al., Regulation of polyphosphoinositide-specific phospholipase C activity by purified Gq, *Science*, 251, 804, 1991.
16. Taylor, S.J. et al., Activation of the β1 isozyme of phospolipase C by α subunits of the Gq class of G proteins, *Nature*, 350, 516, 1991.
17. Malenka, R.C. and Nicoll, R.A., Long-term potentiation — a decade of progress? *Science*, 285, 1870, 1999.

18. Smith, T.D., Gallagher, M., and Leslie, F.M., Cholinergic binding sites in rat brain: analysis by age and cognitive status, *Neurobiol. Aging*, 16, 161, 1995.
19. Aubert, I. et al., Cholinergic markers in aged cognitively impaired Long-Evans rats, *Neuroscience*, 67, 277, 1995.
20. Schutz-Geschwender, A. et al., Quantitative, two-color western blot detection with infrared fluorescence. www.licor.com, 2004.
21. Van Der Zee, E.A., Luiten, P.G.M., and Disterhoft, J.F., Learning-induced alterations in hippocampal PKC-immunoreactivity: a review and hypothesis of its functional significance, *Prog. Neuropsychopharmcol. Biol. Psychiatry*, 21, 531, 1997.
22. Micheau, J., Protein kinases: which one is the memory molecule? Molecular mechanisms of memory formation: from receptor activation to synaptic changes, *Cell. Mol. Life Sci.*, 55, 534, 1999.
23. Colombo, P.J., Wetsel, W.C., and Gallagher, M., Spatial memory is related to hippocampal subcellular concentrations of calcium-dependent protein kinase C isoforms in young and aged rats, *Proc. Natl. Acad. Sci. U.S.A.*, 94, 14195, 1997.
24. Kendall, D.A. and Whitworth, P., Lithium amplifies inhibitions of inositol phospholipid hydrolysis in mammalian brain slices, *Br. J. Pharmacol.*, 100, 723, 1990.
25. Frang, H. et al., Nonradioactive GTP binding assay to monitor activation of G protein-coupled receptors, *Assay Drug Dev. Technol.*, 1, 275, 2003.
26. Zhang, H.Y. et al., Muscarinic receptor-mediated GTP-Eu binding in the hippocampus and prefrontal cortex is correlated with spatial memory impairment in aged rats, *Neurobiol. Aging*, in press, 2007.
27. Sim-Selley, L.J. and Childers, S.R., Neuroanatomical localization of receptor-activated G proteins in brain, *Meth. Enzymol.*, 344, 42, 2002.
28. Sim, L.J., Selley, D.E., and Childers, S.R., *In vitro* autoradiography of receptor-activated G proteins in rat brain by agonist-stimulated guanylyl 5'-[γ-[^{35}s]thio]-triphosphate binding, *Proc. Natl. Acad. Sci. U.S.A.*, 92, 7242, 1995.
29. Sim, L.J. et al., Effects of chronic morphine administration on μ opioid receptor-stimulated [^{35}S]GTPγS autoradiography in rat brain, *J. Neurosci.*, 16, 2684, 1996.
30. Nicolle, M.M., Gallagher, M., and McKinney, M., Visualization of muscarinic receptor-mediated phosphoinositide turnover in the hippocampus of young and aged, learning impaired Long-Evans rats, *Hippocampus*, 11, 741, 2001.
31. Hwang, P.M., Bredt, D.S., and Snyder, S.H., Autoradiographic imaging of phosphoinositide turnover in the brain, *Science*, 249, 802, 1990.
32. Godfrey, P.P., Potentiation by lithium of CMP-phosphatidate formation in carbachol-stimulated rat cerebral-cortical slices and its reversal by myo-inositol, *Biochem. J.*, 258, 621, 1989.
33. Zarbin, M.A. et al., Axonal transport of beta-adrenergic receptors. Antero- and retrogradely transported receptors differ in agonist affinity and nucleotide sensitivity, *Mol. Pharmacol.*, 24, 341, 1983.
34. O'Neill, C. et al., Assay of a phosphatidylinositol bisphosphate phospholipase C activity in postmortem human brain, *Brain Res.*, 543, 307, 1991.

10 Neurophysiology of Old Neurons and Synapses

Ashok Kumar and Thomas C. Foster

CONTENTS

I.   INTRODUCTION

Aging is associated with multiple sensory and motor impairments, including hearing loss, poor eyesight, reduced muscle strength, and increased reaction time. In many cases, sensory-motor deficits involve changes in the transduction or output systems and the knowledge concerning senescence of the processing mechanisms permits compensation through adjuncts, such as hearing aids and corrective lenses. In contrast, senescence of the central nervous system mechanisms involved in cognition is not well understood, creating a challenge for treating the impairment in short-term memory and increased forgetting associated with normal aging. In addition, overlaid upon the memory deficits and response slowing, is dementia linked to Alzheimer's or Parkinson's disease. In considering the mechanisms of aging-related changes in cognitive function, several questions arise:

- How do the cellular properties of neurons change during normal aging?
- Do the changes represent the decline in neural function per se, or compensation for senescence of a more fundamental process?

- Are these properties different from age-related disease, or is Alzheimer's disease an inevitable consequence of a long life?

Certainly there is some interaction between diseases of the elderly and normal aging, because the appearance of these diseases increases with age. Nevertheless, there are important differences between the cognitive decline due to neurodegenerative ailments, which are more prevalent in the elderly, and memory deficits that arise in healthy elderly individuals. Unlike neurodegenerative diseases, cognitive changes associated with senescence are not linked to overt brain lesions or a significant loss of neurons [1, 2], although normal aging may be accompanied by some loss of neuronal elements, including changes in the branching of axons and in the number or size of synaptic contacts [3]. More important may be the fact that aging is associated with a shift in the timing or level of transmission through neural structures. The transmission properties of neurons and the functional connectivity between neurons determine the fidelity of sensory processing, computational capability, and the reliability of motor output. In turn, changes in transmission properties or functional connectivity can provide developmental control on the emergence of behavior, and may represent a mechanism for recording and integrating experience. As such, a decrease in transmission through a brain structure or a shift in the ability to modify synaptic connections could constitute a functional lesion that may form the basis for cognitive decline during aging.

Due to the invasive nature of studies that directly record cell discharges and synaptic responses from brain structures, it currently is not feasible to measure transmission properties in humans. Surface electrodes have been used, however, to detect and characterize age-related changes that may contribute to functional lesions. As humans age, the amplitude of sensory-evoked responses wane and the response latency increases [4]. Changes in the latency of transmission through sensory systems could contribute to age-related impairments in the temporal processing of sensory information [5, 6]. Studies in aged animals indicate that conduction velocity (i.e., the speed at which that an action potential travels down the axon) decreases for neocortical, cerebellar, and peripheral sensory and motor neurons [7–15]. The cause of this reduced conduction velocity is unclear, but it may result from alterations in the myelin sheath [16, 17].

II. CELL EXCITABILITY AND AFTERHYPERPOLARIZATION

Cell excitability, the propensity to elicit an action potential by intracellular injection of current, is reduced in the hippocampus and cerebellum of aged animals [7, 18]. The hippocampus is one of the most intensely studied regions of the brain in terms of aging, due to the fact that memory processes that depend on the hippocampus are highly susceptible to disruption with advanced age [19]. One conspicuous characteristic of aging hippocampal neurons is an increase in the magnitude of the Ca^{2+}-dependent, K^+-mediated afterhyperpolarization (AHP) (Figure 10.1). The amplitude of the AHP is consistently increased and prolonged in the hippocampal CA1 pyramidal neurons during senescence in male and female rats [20–27] and in rabbits [28–33].

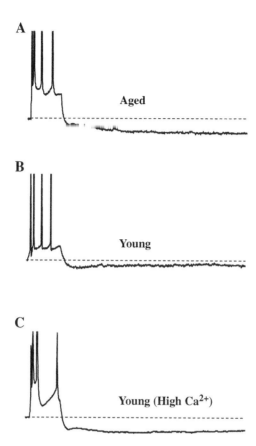

FIGURE 10.1 The amplitude of the AHP increases during aging and as a function of extracellular Ca^{2+}. The figure illustrates representative hyperpolarizing responses recorded intracellularly from CA1 pyramidal cells in aged (A) and young (B) rats. The amplitude of the AHP is measured as the difference between the response and the resting membrane potential (dashed line). (C) The AHP is Ca^{2+} dependent, as such elevation of the Ca^{2+} in the recording medium from 2 mM to 4 mM is associated with a marked increase in the AHP amplitude in young rats. Note that in this and subsequent figures, action potentials are truncated or removed to better show the AHP.

A. REGULATION OF AHP BY Ca^{2+} AND K^+ CHANNELS

Importantly, generation of AHP depends on Ca^{2+}, and altered Ca^{2+} regulation during neural activity is thought to contribute to the age-related increase in AHP. In young animals, the amplitude of AHP can be increased by raising the level of Ca^{2+} in the extracellular recording medium (Figure 10.1C). Indeed, under conditions of elevated extracellular Ca^{2+}, no age difference is observed, suggesting a ceiling effect on the underlying process [27, 34]. An increase in AHP can also be observed by application of L-type Ca^{2+} channel agonists. Reports from various groups have demonstrated that the age-associated augmentation of the AHP is linked to Ca^{2+} influx through voltage-gated Ca^{2+} channels (VGCC) [35, 36], partially the L-type Ca^{2+} channel [27,

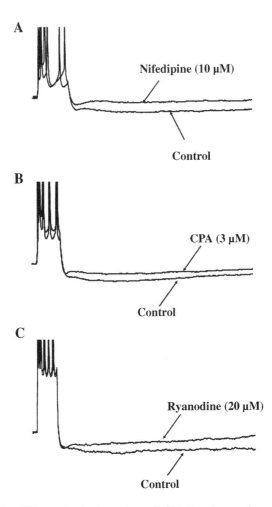

FIGURE 10.2 The AHP amplitude depends on Ca^{2+} influx from voltage-dependent L-type Ca^{2+} channels and release of Ca^{2+} from intracellular Ca^{2+} stores. Each panel shows a relatively large AHP recorded from a CA1 pyramidal neuron from aged rats and elicited by a train of five action potentials (Control). In each case, the AHP is reduced by application of (A) the L-channel blocker nifedipine; (B) depletion of intracellular stores by cyclopiazonic acid (CPA); or blockade of Ca^{2+} release from intracellular stores by ryanodine (C).

30, 37–40]. In addition, a recent report demonstrated that Ca^{2+} release from intracellular calcium stores contributes to the enhanced AHP amplitude during aging [25]. Finally, age-related changes in Ca^{2+} buffering or extrusion could contribute to altered Ca^{2+} homeostasis [41, 42], leading to a prolonged Ca^{2+} response [43]. Taken together, the results indicate that Ca^{2+} from several sources could contribute to the larger AHP during aging (Figure 10.2).

In addition to the Ca^{2+}-dependent triggering of AHP, changes in K^+ channels that underlie AHP could be altered with advanced age. The AHP has at least three temporally distinct components that depend on Ca^{2+} and involve distinct K^+ currents.

The AHP is a composition of fast (fAHP), medium (mAHP), and slow (sAHP) components [44]. In turn, these components are mediated by three outward K+ currents (I_C, I_{AHP}, and sI_{AHP}) [45–48]. The fAHP is of short duration (1 to 10 ms) and follows closely after the initiation of the action potential [44, 49, 50]. The current underlying the fAHP, I_C, is due to the activation of large conduction Ca^{2+}-dependent BK channels. BK channel activity contributes to repolarization of the action potential, and inhibition of this channel following multiple action potentials results in spike broadening and a reduction in the fAHP [44, 50, 51]. An examination of the fAHP in aged animals indicates, however, that this component is not altered and thus does not contribute to the enhancement of later components [31].

The fAHP is followed by a prolonged phase of hyperpolarization that involves the opening of other Ca^{2+}-dependent K+ channels; an increase in this later stage underlies the enhancement of the AHP in the aging neurons [30, 33]. This later phase is the result of two overlapping components: mAHP and sAHP. The mAHP commences within 5 ms of the generation of the action potential, is mediated by I_{AHP}, and lasts for hundreds of milliseconds (100 to 300 ms). This hyperpolarizing response results from the activation of several K+ channels, including M-channels, h-channels, and calcium-activated small conductance SK channels [45, 52, 53]. Apamin, a selective blocker of SK channels, selectively suppresses a component of the mAHP and increases excitability by shortening the interspike interval [45, 54]. In aged animals, apamin reduces the AHP by approximately the same magnitude as that observed following L-channel blockade [55].

Relative to the mAHP, the sAHP has a slower onset and an extended duration, up to several seconds [44–46, 56]. While the properties of the K+ channels underlying the sI_{AHP} have been described, the exact identity of the channel remains unknown. The sI_{AHP} is carried by K+-selective channels that are voltage independent and require Ca^{2+} for their activation [44, 49, 53]. Furthermore, the sAHP is reduced by activation of a number of G-protein coupled receptors, including dopamine [57–60], acetylcholine [31, 61–63], serotonin [61, 64, 65], norepinephrine [61, 66], histamine [67], and metabotropic glutamate receptors [68, 69]. In addition to local neuromodulators, the amplitude of the AHP is under hormonal regulation [27, 70]. In considering the mechanism for the age-associated increase in the AHP, it may be important that the responsiveness to many neuromodulators that act through G-protein coupled signaling appears to decrease with advanced age [19, 71–76]. As such, the increase in this delayed hyperpolarization may not be due to changes in extrinsic modulators, per se. Rather, the age-related growth of the AHP probably is linked to factors intrinsic to the cell involving the regulation of Ca^{2+}, expression or function of various K+ channels, and G-protein coupled signaling. Advancement in this area will depend on better characterization of how these processes or channels change with age.

B. FUNCTIONAL SIGNIFICANCE OF SENESCENT CHANGES IN AHP

The larger AHP of older animals has important ramifications for the induction of synaptic plasticity and the transmission of information through the hippocampus. For example, the AHP hinders the membrane potential from reaching the threshold for generating an action potential. As such, the hyperpolarization acts to restrain the

postsynaptic depolarization to remove a Mg^{2+} block of the NMDA receptor channel. In turn, impairments in LTP induction could arise due to weakened synaptic depolarization or disruption of NMDA receptors. Evidence has been provided that NMDA receptor function may be compromised due to altered Ca^{2+} homeostasis leading to increased activity of the Ca^{2+}-dependent phosphatase, calcineurin [25]. Calcineurin activity depends on a modest rise in intracellular Ca^{2+}, and aged memory impaired animals exhibit an increase in calcineurin activity [134]. In turn, calcineurin can act on NMDA receptors to reduce Ca^{2+} influx [135, 136].

The idea that induction of LTP is subdued as a result of a reduction in NMDA receptor activation is supported by research showing that induction deficits can be overcome by strong postsynaptic depolarization [124]. Indeed, there are several reasons to believe that an inability to achieve sufficient postsynaptic depolarization, a prerequisite for NMDA receptor activation, may be more problematic for LTP induction during aging. First, the reduced synaptic strength of aged animals may result in a reduced afferent cooperativity in depolarizing the postsynaptic neuron and an inability to reach the level of depolarization needed for NMDA receptor activation. Moreover, we have proposed that the inability to depolarize the cell is compounded during patterned stimulation due to the larger AHP (Figure 10.4). In fact, we suggest that it is the large AHP that underlies much of the LTP impairment [19, 91], and may even mask a propensity for enhanced LTP induction during aging [25]. Normally, there is a relationship between the frequency of afferent stimulation required for LTP induction and the level of depolarization [137] but, as noted above, a large and long-lasting AHP is observed following an action potential in older animals. The large AHP disrupts the integration of depolarizing postsynaptic potentials and the duration of this disruption is a function of the extent and duration of the AHP [19, 91, 115]. The disruption would increase the level of stimulation needed for LTP, resulting in the plateau in the frequency response function (Figure 10.3). Our research shows that pharmacological manipulations that reduce the AHP shift the frequency response functions such that LTP can be observed for much lower stimulation frequencies that would normally not elicit LTP in young or aged animals. For example, blockade of VGCCs [54] or inhibition of Ca^{2+} stores [25] reduces the AHP and facilitates induction of LTP (Figure 10.5). The process can be reversed such that an increase in the AHP following the addition of an L-channel agonist prevents LTP induction by 5-Hz stimulation [25]. Thus, an interesting aspect of this work is the fact that while induction of LTP depends on a large rise in intracellular Ca^{2+}, LTP induction is facilitated by blocking several Ca^{2+} sources that contribute to the AHP.

A complementary method for investigating the relationship between the AHP and LTP threshold is to reduce the AHP through manipulation of the potassium channels. For example, blockade of SK channels by apamin increases cell excitability and facilitates LTP-induction [54]. Moreover, deletion of the $Kv\beta1.1$ subunit results in enhanced cell repolarization during repetitive firing by preventing A-type potassium channel inactivation. In turn, the normal spike broadening and increased Ca^{2+} influx through VGCCs is impaired by rapid repolarization. In aged $Kv\beta1.1$ knockout mice, the AHP is reduced, LTP is facilitated, and spatial memory is enhanced [138].

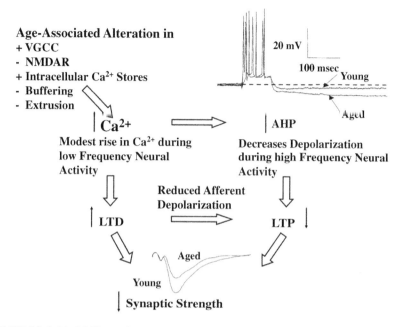

FIGURE 10.4 Model illustrating the relationship between altered Ca^{2+} regulation and synaptic function during aging. The filled arrows indicate the direction of physiological alteration occurring during aging, and the open arrows indicate how age-related changes interact with other physiological processes. An age-related change in Ca^{2+} regulation (decreased NMDAR function and increased contribution from VGCCs and intracellular stores) increases intracellular Ca^{2+} during low-frequency neural activity, which facilitates LTD induction and increases the amplitude and duration of the AHP. In turn, a reduction in the level of depolarization due to a decline in cooperativity as a result of decreased strength of synaptic contacts and a larger AHP acts to impair NMDAR activation and subsequent LTP induction. The shift in the balance of LTP/LTD, favoring LTD, acts to decrease synaptic transmission. The insets illustrate the increase in the AHP (upper right) and decrease in synaptic strength (bottom) observed for aged animals.

The results emphasize that the source of Ca^{2+} provides an overriding control of synaptic modifiability, shifting the threshold frequency of LTP induction.

The shift in Ca^{2+} sources, increased AHP, and altered Ca^{2+} signaling involving a shift in the activity of phosphatases and kinases, also give rise to increased susceptibility to induction of LTD during aging. The induction of LTD depends on a modest rise in Ca^{2+}, which activates a signaling cascade to dephosphorylate glutamate receptors. Recent studies indicate that induction of LTD depends on suppression of NMDA receptors through a process in which Ca^{2+} influx through L-channels activates the Ca^{2+}-dependent phosphatase, calcineurin, resulting in reduced NMDA receptor function [137]. In aged animals, blockade of NMDA receptors can reduce, but does not necessarily prevent, LTD [54]. In fact, LTD induction is facilitated by treatments that enhance potassium channel currents, hyperpolarizing the cell and limiting NMDA receptor activity [139]. Treatments that reduce the AHP, including blockade of L-channels [54], depletion of Ca^{2+} stores [133], or treatment

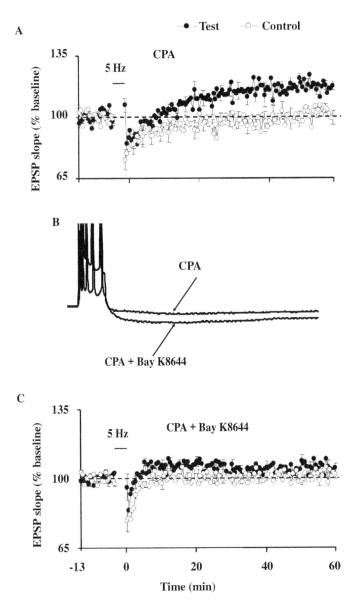

FIGURE 10.5 The LTP threshold is regulated by the AHP amplitude in aged animals. Normally, no change is observed following 5-Hz stimulation (Figure 10.3). However, LTP is induced by treatments that reduce the AHP, such as L-channel blockade or inhibition of Ca^{2+} release from intracellular Ca^{2+} stores (Figure 10.2). (A) Time course of the synaptic response, including induction of LTP following 5-Hz pattern stimulation for aged rats during depletion of Ca^{2+} stores by CPA. (B) The reduction in the AHP by CPA can be reversed by application of the L-channel agonist, Bay K8644. (C) Under conditions in which the AHP is once again increased by Bay K8644, induction of LTP by 5-Hz stimulation is blocked.

with estrogen [27, 130], impair LTD induction in aged animals. Thus, as for LTP, the source of Ca^{2+} is important in determining synapse modifiability and LTD depends on Ca^{2+} from VGCCs and intracellular stores rather than NMDA receptors.

The results paint a picture of a shift in Ca^{2+} homeostasis (Figure 10.4), such that aging cells exhibit reduced Ca^{2+} influx from NMDA receptors and an increased contribution from VGCCs and intracellular stores to intracellular Ca^{2+} during neural activity [19]. In addition, it is likely that aged neurons exhibit changes in intracellular buffering and processes for extrusion of Ca^{2+}. Collectively, this shift results in changes in Ca^{2+}-related physiology, including an increase in the AHP and impaired LTP induction, at least under physiological $Ca^{2+}:Mg^{2+}$ conditions.

The change in homeostasis, which shifts the cell away from Ca^{2+} influx through NMDA receptors, may be neuroprotective against Ca^{2+}-mediated damage and thus act as compensation for increased vulnerability to neurotoxicity [140]. Alternatively, the shift in Ca^{2+} homeostasis could result from an age-related increase in oxidative stress [141–143]. Reactive oxygen species could induce a rise in intracellular Ca^{2+} through release of Ca^{2+} from Ca^{2+} binding proteins (i.e., decreased buffering), and oxidation of calcium regulatory proteins (calmodulin, SERCA, PMCA) would disrupt intracellular stores, and increase entry through Ca^{2+} channels [142, 144]. In the hippocampus, oxidative stress has effects that mimic aging: increasing Ca^{2+} influx through L-channels [145, 146], increasing the function of Ca^{2+}-dependent K^+ channels [23, 147], and decreasing NMDAR function [148]. Furthermore, oxygen radicals can influence the activity of Ca^{2+}-dependent enzymes. The unstable superoxide (O^-) or high levels of H_2O_2 (beyond the physiological range) inhibit calcineurin in tissue homogenates [149, 150]. However, in intact tissue, reactive oxygen species increase calcineurin activity, either through changes in the calcineurin inhibitory protein [151] or altered Ca^{2+} regulation involving increased Ca^{2+} from intracellular stores and VGCCs, leading to impaired induction of LTP [149]. Future research will be required to determine whether treatments designed to reduce oxidative stress can reverse senescent physiology or ameliorate cognitive decline (see Chapter 15).

IV. THE RELATIONSHIP BETWEEN SENESCENT PHYSIOLOGY AND COGNITION

Extensive research has been put forth to ascertain a role for LTP in encoding memory and the role of LTD in memory processes now is being examined. Although the relationship between synaptic plasticity and memory function is far from clear, the available data suggest that aged memory-impaired animals exhibit alterations in hippocampal morphology, biochemistry, and physiology that are linked to a shift in the susceptibility to induction of synaptic plasticity [3, 19]. It is probable that LTD-like processes are involved in hippocampal-dependent cognition; however, the exact role is unclear. Behavioral studies offer at least two possibilities: (1) an essential role for LTD in encoding memory and (2) LTD as a mechanism for degradation of memory consolidation. Evidence that exposure to novel environments can promote the induction of LTD and reversal of LTP [152, 153] led to the suggestion that LTD contributes to memory storage. In contrast, reports that behavioral stress also promotes the induction of LTD and reversal of LTP [154, 155] suggest that LTD contributes to memory impairment. Interestingly, several animal models of diseases associated with impaired memory exhibit enhanced susceptibility to LTD induction, supporting the idea that increased susceptibility to LTD is linked to memory impairments [156–159]. Similarly, behavioral characterization of mice with genetic manipulations of phosphatases involved in the LTD signaling pathway suggests a role for LTD in memory [160–163]. Unfortunately, the relatively brief temporal window for memory encoding or consolidation and a lack of regional specificity for genetic manipulations has made it difficult to provide a precise correlate of hippocampal LTD mechanisms with specific phases of memory [164, 165].

In contrast to genetic models that manipulate protein expression, aging is associated with Ca^{2+} dysregulation, which encourages the activation of signaling cascades that mediate LTD. Thus, it might be concluded that aging results in altered Ca^{2+} regulation leading to an increase in the AHP, and that the reduced cell excitability and increased susceptibility to LTD represent a functional lesion in the memory system. Furthermore, these data point to the importance of mechanisms inherent in the cell (e.g., Ca^{2+} and K^+ channels) in regulating the synaptic plasticity threshold. Related to this is the possibility that aged animals exhibit deficits in metaplasticity. Metaplasticity refers to the process by which previous neural activity modifies subsequent synaptic plasticity [166]. Tangential evidence is provided by studies demonstrating that learning is associated with a reduction in the amplitude of the Ca^{2+}-dependent AHP [26, 55, 167, 168]. In addition, several reports indicate that learning or behavioral conditioning modifies synaptic function [169–171]. Together, the results imply that prior neural activity associated with training can influence the AHP. In turn, a decrease in the AHP would shift synaptic plasticity thresholds, promoting LTP. Thus, memory-impaired animals may be unable to activate metaplasticity processes to influence cell excitability and synaptic function. This idea remains to be tested.

ACKNOWLEDGMENTS

This work was supported by National Institutes of Health Grants AG14979, MH59891, and an Evelyn F. McKnight Brain Research Grant.

REFERENCES

1. Hof, P.R. et al., Age-related changes in GluR2 and NMDAR1 glutamate receptor subunit protein immunoreactivity in corticocortically projecting neurons in macaque and patas monkeys, *Brain Res.*, 928, 175, 2002.
2. Hof, P.R. and Morrison, J.H., The aging brain: morphomolecular senescence of cortical circuits, *Trends Neurosci.*, 27, 607, 2004.
3. Foster, T.C., Regulation of synaptic plasticity in memory and memory decline with aging, *Prog. Brain Res.*, 138, 283, 2002.
4. Onofrj, M. et al., Age-related changes of evoked potentials, *Neurophysiol. Clin.*, 31, 83, 2001.

5. Pickora-Fuller, M.K., Processing speed and timing in aging adults: psychoacoustics, speech perception, and comprehension, *Int. J. Audiol.*, 42 Suppl, S59, 2003.

6. Jackson, G.R. and Owsley, C., Visual dysfunction, neurodegenerative diseases, and aging, *Neurol. Clin.*, 21, 709, 2003.

7. Rogers, J. et al., Senescent pathology of cerebellum: Purkinje neurons and their parallel fiber afferents, *Neurobiol. Aging*, 2, 15, 1981.

8. Boxer, P.A. et al., Alterations of group Ia-motoneuron monosynaptic EPSPs in aged cats, *Exp. Neurol.*, 100, 583, 1988.

9. Chase, M.H. et al., Aging of motoneurons and synaptic processes in the cat, *Exp. Neurol.*, 90, 471, 1985.

10. Kanda, K. et al., The effects of aging on physiological properties of fast and slow twitch motor units in the rat gastrocnemius, *Neurosci. Res.*, 3, 242, 1986.

11. Lamour, Y. et al., Cerebral neocortical neurons in the aged rat: spontaneous activity, properties of pyramidal tract neurons and effect of acetylcholine and cholinergic drugs, *Neuroscience,* 16, 835, 1985.

12. Wheeler, S.J., Effect of age on sensory nerve conduction velocity in the horse, *Res. Vet. Sci.*, 48, 141, 1990.

13. Xi, M.C. et al., Changes in the axonal conduction velocity of pyramidal tract neurons in the aged cat, *Neuroscience*, 92, 219, 1999.

14. Morales, F.R. et al., Basic electrophysiological properties of spinal cord motoneurons during old age in the cat, *J. Neurophysiol.*, 58, 180, 1987.

15. Aston-Jones, G. et al., Age-impaired impulse flow from nucleus basalis to cortex, *Nature,* 318, 462, 1985.

16. Peters, A., The effects of normal aging on myelin and nerve fibers: a review, *J. Neurocytol.*, 31, 581, 2002.

17. Peters, A. et al., Neurobiological bases of age-related cognitive decline in the rhesus monkey, *J. Neuropathol. Exp. Neurol.*, 55, 861, 1996.

18. Turner, D.A. and Deupree, D.L., Functional elongation of CA1 hippocampal neurons with aging in Fischer 344 rats, *Neurobiol. Aging*, 12, 201, 1991.

19. Foster, T.C., Involvement of hippocampal synaptic plasticity in age-related memory decline, *Brain Res. Rev.*, 30, 236, 1999.

20. Landfield, P.W. and Pitler, T.A., Prolonged Ca^{2+}-dependent afterhyperpolarizations in hippocampal neurons of aged rats, *Science,* 226, 1089, 1984.

21. Kerr, D.S. et al., Corticosteroid modulation of hippocampal potentials: increased effect with aging, *Science,* 245, 1505, 1989.

22. Pitler, T.A. and Landfield, P.W., Aging-related prolongation of calcium spike duration in rat hippocampal slice neurons, *Brain Res.*, 508, 1, 1990.

23. Gong, L.W. et al., Transient forebrain ischemia induces persistent hyperactivity of large conductance Ca^{2+}-activated potassium channels via oxidation modulation in rat hippocampal CA1 pyramidal neurons, *Eur. J. Neurosci.*, 15, 779, 2002.

24. Hsu, K.S. et al., Alterations in the balance of protein kinase and phosphatase activities and age-related impairments of synaptic transmission and long-term potentiation, *Hippocampus,* 12, 787, 2002.

25. Kumar, A. and Foster, T.C., Enhanced long-term potentiation during aging is masked by processes involving intracellular calcium stores, *J. Neurophysiol.*, 91, 2437, 2004.

26. Tombaugh, G.C. et al., The slow afterhyperpolarization in hippocampal CA1 neurons covaries with spatial learning ability in aged Fisher 344 rats, *J. Neurosci.*, 25, 2609, 2005.

27. Kumar, A. and Foster, T.C., 17beta-Estradiol benzoate decreases the AHP amplitude in CA1 pyramidal neurons, *J. Neurophysiol.*, 88, 621, 2002.

28. Disterhoft, J.F. et al., Functional aspects of calcium-channel modulation, *Clin. Neuropharmacol.*, 16 S12, 1993.

29. Disterhoft, J.F. et al., Calcium-dependent afterhyperpolarization and learning in young and aging hippocampus, *Life Sci.*, 59, 413, 1996.

30. Moyer, J.R., Jr. et al., Nimodipine increases excitability of rabbit CA1 pyramidal neurons in an age- and concentration-dependent manner, *J. Neurophysiol.*, 68, 2100, 1992.

31. Power, J.M. et al., Metrifonate decreases sI(AHP) in CA1 pyramidal neurons *in vitro*, *J. Neurophysiol.*, 85, 319, 2001.

32. Moyer, J.R., Jr. et al., Increased excitability of aged rabbit CA1 neurons after trace eyeblink conditioning, *J. Neurosci.*, 20, 5476, 2000.

33. Power, J.M. et al., Age-related enhancement of the slow outward calcium-activated potassium current in hippocampal CA1 pyramidal neurons in vitro, *J. Neurosci.*, 22, 7234, 2002.

34. Potier, B. et al., Alterations in the properties of hippocampal pyramidal neurons in the aged rat, *Neuroscience*, 48, 793, 1992.

35. Kaczorowski, C.C. et al., Effects of conotoxin MVIIC on the afterhyperpolarization in hippocampal CA1 pyramidal neurons. *Soc. Neurosc. Abst.*, 28, Prgm. #340.19, 2002.

36. Tanabe, M. et al., L-Type $Ca2+$ channels mediate the slow $Ca2+$-dependent afterhyperpolarization current in rat CA3 pyramidal cells *in vitro*, *J. Neurophysiol.*, 80, 2268, 1998.

37. Chen, K.C. et al., Expression of alpha 1D subunit mRNA is correlated with L-type $Ca2+$ channel activity in single neurons of hippocampal "zipper" slices, *Proc. Natl. Acad. Sci. U.S.A.*, 97, 4357, 2000.

38. Thibault, O. and Landfield, P.W., Increase in single L-type calcium channels in hippocampal neurons during aging, *Science*, 272, 1017, 1996.

39. Thibault, O. et al., Elevated postsynaptic [Ca2+]i and L-type calcium channel activity in aged hippocampal neurons: relationship to impaired synaptic plasticity, *J. Neurosci.*, 21, 9744, 2001.

40. Moyer, J.R., Jr. and Disterhoft, J.F., Nimodipine decreases calcium action potentials in rabbit hippocampal CA1 neurons in an age-dependent and concentration-dependent manner, *Hippocampus*, 4, 11, 1994.

41. Satrustegui, J. et al., Cytosolic and mitochondrial calcium in synaptosomes during aging, *Life Sci.*, 59, 429, 1996.

42. Murchison, D. et al., Reduced mitochondrial buffering of voltage-gated calcium influx in aged rat basal forebrain neurons, *Cell. Calcium*, 36, 61, 2004.

43. Toescu, E.C. and Verkhratsky, A., Parameters of calcium homeostasis in normal neuronal ageing, *J. Anat.*, 197, 563, 2000.

44. Sah, P. and Faber, E.S., Channels underlying neuronal calcium-activated potassium currents, *Prog. Neurobiol.*, 66, 345, 2002.

45. Stocker, M. et al., An apamin-sensitive $Ca2+$-activated $K+$ current in hippocampal pyramidal neurons, *Proc. Natl. Acad. Sci. U.S.A.*, 96, 4662, 1999.

46. Sah, P., $Ca(2+)$-activated $K+$ currents in neurones: types, physiological roles and modulation, *Trends Neurosci.*, 19, 150, 1996.

47. Storm, J.F., Potassium currents in hippocampal pyramidal cells, *Prog. Brain Res.*, 83, 161, 1990.

48. Maccaferri, G. et al., Properties of the hyperpolarization-activated current in rat hippocampal CA1 pyramidal cells, *J. Neurophysiol.*, 69, 2129, 1993.

49. Lancaster, B. and Adams, P.R., Calcium-dependent current generating the afterhyperpolarization of hippocampal neurons, *J. Neurophysiol.,* 55, 1268, 1986.

50. Shao, L.R. et al., The role of BK-type Ca2+-dependent K+ channels in spike broadening during repetitive firing in rat hippocampal pyramidal cells, *J. Physiol.,* 521 Pt 1, 135, 1999.

51. Lancaster, B. and Nicoll, R.A., Properties of two calcium-activated hyperpolarizations in rat hippocampal neurones, *J. Physiol.,* 389, 187, 1987.

52. Gu, N. et al., Kv7/KCNQ/M and HCN/h, but not KCa2/SK channels, contribute to the somatic medium after-hyperpolarization and excitability control in CA1 hippocampal pyramidal cells, *J. Physiol.,* 566 Pt 3, 689, 2005.

53. Bond, C.T. et al., Small conductance Ca2+-activated K+ channel knock-out mice reveal the identity of calcium-dependent afterhyperpolarization currents, *J. Neurosci.,* 24, 5301, 2004.

54. Norris, C.M. et al., Reversal of age-related alterations in synaptic plasticity by blockade of L-type Ca2+ channels, *J. Neurosci.,* 18, 3171, 1998.

55. Disterhoft, J.F. et al., Biophysical alterations of hippocampal pyramidal neurons in learning, ageing and Alzheimer's disease, *Ageing Res. Rev.,* 3, 383, 2004.

56. Gerlach, A.C. et al., Activation kinetics of the slow afterhyperpolarization in hippocampal CA1 neurons, *Pflugers Arch.,* 448, 187, 2004.

57. Pedarzani, P. and Storm, J.F., Dopamine modulates the slow Ca(2+)-activated K+ current IAHP via cyclic AMP-dependent protein kinase in hippocampal neurons, *J. Neurophysiol.,* 74, 2749, 1995.

58. Pedarzani, P. and Storm, J.F., Evidence that Ca/calmodulin-dependent protein kinase mediates the modulation of the Ca2+-dependent K+ current, IAHP, by acetylcholine, but not by glutamate, in hippocampal neurons, *Pflugers Arch.,* 431, 723, 1996.

59. Malenka, R.C. and Nicoll, R.A., Dopamine decreases the calcium-activated afterhyperpolarization in hippocampal CA1 pyramidal cells, *Brain Res.,* 379, 210, 1986.

60. Malenka, R.C. et al., Phorbol esters mimic some cholinergic actions in hippocampal pyramidal neurons, *J. Neurosci.,* 6, 475, 1986.

61. Nicoll, R.A., The coupling of neurotransmitter receptors to ion channels in the brain, *Science,* 241, 545, 1988.

62. Weiss, C. et al., The M1 muscarinic agonist CI-1017 facilitates trace eyeblink conditioning in aging rabbits and increases the excitability of CA1 pyramidal neurons, *J. Neurosci.,* 20, 783, 2000.

63. Saar, D. et al., Long-lasting cholinergic modulation underlies rule learning in rats, *J. Neurosci.,* 21, 1385, 2001.

64. Colino, A. and Halliwell, J.V., Differential modulation of three separate K-conductances in hippocampal CA1 neurons by serotonin, *Nature,* 328, 73, 1987.

65. Grunnet, M. et al., 5-HT1A receptors modulate small-conductance Ca2+-activated K+ channels, *J. Neurosci. Res.,* 78, 845, 2004.

66. Haas, H.L. and Konnerth, A., Histamine and noradrenaline decrease calcium-activated potassium conductance in hippocampal pyramidal cells, *Nature,* 302, 432, 1983.

67. Haas, H.L. and Greene, R.W., Effects of histamine on hippocampal pyramidal cells of the rat *in vitro, Exp. Brain Res.,* 62, 123, 1986.

68. Mannaioni, G. et al., Metabotropic glutamate receptors 1 and 5 differentially regulate CA1 pyramidal cell function, *J. Neurosci.,* 21, 5925, 2001.

69. Tan, Y. et al., The mechanism of presynaptic long-term depression mediated by group I metabotropic glutamate receptors, *Cell. Mol. Neurobiol.,* 23, 187, 2003.

70. Joels, M. and de Kloet, E.R., Effects of glucocorticoids and norepinephrine on the excitability in the hippocampus, *Science,* 245, 1502, 1989.

71. Bickford, P.C. et al., Diminished interaction of norepinephrine with climbing fiber inputs to cerebellar Purkinje neurons in aged Fischer 344 rats, *Brain Res.*, 385, 405, 1986.

72. Bickford-Wimer, P.C. et al., Age-related reduction in responses of rat hippocampal neurons to locally applied monoamines, *Neurobiol. Aging*, 9, 173, 1988.

73. Stern, W.C. et al., Single unit activity in frontal cortex and caudate nucleus of young and old rats, *Neurobiol. Aging*, 6, 245, 1985.

74. Ayyagari, P.V. et al., Uncoupling of muscarinic cholinergic phosphoinositide signals in senescent cerebral cortical and hippocampal membranes, *Neurochem. Int.*, 32, 107, 1998.

75. Shen, J. and Barnes, C.A., Age-related decrease in cholinergic synaptic transmission in three hippocampal subfields, *Neurobiol. Aging*, 17, 439, 1996.

76. Nicolle, M.M. et al., Metabotropic glutamate receptor-mediated hippocampal phosphoinositide turnover is blunted in spatial learning-impaired aged rats, *J. Neurosci.*, 19, 9604, 1999.

77. Madison, D.V. and Nicoll, R.A., Control of the repetitive discharge of rat CA 1 pyramidal neurones in vitro, *J. Physiol.*, 354, 319, 1984.

78. Him, A. et al., Tonic activity and GABA responsiveness of medial vestibular nucleus neurons in aged rats. *Neuroreport*, 12, 3965, 2001.

79. Palombi, P.S. and Caspary, D.M., Physiology of the aged Fischer 344 rat inferior colliculus: responses to contralateral monaural stimuli, *J. Neurophysiol.*, 76, 3114, 1996.

80. Shen, J. et al., The effect of aging on experience-dependent plasticity of hippocampal place cells, *J. Neurosci.*, 17, 6769, 1997.

81. Smith, A.C. et al., Effect of age on burst firing characteristics of rat hippocampal pyramidal cells, *Neuroreport*, 11, 3865, 2000.

82. Wilson, I.A. et al., Age-associated alterations of hippocampal place cells are subregion specific, *J. Neurosci.*, 25, 6877, 2005.

83. Oler, J.A. and Markus, E.J., Age-related deficits in the ability to encode contextual change: a place cell analysis, *Hippocampus*, 10, 338, 2000.

84. Barnes, C.A. et al., Multistability of cognitive maps in the hippocampus of old rats, *Nature*, 388, 272, 1997.

85. Papatheodoropoulos, C. and Kostopoulos, G., Age-related changes in excitability and recurrent inhibition in the rat CA1 hippocampal region, *Eur. J. Neurosci.*, 8, 510, 1996.

86. Barnes, C.A. and McNaughton, B.L., Physiological compensation for loss of afferent synapses in rat hippocampal granule cells during senescence, *J. Physiol.*, 309, 473, 1980.

87. Ekstrom, A.D. et al., NMDA receptor antagonism blocks experience-dependent expansion of hippocampal "place fields," *Neuron*, 31, 631, 2001.

88. Barnes, C.A., Effects of aging on the dynamics of information processing and synaptic weight changes in the mammalian hippocampus, *Prog. Brain Res.*, 86, 89, 1990.

89. Rosenzweig, E.S. and Barnes, C.A., Impact of aging on hippocampal function: plasticity, network dynamics, and cognition, *Prog. Neurobiol.*, 69, 143, 2003.

90. Geinisman, Y. et al., Hippocampal markers of age-related memory dysfunction: behavioral, electrophysiological and morphological perspectives, *Prog. Neurobiol.*, 45, 223, 1995.

91. Foster, T.C. and Norris, C.M., Age-associated changes in $Ca2+$-dependent processes: relation to hippocampal synaptic plasticity, *Hippocampus*, 7, 602, 1997.

92. Landfield, P.W. et al., The effects of high $Mg2+$-to-$Ca2+$ ratios on frequency potentiation in hippocampal slices of young and aged rats, *J. Neurophysiol.*, 56, 797, 1986.

93. Deupree, D.L. et al., Age-related alterations in potentiation in the CA1 region in F344 rats, *Neurobiol. Aging,* 14, 249, 1993.

94. Barnes, C.A. et al., Region-specific age effects on AMPA sensitivity: electrophysiological evidence for loss of synaptic contacts in hippocampal field CA1, *Hippocampus,* 2, 457, 1992.

95. Jouvenceau, A. et al., Alteration of NMDA receptor-mediated synaptic responses in CA1 area of the aged rat hippocampus: contribution of GABAergic and cholinergic deficits, *Hippocampus,* 0, 627, 1990.

96. Barnes, C.A. et al., Age-related decrease in the Schaffer collateral-evoked EPSP in awake, freely behaving rats, *Neural Plast.,* 7, 167, 2000.

97. Foster, T.C. et al., Increase in perforant path quantal size in aged F-344 rats, *Neurobiol. Aging,* 12, 441, 1991.

98. Levkovitz, Y. and Segal, M., Age-dependent local modulation of hippocampal-evoked responses to perforant path stimulation, *Neurobiol. Aging,* 19, 317, 1998.

99. Talmi, M. et al., Similar effects of aging and corticosterone treatment on mouse hippocampal function, *Neurobiol. Aging,* 14, 239, 1993.

100. Smith, T.D. et al., Circuit-specific alterations in hippocampal synaptophysin immunoreactivity predict spatial learning impairment in aged rats, *J. Neurosci.,* 20, 6587, 2000.

101. Saito, S. et al., Decreased synaptic density in aged brains and its prevention by rearing under enriched environment as revealed by synaptophysin contents, *J. Neurosci. Res.,* 39, 57, 1994.

102. Casoli, T. et al., Neuronal plasticity in aging: a quantitative immunohistochemical study of GAP-43 distribution in discrete regions of the rat brain, *Brain Res.,* 714, 111, 1996.

103. Chen, Y.C. et al., Physical training modifies the age-related decrease of GAP-43 and synaptophysin in the hippocampal formation in C57BL/6J mouse, *Brain Res.,* 806, 238, 1998.

104. Geinisman, Y. et al., Age-related loss of axospinous synapses formed by two afferent systems in the rat dentate gyrus as revealed by the unbiased stereological dissector technique, *Hippocampus,* 2, 437, 1992.

105. Eastwood, S.L. et al., Synaptophysin gene expression in human brain: a quantitative in situ hybridization and immunocytochemical study, *Neuroscience,* 59, 881, 1994.

106. Tigges, J. et al., Preservation into old age of synaptic number and size in the supragranular layer of the dentate gyrus in rhesus monkeys, *Acta Anat. (Basel),* 157, 63, 1996.

107. Curcio, C.A. and Hinds, J.W., Stability of synaptic density and spine volume in dentate gyrus of aged rats, *Neurobiol. Aging,* 4, 77, 1983.

108. Nicolle, M.M. et al., No loss of synaptic proteins in the hippocampus of aged, behaviorally impaired rats, *Neurobiol. Aging,* 20, 343, 1999.

109. Lippa, C.F. et al., Alzheimer's disease and aging: effects on perforant pathway perikarya and synapses, *Neurobiol. Aging,* 13, 405, 1992.

110. Nicholson, D.A. et al., Reduction in size of perforated postsynaptic densities in hippocampal axospinous synapses and age-related spatial learning impairments, *J. Neurosci.,* 24, 7648, 2004.

111. Schweizer, T. et al., 3,4-DAP-evoked transmitter release in hippocampal slices of aged rats with impaired memory, *Brain Res. Bull.,* 62, 129, 2003.

112. Geinisman, Y. et al., Aging, spatial learning, and total synapse number in the rat CA1 stratum radiatum, *Neurobiol. Aging,* 25, 407, 2004.

113. Calhoun, M.E. et al., Hippocampal neuron and synaptophysin-positive bouton number in aging C57BL/6 mice, *Neurobiol. Aging*, 19, 599, 1998.

114. Segovia, G. et al., Glutamatergic neurotransmission in aging: a critical perspective, *Mech. Ageing Dev.*, 122, 1, 2001.

115. Foster, T.C. and Kumar, A., Calcium dysregulation in the aging brain, *Neuroscientist*, 8, 297, 2002.

116. Potier, B. et al., NMDA receptor activation in the aged rat hippocampus, *Exp. Gerontol.*, 35, 1185, 2000.

117. Barnes, C.A. et al., Age-related decrease in the N-methyl-D-aspartate-mediated excitatory postsynaptic potential in hippocampal region CA1, *Neurobiol. Aging*, 18, 445, 1997.

118. Bienenstock, E.L. et al., Theory for the development of neuron selectivity: orientation specificity and binocular interaction in visual cortex, *J. Neurosci.*, 2, 32, 1982.

119. Artola, A. and Singer, W., Long-term depression of excitatory synaptic transmission and its relationship to long-term potentiation, *Trends Neurosci.*, 16, 480, 1993.

120. Rex, C.S. et al., Long-term potentiation is impaired in middle-aged rats: regional specificity and reversal by adenosine receptor antagonists, *J. Neurosci.*, 25, 5956, 2005.

121. Norris, C.M. et al., Increased susceptibility to induction of long-term depression and long- term potentiation reversal during aging, *J. Neurosci.*, 16, 5382, 1996.

122. Shankar, S. et al., Aging differentially alters forms of long-term potentiation in rat hippocampal area CA1, *J. Neurophysiol.*, 79, 334, 1998.

123. Diana, G. et al., Age and strain differences in rat place learning and hippocampal dentate gyrus frequency-potentiation, *Neurosci. Lett.*, 171, 113, 1994.

124. Barnes, C.A. et al., Functional integrity of NMDA-dependent LTP induction mechanisms across the lifespan of F-344 rats, *Learn. Mem.*, 3, 124, 1996.

125. Watabe, A.M. and O'Dell, T.J., Age-related changes in theta frequency stimulation-induced long-term potentiation, *Neurobiol. Aging*, 24, 267, 2003.

126. Zamani, M.R. et al., Estradiol modulates long-term synaptic depression in female rat hippocampus, *J. Neurophysiol.*, 84, 1800, 2000.

127. Kemp, N. et al., Different forms of LTD in the CA1 region of the hippocampus: role of age and stimulus protocol, *Eur. J. Neurosci.*, 12, 360, 2000.

128. Thinschmidt, J.S. et al., Aging effects on asymptotic long-term depression and long-term potentiation, *Society Neuroscience Abstract* 974.10, 2004.

129. Dudek, S.M. and Bear, M.F., Bidirectional long-term modification of synaptic effectiveness in the adult and immature hippocampus, *J. Neurosci.*, 13, 2910, 1993.

130. Vouimba, R.M. et al., 17beta-estradiol suppresses expression of long-term depression in aged rats, *Brain Res. Bull.*, 53, 783, 2000.

131. Moore, C.I. et al., Hippocampal plasticity induced by primed burst, but not long-term potentiation, stimulation is impaired in area CA1 of aged Fischer 344 rats, *Hippocampus*, 3, 57, 1993.

132. Rosenzweig, E.S. et al., Role of temporal summation in age-related long-term potentiation- induction deficits, *Hippocampus*, 7, 549, 1997.

133. Kumar, A. and Foster, T.C., Intracellular calcium stores contribute to increased susceptibility to LTD induction during aging, *Brain Res.*, 1031, 125, 2005.

134. Foster, T.C. et al., Calcineurin links Ca2+ dysregulation with brain aging, *J. Neurosci.*, 21, 4066, 2001.

135. Tong, G. and Jahr, C.E., Regulation of glycine-insensitive desensitization of the NMDA receptor in outside-out patches, *J. Neurophysiol.*, 72, 754, 1994.

136. Lieberman, D.N. and Mody, I., Regulation of NMDA channel function by endogenous Ca(2+)-dependent phosphatase, *Nature,* 369, 235, 1994.

137. Froemke, R.C. et al., Spike-timing-dependent synaptic plasticity depends on dendritic location, *Nature,* 434, 221, 2005.

138. Murphy, G.G. et al., Increased neuronal excitability, synaptic plasticity, and learning in aged Kvbeta1.1 knockout mice, *Curr. Biol.,* 14, 1907, 2004.

139. Azad, S.C. et al., The potassium channel modulator flupirtine shifts the frequency-response function of hippocampal synapses to favour LTD in mice, *Neurosci. Lett.,* 370, 186, 2004.

140. Phillips, R.G. et al., Calbindin D28K gene transfer via herpes simplex virus amplicon vector decreases hippocampal damage in vivo following neurotoxic insults, *J. Neurochem.,* 73, 1200, 1999.

141. Annunziato, L. et al., Apoptosis induced in neuronal cells by oxidative stress: role played by caspases and intracellular calcium ions, *Toxicol. Lett.,* 139, 125, 2003.

142. Squier, T.C., Oxidative stress and protein aggregation during biological aging, *Exp. Gerontol.,* 36, 1539, 2001.

143. Serrano, F. and Klann, E., Reactive oxygen species and synaptic plasticity in the aging hippocampus, *Ageing Res. Rev.,* 3, 431, 2004.

144. Suzuki, Y.J. et al., Oxidants as stimulators of signal transduction, *Free Radic. Biol. Med.,* 22, 269, 1997.

145. Lu, C. et al., The lipid peroxidation product 4-hydroxynonenal facilitates opening of voltage-dependent Ca2+ channels in neurons by increasing protein tyrosine phosphorylation, *J. Biol. Chem.,* 277, 24368, 2002.

146. Akaishi, T. et al., Hydrogen peroxide modulates whole cell Ca2+ currents through L-type channels in cultured rat dentate granule cells, *Neurosci. Lett.,* 356, 25, 2004.

147. Gong, L. et al., Redox modulation of large conductance calcium-activated potassium channels in CA1 pyramidal neurons from adult rat hippocampus, *Neurosci. Lett.,* 286, 191, 2000.

148. Lu, C. et al., Selective and biphasic effect of the membrane lipid peroxidation product 4-hydroxy-2,3-nonenal on N-methyl-D-aspartate channels, *J. Neurochem.,* 78, 577, 2001.

149. Kamsler, A. and Segal, M., Hydrogen peroxide as a diffusible signal molecule in synaptic plasticity, *Mol. Neurobiol.,* 29, 167, 2004.

150. Ullrich, V. et al., Superoxide as inhibitor of calcineurin and mediator of redox regulation, *Toxicol. Lett.,* 139, 107, 2003.

151. Lin, H.Y. et al., Oxidative and calcium stress regulate DSCR1 (Adapt78/MCIP1) protein, *Free Radic. Biol. Med.,* 35, 528, 2003.

152. Xu, L. et al., Behavioural stress facilitates the induction of long-term depression in the hippocampus, *Nature,* 387, 497, 1997.

153. Manahan-Vaughan, D. et al., Presynaptic group 1 metabotropic glutamate receptors may contribute to the expression of long-term potentiation in the hippocampal CA1 region, *Neuroscience,* 94, 71, 1999.

154. Xu, L. et al., Glucocorticoid receptor and protein/RNA synthesis-dependent mechanisms underlie the control of synaptic plasticity by stress, *Proc. Natl. Acad. Sci. U.S.A.,* 95, 3204, 1998.

155. Kim, J.J. et al., Behavioral stress modifies hippocampal plasticity through N-methyl-D-aspartate receptor activation, *Proc. Natl. Acad. Sci. U.S.A.,* 93, 4750, 1996.

156. Artola, A. et al., Diabetes mellitus concomitantly facilitates the induction of long-term depression and inhibits that of long-term potentiation in hippocampus, *Eur. J. Neurosci.,* 22, 169, 2005.

neural changes that correspond to those behavioral differences, and eventually, to discover which of the myriad developmental changes that occur during aging are responsible for the beneficial and detrimental aspects of the aging process. Although the emphasis is on the developmental processes that occur during normal aging, this chapter addresses, to some extent, the manner in which these methods also make possible investigations of the pathological changes that often accompany aging, including those associated with Alzheimer's disease, and may allow discrimination between such pathological processes and normal processes. In turn, such discrimination will make possible more accurate and earlier diagnosis of these pathologies and allow more targeted treatment for the individuals most at risk.

It should be stated at the outset that there is not presently (and there may never be) a single encompassing theory of the neurocognitive changes that occur during aging. Several reviews, however, have suggested a two-component view of aging in which one component is associated with normal aging processes, while a second component is associated with pathological processes [1–4]. The first of these components revolves around changes in the volume and function of the prefrontal cortex (PFC), related frontal-striatal and frontal-parietal circuits, and their associated neurotransmitter systems, including dopamine [5, 6]. The neural circuits in this component are associated with high-level cognitive operations referred to as executive control or attentional control [7–9]. Attentional control refers to the ability to modulate and coordinate multiple component processes to maintain focus on task-relevant information in the face of distraction, an ability at which normal older adults can perform notoriously poorly [10–12]. The effects of aging on this component are supported by evidence that age-related structural declines in the PFC are among the largest in the brain, that functional measures consistently observe large age-related changes in the PFC and related structures, that behavioral measures of cognitive functions such as strategic attentional control are disproportionately impaired during aging, and that neurotransmitter systems active in the PFC show large age-related changes [13–15]. Additionally, white matter tracts in the frontal lobes exhibit an age-related loss of integrity that might affect memory circuits involving the frontal cortices [16, 17]. Developmental changes in this component appear to be a consequence of normal aging, as such changes are observed even in individuals without dementia symptoms, develop gradually throughout adulthood, and are correlated with age-related declines in behavioral memory measures.

The second component, in contrast to the changes observed during normal aging, involves pathological age-related changes centered in the medial temporal lobes (MTL) that are primarily associated with Alzheimer's disease. These appear to begin with volume losses in the entorhinal cortex, an important relay between the hippocampus and association cortices, and progressively affect the hippocampus proper. The progression from normal aging to frank Alzheimer's dementia can occur in a graded fashion, lasting perhaps a decade or longer. However, pathological changes in entorhinal cortex often occur prior to clinical diagnosis of Alzheimer's disease [18, 19]. Therefore, individuals in a prodromal stage of pathology may be inadvertently included in samples of apparently normal elderly participants [20]. Fortunately, behavioral measures of cognitive impairment can be used to predict progression from normal aging to mild cognitive impairment (MCI) to Alzheimer's disease so that individuals with pathology can be selectively excluded on the basis of such performance.

This chapter focuses primarily on recent advances in the functional neuroimaging of human cognition that have led toward a converging view that neural circuits involving prefrontal function and the related capacity for attentional control are key components of the developmental changes associated with normal aging. Along the way, this chapter discusses the neurocognitive correlates of attentional control, how aging affects these behavioral and neurological relationships, how these effects differ from those seen in age-associated pathology, how individuals vary in their susceptibility to such effects of aging, and what implications such individual differences hold for our understanding of the aging brain.

II. STRUCTURE-FUNCTION RELATIONSHIPS

In its own way, the cognitive neuroscience of aging is primarily a methodological enterprise, relying almost entirely on continually evolving techniques of *in vivo* imaging, each with its own limits and advantages. As such, any discussion of the cognitive neuroscience of aging must address a number of methodological challenges faced by the field. Because the emphasis of this volume is as much on methods as it is on models and mechanisms, this chapter largely treats these methodological issues within the context of discussions regarding the theoretical issues that those methods help to address. However, to better understand the most basic methodological issues faced by the application of methods of functional neuroimaging to the study of aging, we first address the relationship of age-related changes in structure to age-related changes in function.

A. Volumetric Changes in Frontal-Striatal Gray Matter

Although both postmortem and *in vivo* studies have found the brains of older adults to have lower volumes of gray matter than the brains of younger adults [21, 22], the changes in regional volume are not uniform. Some regions, such as the PFC, show particularly dramatic changes in volume, while other regions, such as the occipital cortex, are relatively unaffected by normal aging [5, 14, 22, 23]. The largest age-related volumetric changes in older adulthood appear to occur in the PFC [21, 22, 24], with cross-sectional estimates of average volume loss of approximately 5% per decade after the age of 20 [23]. The largest age correlation with regional volume, both at baseline and follow-up in a longitudinal study, was in the lateral PFC, with an estimated rate of loss of 0.91% per year [5]. Orbito-frontal PFC declines were nearly as large, with an estimated annual loss of 0.85% [5]. In contrast, patients with Alzheimer's disease show the greatest degeneration in the inferior PFC [25], although deterioration of PFC is not observed early in the disease [26]. Somewhat smaller age-related declines are observed in the striatum, a subregion of the basal ganglia that includes the caudate and putamen and is heavily involved in dopaminergic circuits connecting to the PFC. Cross-sectional estimates place striatal volume declines at about 3% per decade [27], while longitudinal estimates of caudate volume declines are approximately 0.75% per year [5, 28].

C.   REGIONAL BLOOD FLOW AND FUNCTIONAL NEUROIMAGING

Although the methods of functional neuroimaging are many and varied, this chapter focuses primarily on two of the most widely used: (1) positron emission tomography (PET) and (2) functional magnetic resonance imaging (fMRI). Briefly, both PET, which usually uses injections of radioactively labeled oxygen, and fMRI, which relies on the natural blood oxygen-level dependent (BOLD) response, are measures of regional cerebral blood flow, and are therefore indirect measures of neuronal activity. Recent studies using simultaneous population cell recording and fMRI have shown a strong correlation between local population firing and regional BOLD responses [38–40]. Because these measurements depend on small changes in regional blood flow, vascular changes throughout the body may affect the results from these techniques. Of special concern are the effects of vascular conditions prevalent among older adults, including hypertension, atherosclerosis and arteriosclerosis, and prior incidence of heart attack or stroke. Most studies of normal older adults exclude participants with any such conditions, but it is nearly impossible to guarantee that no participants with undiagnosed vascular conditions are admitted. It is therefore important to characterize the hemodynamic response function (HRF) exhibited by older adults and to compare this HRF with that of younger adults. The results of such methodological studies are particularly important for the interpretation of age differences in functional imaging studies, as group differences in HRF characteristics, if not properly accounted for, could conceivably affect any conclusions regarding age-related differences in regional cerebral blood flow.

A number of studies have examined precisely this issue, primarily using fMRI to determine age differences in the timing and shape of the BOLD response during simple sensory or motor tasks (reviewed in [41]). Across several studies, older adults display a smaller spatial extent, or the number of above-threshold voxels, compared to younger adults, often accompanied by a lower signal-to-noise ratio for older adults [42–47]. However, when comparable above-threshold voxels were examined, the majority of studies have observed no differences between younger and older adults in the amplitude or in the variance of the BOLD response in primary motor cortex and/or primary visual cortex [42–44, 46–48]. Several studies have reported a slower return to baseline in older than in younger adults in either the visual or motor cortex [42–44]. In studies directly comparing BOLD responses in the visual and motor cortices, age differences appear to be moderately larger in visual than in motor cortex [42, 43]. In general, the pattern of results across studies indicates that age differences in hemodynamic responsivity in sensory-motor brain regions are relatively slight [41].

Two specific studies are of particular interest. First, when direct stimulation was applied to the motor cortex using transcranial magnetic stimulation, no age differences in the BOLD response were observed, indicating that the regional vascular response to direct neural stimulation is not affected by aging [49]. Second, a study that investigated BOLD responses during a cognitive inhibition task found no significant age differences across a variety of prefrontal and other cortical sites [50]. This study demonstrated that the lack of age differences in BOLD reactivity generalizes to cortical regions that are more directly associated with cognition, and is not constrained to sensory-motor areas.

Although age differences in the HRF appear to be relatively slight, most of the studies have investigated responses within primary sensory and motor cortices, rather than in the prefrontal, parietal, and striatal regions that appear to be most age sensitive. Despite limited evidence that HRFs in these regions do not change with normal aging [50], it remains possible that some critical regions exhibit different HRF profiles in older and younger adults. To make plausible inferences about the effects of aging, researchers look for age by condition and age by region interactions to show that age is related to some, but not other, neurocognitive functions. Such interactions cannot be explained by HRF differences alone, unless one assumes that the regions differ in their HRFs to precisely the degree that age differences are apparent.

III. ATTENTIONAL CONTROL

As previously noted, attentional control (or executive control) refers to the ability to modulate and coordinate multiple component processes in an effort to maintain focus on task-relevant information in the presence of distraction. There is presently a large literature regarding the nature and potential numerosity of such attentional control mechanisms [10–12]. For present purposes, the discussion is restricted to several of the most commonly studied attentional control processes in which the effects of aging have been addressed using functional neuroimaging methods. These include working memory (sometimes more specifically referred to as updating), inhibition, and task switching (or shifting).

Numerous studies have described age-related declines in a variety of control processes in normal elderly populations [10, 12]. In large part because normal older adults exhibit deficits in attentional control processes that are similar to those displayed by patients with frontal lesions, neuropsychologists have long speculated that deficits in prefrontal cortical function are a main cause of age-related declines in cognitive function, including failures to suppress interfering information, commission of perseverative errors, and an inability to organize the contents of working memory [13, 14].

A.   ATTENTIONAL CONTROL AND PFC FUNCTION

In studies involving younger adults, a consistent network of regions involved in attentional control has been identified [51]. Collette and Van der Linden [52] summarized the results of PET and fMRI studies of the control processes of updating, inhibition, shifting, and dual-task coordination. Their review found that several regions in prefrontal and parietal cortices were activated across many studies, despite the diversity of tasks and control processes sampled. Prefrontal regions included dorsolateral PFC [Brodmann area (BA) 9 and 46], ventrolateral PFC (BA 44 and 45, sometimes including BA 47), frontopolar cortex (BA 10), middle frontal cortex (BA 6 and 8), and anterior cingulate cortex (ACC, primarily BA 32). Parietal regions included the inferior parietal lobule (BA 7), superior parietal lobule (BA 40), and the temporal-parietal junction (BA 39). Although not every control process activated all these regions, and not every study of a particular process found the same set of regions, there was enough overlap among process-to-activation associations for the authors to conclude that "executive functioning seems to be better conceptualized in terms of interrelationships within a network of cerebral areas rather than associations between one executive function and a few specific prefrontal cerebral areas." [52, p. 122]. A meta-analysis of activations across studies of executive working memory (or updating) and switching processes came to a similar conclusion. That study found that while both types of processes activated dorsolateral PFC, ACC, and parietal cortex, certain areas tended to show more activation during switching than in working memory (primarily ACC and left-lateralized parietal cortex), while other areas tended to show more activation during working memory than switching (primarily dorsolateral PFC, medial parietal cortex, and frontopolar cortex) [8]. These results suggest that a prefrontal-parietal network underlies attentional control, with component processes being more or less dependent on particular regions within this network.

B. WORKING MEMORY

Working memory refers to those processes used to maintain and manipulate information online for short periods of time, such as when holding several digits and the results of carrying operations in mind while performing mental arithmetic. Many neuroimaging studies have associated activation within the PFC with working memory processes, finding that the maintenance of information is associated with ventrolateral PFC activation, while the manipulation of information is associated with activation in the dorsolateral PFC [53–55]. Additionally, activation in these PFC regions during working memory performance is associated with activation in posterior regions, particularly within the parietal cortex, so that working memory function appears to be subserved by a larger frontal-parietal network [56].

Older adults exhibit declines in working memory performance, and several neuroimaging studies have observed concomitant age-related changes in prefrontal and parietal activation [57–61]. Of interest, behavioral studies revealed that older adults perform nearly as well as their younger counterparts on maintenance tasks, but that steep age-related declines are observed during tasks requiring online manipulation of information [62]. In keeping with this pattern and with the association between maintenance and ventrolateral PFC and between manipulation and dorsolateral PFC, one study found that older adults had activation similar to younger adults in ventrolateral PFC, but reduced activation in dorsolateral PFC at high memory loads [61]. Another study, which investigated the ability to intentionally refresh information held in working memory, found an age-related decline in a region of dorsolateral PFC (BA 9), although age equivalence was also observed in several other PFC sites [63]. In a recent review that included nine studies of age-related effects on PFC activation during working memory, the main pattern was one of increased activation in older compared to younger adults in left dorsolateral PFC regions [64] (Figure 11.2). This age-related increase in activation primarily occurred during conditions of short delay periods or when older adults performed as well as younger adults. In the same review, ventrolateral PFC regions were found to exhibit somewhat more activation in younger compared to older adults, although this pattern

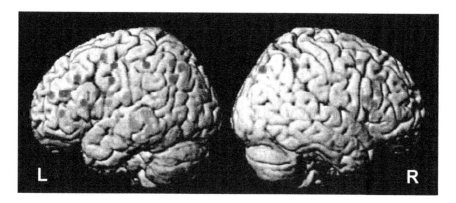

FIGURE 11.2 (SEE COLOR INSERT FOLLOWING PAGE 204) Summary of age-related effects on functional activation in prefrontal and parietal cortex during working memory. In blue: sites of decreased activation during aging (younger > older); in red: sites of increased activation during aging (older > younger). It can be noted that sites of increased activation in the PFC during aging are predominantly left-lateralized in dorsolateral and posterior ventrolateral PFC. Sites of decreased activation during aging are bilateral and predominantly located in more anterior sites in ventrolateral PFC. Activation sites were taken from studies using various working memory tasks, both verbal and nonverbal. Activations were included only if the source study unambiguously indicated the peak voxel of activation and a significant age effect at that voxel. Points indicate a spherical region 6 mm in diameter around each peak voxel. Activations are summarized from [57, 58, 61, 125, 126, 149, 150].

was slight, with several studies observing similar activations in younger and older adults [64].

Given the general pattern of age-related declines in working memory performance, it may seem counter-intuitive that older adults sometimes exhibit greater activation in dorsolateral PFC regions. One study, in which reaction times during retrieval from working memory were correlated with activation in the dorsolateral PFC across participants, found a positive correlation in younger adults (i.e., slower latencies were accompanied by greater activation) and a negative correlation in older adults (i.e., faster latencies were accompanied by greater activation) [60]. The authors suggested that such reversed correlations could occur if there is a sigmoid relationship between neural activation and performance and if aging is accompanied by a decrease in neural efficiency (resulting in a rightward shift in this sigmoid function), so that older adults require more activation than younger adults to achieve optimal levels of performance [60]. A subsequent study has also observed reversed relationships between activation and working memory performance across age groups, again suggesting that normal aging is accompanied by decreased neural efficiency, and hence increased activation, in PFC regions during working memory tasks [65].

In general, older adults appear to exhibit similar or increased activations in PFC and parietal regions compared to younger adults when performing easier task conditions in which their behavioral performance is similar to that of younger adults. In contrast, under more difficult task conditions in which their behavioral performance is worse than younger adults, older adults tend to exhibit reduced levels of activation in working memory-related regions of PFC and parietal cortex. This suggests that the reduced neural efficiency experienced by older adults leads them to recruit attentional control processes to support performance at the same level as younger adults, but that once task demands exceed the capacity limits of older adults, they can no longer effectively use attentional control in the service of task performance.

C.   INHIBITORY CONTROL

The concept of inhibitory function has come to play a large role in understanding age-related differences in cognition. Hasher and Zacks [66] proposed that older adults experience a selective deficit in the ability to inhibit distracting task-irrelevant information, and that this deficit could potentially account for a wide range of age differences in memory and attention. Many studies were subsequently conducted that support this view, including a number of studies that implicate an age-related inhibitory deficit in the working memory failures of older adults [67–70]. However, this overarching theory remains controversial, as a number of studies have failed to find age-related differences in several hallmark inhibitory tasks [71, 72].

It is important to distinguish this type of cognitive inhibition from inhibition at the neural level. In particular, this theory does not propose that normal aging is accompanied by a decline in the function of inhibitory neural connections or in inhibitory neurotransmitters. Rather, the theory would predict that certain neural mechanisms supporting the identification and suppression of task-irrelevant information will be adversely affected during normal aging. One such mechanism involves the function of an area of right ventrolateral PFC, namely the inferior frontal gyrus (BA 47, sometimes extending into BA 45). This region has been implicated in both human and primate studies in the suppression of previously attended information that, due to changing task contexts, is currently task irrelevant [73]. Surprisingly, very few studies of normal older adults have investigated the effects of aging on neural correlates of inhibition, and only a limited number of these have specifically investigated the right inferior frontal gyrus.

One of the most commonly used inhibitory tasks is the Stroop color-word task [74], in which participants must name the color of ink in which a word is printed while simultaneously suppressing the impulse to read the color represented by the word's content (e.g., respond "blue" to the word RED printed in blue ink). Two functional imaging studies have investigated the neural correlates of age-related effects in this task [75, 76]. While Langenecker and colleagues [75] found no activations in the PFC and parietal cortices that were larger in younger than in older adults, Milham and colleagues [76] reported a number of such activations in bilateral regions of ventrolateral and dorsolateral PFC and parietal cortex. However, both studies observed activations in ventrolateral PFC and in parietal cortex that were larger in older than in younger adults. Of special interest, both studies observed that older adults exhibited greater activation than did younger adults in right inferior frontal gyrus (BA 47). In the study by Milham and co-workers, this pattern was also observed in the homologous left inferior frontal gyrus. This increased activation was observed despite larger behavioral interference effects in the older adults [75, 76]. These results suggest that increased activation in this region does not accompany better inhibition, but that, similar to the age-related effects on working memory, older adults may experience decreased neural efficiency in regions related to attentional control and therefore require greater activation of these areas in efforts to support task performance.

In another study, age differences in inhibitory control were investigated in a paradigm wherein participants generated verbs to nouns that had either few or many appropriate verb pairings, finding that older adults exhibited greater activation than younger adults in the right inferior frontal gyrus [77]. The verb generation task involves selection among competing alternatives when many appropriate verbs come to mind, but this selection may, in part, invoke inhibitory processes that are engaged to suppress the non-selected items. Of interest, the left inferior frontal gyrus (BA 45) has been implicated in the selection process, specifically in the capacity to resolve interference among competing responses [78]. In the verb generation task, younger adults exhibited greater activation than older adults in this region of left inferior frontal gyrus [77]. Similarly, older adults' failures to resolve interference from irrelevant, but recently encountered, responses have been found to be accompanied by decreased activation in left inferior frontal gyrus (BA 45) [79]. In the same study, however, older adults exhibited increased activation in right inferior frontal gyrus (BA 47) [79]. Together, these results suggest an age-related deficit in attentional control mechanisms related to selection among interfering alternatives that is correlated with activation in left inferior frontal gyrus, while simultaneously implicating an inefficient inhibitory mechanism that results in increased activation in right inferior frontal gyrus. One intriguing possibility, suggested by age-related degradation in frontal white matter tracts that connect the left and right hemispheres, is that aging may be associated with an inability to coordinate between these two normally related control capacities, such that neural systems that inhibit irrelevant representations become hyper-activated as those systems that select among competing alternatives fail to provide appropriate interference resolution.

D.   TASK SWITCHING

Task switching, sometimes known as *shifting,* refers to the ability to fluidly and accurately alternate between multiple rule sets that govern task responding [80]. Switching has been associated with a prefrontal-parietal network similar to that involved in working memory, although it appears to rely somewhat more heavily on activation in parietal regions of this network [8, 81]. Numerous studies have investigated the behavioral effects of aging on task switching, generally finding that older adults exhibit disproportionately large dual-task or switch costs relative to younger adults, although these age differences tend to be most pronounced for between-block switch costs rather than for within-block switch costs [82–84]. Despite the natural translation of task switching paradigms into blocked and event-related functional imaging methods, imaging studies of age differences on task switching are remarkably scarce.

DiGirolamo and colleagues [85] conducted a study in which participants were trained to respond (based on a color cue) to a digit stimulus consisting of several copies of a single digit (e.g., 7777); participants either determined whether the digit's value or the number of copies of the digit was greater than or less than 5. Switch costs were measured across blocks — participants responded to both single-task (nonswitch) blocks and dual-task (switch) blocks. Older adults were slower to perform each single task, but also exhibited a larger switch cost than younger adults. When directly comparing activation in switch blocks to nonswitch blocks, younger adults displayed activation in a large number of regions, many of them in the prefrontal-parietal network associated with attentional control. These regions included bilateral ventrolateral and dorsolateral PFC, left-lateralized inferior frontal gyrus (BA 47), and bilateral parietal cortex (BA 7/40). In the same contrast, older adults did not display any above-threshold regions of activation. However, this was not because these regions were under-activated in older adults; rather, when compared to fixation, the older adults were found to display activation in these regions during both switch and non-switch blocks [85]. In contrast, younger adults displayed above-threshold activation in these regions almost solely during switch blocks. That is, the older adults were utilizing the PFC and parietal regions involved in attentional control to almost the same extent during both switch and non-switch conditions. The authors interpreted this as evidence that older adults relied on attentional control even in the easier non-switch conditions to support task performance, whereas younger adults only required such control processes during the switch condition [85].

In a study involving dual-task performance of an operation span working memory task, younger and older adults performed single-task or dual-task blocks in which they either attended to a memory or arithmetic task, or simultaneously performed both task types [86]. In this study, when comparing dual-task performance to single-task performance, older adults exhibited activation in left hemisphere dorsolateral PFC (BA 9) and ventrolateral PFC (BA 44) sites, as well as in parietal cortex (BA 7). In contrast, younger adults did not exhibit activation in any of these regions, suggesting that they did not require activation of the attentional control network to switch attention during a sub-span working memory task. However, when the group of younger adults was split into relatively good and poor performers according to memory accuracy in the dual-task condition, an interesting pattern emerged. The young poor performers, but not the good performers, exhibited increased activation in the same region of dorsolateral PFC (BA 9) as did the older adults [86]. This suggests that this region of PFC underlies task switching, but is only required when participants are challenged by the difficulty of the alternating tasks. Although the authors did not discuss it, young poor performers and older adults both exhibited activation in areas of left superior parietal cortex (BA 7), suggesting that this region may play a similar role in supporting task switching [86].

E.   RELATIONS AMONG ATTENTIONAL CONTROL PROCESSES

Throughout the discussions of working memory, inhibition, and task switching, it can be observed that age differences appear in a number of recurring PFC and parietal regions. Although these different types of attentional control have been found to be distinct from one another in behavioral studies [11], it can often be difficult to disentangle their involvement in various task domains. For example, it can be argued that task switching is required during the performance of any complex working memory task, in that participants must constantly shift between maintaining the current contents of working memory and updating those contents as new information becomes available from each aspect of the task or tasks being attended. In a similar fashion, one can argue that inhibition is required during task switching, in that each shift requires not only the reactivation of the now-current rule set to govern task responding, but also invokes the suppression (or inhibition) of the just-prior rule set. Indeed, each of these attentional control processes appears to rely on the same general prefrontal-parietal network [8, 52, 81]. However, each control process may rely to a greater or lesser extent on certain regions within this network. For example, working memory manipulation appears to involve the dorsolateral PFC (BA 46), while inhibition relies upon the inferior frontal gyrus (BA 47), and task switching involves regions of the dorsolateral PFC (BA 9) and parietal cortex (BA 7). Such differences among various attentional control processes may provide important clues to specialized functions within this network and within individual regions of the PFC [64]. A common thread appears to be that older adults exhibit declines in such attentional control regions when task difficulty exceeds their capacity for successful responding, but exhibit increases in control regions under conditions where they are able to successfully perform the task. Such age-related increases in activation can occur even when these conditions do not appear to require control processes in younger adults.

F. THE ROLE OF DOPAMINERGIC CIRCUITS IN ATTENTIONAL CONTROL

In addition to the volumetric and functional age-related changes in the PFC, various neurotransmitter systems in the PFC and striatum undergo age-associated changes. Of these, one of the most important, in that it has been repeatedly associated with attentional control and displays large age-related changes, is the dopamine system. Age-related declines have been observed in dopamine concentration, transporter availability, and D2 and D3 receptor density [15, 87–91]. Age-related declines of about 8% per decade in D2 receptors begin by age 40 and are associated with lower glucose metabolism in the PFC, the anterior cingulate, and caudate nucleus [89, 92]. By age 60, normal older adults display 58% declines relative to younger adults in striatal uptake of a dopaminergic analogue (Parkinson's patients exhibit declines of 85%) [93]. Dopamine transporter availability has been estimated to decline at a rate of 4.9% per decade in the caudate and 4.2% per decade in the putamen [15] (Figure 11.3). These declines in dopaminergic function are highly related to performance in episodic memory and attentional control tasks, accounting for up to 96% of the age-related variance in these tasks [6, 15, 94]. Computational models have found that age-related cognitive deficits can be accounted for by changes in a gain parameter modeled after declines in dopamine levels in PFC [95, 96]. Such results suggest that treatment with dopaminergic agents similar to those given to Parkinson's patients might also benefit individuals experiencing the undesirable effects of normal aging on memory and attentional control.

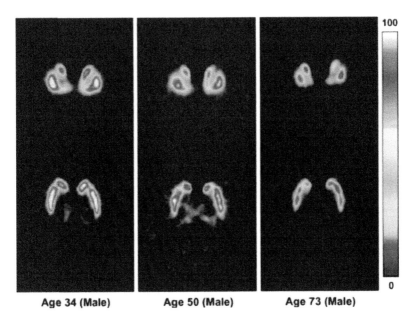

Age 34 (Male)   **Age 50 (Male)**   **Age 73 (Male)**

FIGURE 11.3 (SEE COLOR INSERT FOLLOWING PAGE 204) Striatal dopamine transporter availability in a representative individual from younger, middle, and older age groups. (*Source:* Reproduced from [15]. With permission.)

IV. EPISODIC MEMORY

A. NORMAL AGING AND THE MEDIAL TEMPORAL LOBES

Although this chapter focuses on age-related changes in attentional control, the vast majority of studies regarding the cognitive neuroscience of aging have investigated age-related changes in episodic memory. Age effects on episodic memory are well-documented and several reviews have explored the brain bases of age-related memory deficits [3, 97–99]. The importance of the hippocampus and related medial temporal lobe (MTL) structures to declarative memory makes them of particular interest for understanding developmental and pathological changes [100]. Despite the observation of relatively large decrements in declarative memory function during normal aging, evidence regarding age-related volumetric and functional declines in the MTL has been equivocal. In populations of normal older adults screened to exclude possible early dementia or MCI, age-related declines in hippocampal volume are often minimal. In recent cross-sectional studies, no significant correlation between hippocampal volume and age was observed [101, 102]. However, longitudinal estimates of MTL volume declines during normal aging tend to be somewhat larger than cross-sectional estimates. Adult lifespan studies (with participants in their 20s to 80s) with intervals of 5 years have estimated the rate of decline in hippocampal volume at 0.79 to 0.86% per year [5, 103]. Declines in entorhinal cortex volume were smaller, with the estimated rate of change being approximately 0.33%, although this accelerates somewhat in later life [103]. Recent advances in MRI resolution and analytic techniques are beginning to allow closer examination of age-related effects on volumetric measurements within individual hippocampal subregions. Such studies have found that although the entorhinal cortex and CA1 region appear to be preserved during normal aging, the subiculum and dentate gyrus do display age-related declines in nondemented individuals [104].

The relatively modest age-related changes in volume are not substantially related to memory function in normal populations. Researchers have failed to find correlations between composite memory scores and the size of the hippocampus or other MTL regions [102]. Similarly, a meta-analysis (primarily of cross-sectional studies), involving 1880 participants across the lifespan, found that in those studies involving older adults, the correlation between hippocampal volume and memory function was small ($r = 0.06$) and nonsignificant [105]. However, a few studies have found that after the age of 60, hippocampal volume does predict performance on some episodic memory tasks [24, 106]. Studies using longitudinal estimates of hippocampal volume loss have generally not observed a correlation with memory function in normal older adults, although rates of decline in entorhinal cortex have been correlated with memory performance [107].

Despite the modest changes in MTL volume during normal aging, functional imaging studies of memory tend to reveal age-related decreases in MTL activation [108–110]. Such age effects on MTL function have been found across a variety of memory tasks, including the maintenance of pictures, encoding of subsequently remembered words, and representing conjunctions of stimulus features [59, 108, 111, 112]. Of particular interest, each of these functional imaging studies also observed age-related changes in PFC activation, suggesting that the MTL functions as part of a circuit involving PFC and this circuit is the locus of age-related effects. Supporting this notion, some studies have observed correlations between MTL measurements and PFC activation that are modulated by aging [109, 113]. One possibility is that reductions in MTL function could be reflected in modulations of PFC activation as older adults attempt to process task information via alternative, possibly compensatory, routes [98, 114].

B.   PATHOLOGY IN THE MEDIAL TEMPORAL LOBES

In contrast to the modest MTL volume changes associated with normal aging, the effects of pathological processes, as in mild cognitive impairment (MCI) and Alzheimer's disease, have large adverse effects on both MTL volumes and memory function. In particular, the entorhinal cortex, which serves as an important information relay for the hippocampus, appears to be especially susceptible to atrophy in individuals with MCI. The entorhinal cortex may therefore provide a basis for identifying individuals with MCI in mixed populations and for further classifying those individuals within MCI populations who are most likely to advance to Alzheimer's status [115–117]. Declines in entorhinal cortex volume in MCI patients relative to age-matched controls are twice as large as declines in hippocampal volume [118]. These rates of decline tend to be largest in those normal and MCI individuals who will later progress to Alzheimer's status [117]. Once an individual has advanced to MCI or Alzheimer's status, volume declines extend into the hippocampus.

One such arena that holds great interest in the study of age-related individual differences is the characterization of those older adults who tend to perform as well as younger adults on cognitive tasks [131, 142, 143]. If the continued optimal performance of such "successful seniors" can be understood, researchers will move closer to determining training programs or treatments that might allow the improvement of lower-performing individuals. Behavioral studies have suggested that individual differences among older adults can be explained by performance on attentional control tasks, and other PFC-related neuropsychological tests, rather than by performance on memory tasks associated with MTL function [12, 142, 144]. As discussed, functional neuroimaging studies have found that elderly individuals often show greater activation in PFC regions associated with attentional control and that such additional activations are often associated with better performance, especially in less-demanding task conditions [60, 98, 114]. Such upregulation of PFC regions might reflect attempts to invoke attentional control processes in the service of task performance.

One important, yet currently unaddressed, issue that will have a large bearing on the understanding of individual differences among older adults involves the reliability of functional activations within individuals across time and how this reliability differs among age groups. Several studies have examined the reliability of functional imaging methods in younger adults, generally finding extremely high levels of intra-individual stability [145–147]. However, the effect of aging on the reliability of functional responses remains unknown. Preliminary evidence from a study of repeated measurements of younger and older adults performing a working memory task indicates that both groups exhibit high levels of reliability in functional imaging measures, with older adults displaying reliability that is as high or higher than in younger adults [148]. If these results are confirmed, then individual differences observed in the functional activation of older adults are likely the result of reliable, task-related differences rather than the result of increased noise in the neural or vascular systems of older adults.

VII. CONCLUSION

The neural correlates of cognitive performance during normal aging are complex and varied. Older adults exhibit declines not only in memory performance, but also in several processes related to attentional control, including working memory, inhibition, and task switching. Normal aging appears primarily associated with changes in the prefrontal cortex and a set of related neural networks, including frontal-parietal and frontal-striatal networks. Age-related changes in volume, dopaminergic neurotransmission, and functional activation within these systems appear to underlie, to a large extent, the behavioral differences observed during normal aging. Memory deficits in normal older adults may be attributable to failures of connections between these prefrontal networks and the medial temporal systems that underlie memory function. In contrast, pathological aging processes associated with MCI and Alzheimer's disease appear to directly and severely affect medial temporal lobe memory systems, while not affecting the prefrontal networks to as large a degree. This dissociation between normal and pathological aging processes allows researchers to better isolate the causes and consequences of normal aging and its relationship to cognition. Further developments in functional and structural imaging methods will undoubtedly bring new answers while raising new questions about the relationships between functional neuroanatomy and behavioral performance during normal aging.

REFERENCES

1. Hedden, T. and Gabrieli, J.D., Healthy and pathological processes in adult development: new evidence from neuroimaging of the aging brain, *Curr. Opin. Neurol.*, 18, 740, 2005.
2. Hedden, T. and Gabrieli, J.D., Insights into the ageing mind: a view from cognitive neuroscience, *Nat. Rev. Neurosci.*, 5, 87, 2004.
3. Gabrieli, J.D., Memory systems analyses of mnemonic disorders in aging and age-related diseases, *Proc. Natl. Acad. Sci. U.S.A.*, 93, 13534, 1996.
4. Buckner, R.L., Memory and executive function in aging and AD: multiple factors that cause decline and reserve factors that compensate, *Neuron*, 44, 195, 2004.
5. Raz, N. et al., Regional brain changes in aging healthy adults: general trends, individual differences and modifiers, *Cereb. Cortex*, 15, 1676, 2005.
6. Volkow, N.D. et al., Association between decline in brain dopamine activity with age and cognitive and motor impairment in healthy individuals, *Am. J. Psychiatry*, 155, 344, 1998.
7. Weissman, D.H. et al., The neural bases of momentary lapses in attention, *Nat. Neurosci.*, 9, 971, 2006.
8. Wager, T.D., Jonides, J., and Reading, S., Neuroimaging studies of shifting attention: a meta-analysis, *Neuroimage*, 22, 1679, 2004.
9. Kane, M.J. and Engle, R.W., The role of prefrontal cortex in working-memory capacity, executive attention, and general fluid intelligence: an individual-differences perspective, *Psychon. Bull. Rev.*, 9, 637, 2002.
10. Salthouse, T.A., Atkinson, T.M., and Berish, D.E., Executive functioning as a potential mediator of age-related cognitive decline in normal adults, *J. Exp. Psychol. Gen.*, 132, 566, 2003.
11. Miyake, A. et al., The unity and diversity of executive functions and their contributions to complex "Frontal Lobe" tasks: a latent variable analysis, *Cognit. Psychol.*, 41, 49, 2000.
12. Hedden, T. and Yoon, C., Individual differences in executive processing predict susceptibility to interference in verbal working memory, *Neuropsychology*, 20, 511, 2006.
13. Moscovitch, M. and Winocur, G., Frontal lobes, memory, and aging, *Ann. N.Y. Acad. Sci.*, 769, 119, 1995.
14. West, R.L., An application of prefrontal cortex function theory to cognitive aging, *Psychological Bull.*, 120, 272, 1996.
15. Erixon-Lindroth, N. et al., The role of the striatal dopamine transporter in cognitive aging, *Psychiatry Res.*, 138, 1, 2005.
16. Head, D. et al., Differential vulnerability of anterior white matter in nondemented aging with minimal acceleration in dementia of the Alzheimer type: evidence from diffusion tensor imaging, *Cereb. Cortex*, 14, 410, 2004.

17. Pfefferbaum, A., Adalsteinsson, E., and Sullivan, E.V., Frontal circuitry degradation marks healthy adult aging: evidence from diffusion tensor imaging, *Neuroimage*, 26, 891, 2005.
18. Killiany, R.J. et al., Use of structural magnetic resonance imaging to predict who will get Alzheimer's disease, *Ann. Neurol.*, 47, 430, 2000.
19. Dickerson, B.C. et al., MRI-derived entorhinal and hippocampal atrophy in incipient and very mild Alzheimer's disease, *Neurobiol. Aging*, 22, 747, 2001.
20. Sliwinski, M. et al., The effects of preclinical dementia on estimates of normal cognitive functioning in aging, *J. Gerontol. B Psychol. Sci. Soc. Sci.*, 51, 217, 1996.
21. Haug, H. and Eggers, R., Morphometry of the human cortex cerebri and corpus striatum during aging, *Neurobiol. Aging*, 12, 336, 1991.
22. Resnick, S.M. et al., Longitudinal magnetic resonance imaging studies of older adults: a shrinking brain, *J. Neurosci.*, 23, 3295, 2003.
23. Raz, N. et al., Aging, sexual dimorphism, and hemispheric asymmetry of the cerebral cortex: replicability of regional differences in volume, *Neurobiol. Aging*, 25, 377, 2004.
24. Raz, N. et al., Neuroanatomical correlates of cognitive aging: evidence from structural magnetic resonance imaging, *Neuropsychology*, 12, 95, 1998.
25. Salat, D.H., Kaye, J.A., and Janowsky, J.S., Selective preservation and degeneration within the prefrontal cortex in aging and Alzheimer disease, *Arch. Neurol.*, 58, 1403, 2001.
26. Thompson, P.M. et al., Dynamics of gray matter loss in Alzheimer's disease, *J. Neurosci.*, 23, 994, 2003.
27. Gunning-Dixon, F.M. et al., Differential aging of the human striatum: a prospective MR imaging study, *Am. J. Neuroradiol.*, 19, 1501, 1998.
28. Raz, N. et al., Differential aging of the human striatum: longitudinal evidence, *Am. J. Neuroradiology*, 24, 1849, 2003.
29. Chen, Z.G., Li, T.Q., and Hindmarsh, T., Diffusion tensor trace mapping in normal adult brain using single-shot EPI technique. A methodological study of the aging brain, *Acta Radiol.*, 42, 447, 2001.
30. Guttmann, C.R. et al., White matter changes with normal aging, *Neurology*, 50, 972, 1998.
31. Basser, P.J., Mattiello, J., and LeBihan, D., MR diffusion tensor spectroscopy and imaging, *Biophys. J.*, 66, 259, 1994.
32. Moseley, M., Bammer, R., and Illes, J., Diffusion-tensor imaging of cognitive performance, *Brain Cogn.*, 50, 396, 2002.
33. Bartzokis, G. et al., White matter structural integrity in healthy aging adults and patients with Alzheimer disease: a magnetic resonance imaging study, *Arch. Neurol.*, 60, 393, 2003.
34. Head, D. et al., Frontal-hippocampal double dissociation between normal aging and Alzheimer's disease, *Cerebral Cortex*, 15, 732, 2005.
35. Gunning-Dixon, F.M. and Raz, N., The cognitive correlates of white matter abnormalities in normal aging: a quantitative review, *Neuropsychology*, 14, 224, 2000.
36. Sullivan, E.V., Adalsteinsson, E., and Pfefferbaum, A., Selective age-related degradation of anterior callosal fiber bundles quantified *in vivo* with fiber tracking, *Cerebral Cortex*, 16, 1030, 2006.
37. Soderlund, H. et al., Cerebral changes on MRI and cognitive function: the CASCADE study, *Neurobio. Aging*, 27, 16, 2006.
38. Logothetis, N.K. and Wandell, B.A., Interpreting the BOLD signal, *Annu. Rev. Physiol.*, 66, 735, 2004.

39. Logothetis, N.K., The underpinnings of the BOLD functional magnetic resonance imaging signal, *J. Neurosci.*, 23, 3963, 2003.

40. Arthurs, O.J. and Boniface, S., How well do we understand the neural origins of the fMRI BOLD signal? *Trends Neurosci.*, 25, 27, 2002.

41. D'Esposito, M., Deouell, L.Y., and Gazzaley, A., Alterations in the BOLD fMRI signal with aging and disease: a challenge for neuroimaging, *Nat. Rev. Neurosci.*, 4, 863, 2003.

42. Aizenstein, H.J. et al., The BOLD hemodynamic response in healthy aging, *J. Cogn. Neurosci.*, 16, 786, 2004.

43. Buckner, R.L. et al., Functional brain imaging of young, nondemented, and demented older adults, *J. Cogn. Neurosci.*, 12, 24, 2000.

44. D'Esposito, M. et al., The effect of normal aging on the coupling of neural activity to the bold hemodynamic response, *Neuroimage*, 10, 6, 1999.

45. Hesselmann, V. et al., Age related signal decrease in functional magnetic resonance imaging during motor stimulation in humans, *Neurosci. Lett.*, 308, 141, 2001.

46. Heuttel, S.A., Singerman, J.D., and McCarthy, G., The effects of aging upon the hemodynamic response measured by functional MRI, *Neuroimage*, 13, 161, 2001.

47. Riecker, A. et al., Relation between regional functional MRI activation and vascular reactivity to carbon dioxide during normal aging, *J. Cereb. Blood Flow Metab.*, 23, 565, 2003.

48. Mehagnoul-Schipper, D.J. et al., Simultaneous measurements of cerebral oxygenation changes during brain activation by near-infrared spectroscopy and functional magnetic resonance imaging in healthy young and elderly subjects, *Hum. Brain Mapp.*, 16, 14, 2002.

49. McConnell, K.A. et al., BOLD fMRI response to direct simulation (transcranial magnetic stimulation) of the motor cortex shows no decline with age, *J. Neural Transm.*, 110, 495, 2003.

50. Nielson, K.A. et al., Comparability of functional MRI response in young and old during inhibition, *Neuroreport*, 15, 129, 2004.

51. Miller, E.K. and Cohen, J.D., An integrative theory of prefrontal cortex function, *Annu. Rev. Neurosci.*, 24, 167, 2001.

52. Collette, F. and Van der Linden, M., Brain imaging of the central executive component of working memory, *Neurosci. Biobehav. Rev.*, 26, 105, 2002.

53. D'Esposito, M. et al., Maintenance versus manipulation of information held in working memory: an event-related fMRI study, *Brain Cogn.*, 41, 66, 1999.

54. D'Esposito, M., Postle, B.R., and Rypma, B., Prefrontal cortical contributions to working memory: evidence from event-related fMRI studies, *Exp. Brain Res*, 133, 3, 2000.

55. Smith, E.E. and Jonides, J., Storage and executive processes in the frontal lobes, *Science*, 283, 1657, 1999.

56. Marshuetz, C. et al., Working memory for order and the parietal cortex: an event-related functional magnetic resonance imaging study, *Neuroscience*, 139, 311, 2006.

57. Cabeza, R. et al., Task-independent and task-specific age effects on brain activity during working memory, visual attention and episodic retrieval, *Cereb. Cortex*, 14, 364, 2004.

58. Grady, C.L. et al., Age-related changes in regional cerebral blood flow during working memory for faces, *Neuroimage*, 8, 409, 1998.

59. Park, D.C. et al., Working memory for complex scenes: age differences in frontal and hippocampal activations, *J. Cogn. Neurosci.*, 15, 1122, 2003.

60. Rypma, B. and D'Esposito, M., Isolating the neural mechanisms of age-related changes in human working memory, *Nat. Neurosci.*, 3, 509, 2000.
61. Rypma, B. et al., Age differences in prefrontal cortical activity in working memory, *Psychol. Aging*, 16, 371, 2001.
62. Gregoire, J. and Van der Linden, M., Effects of age on forward and backward digit spans, *Aging, Neuropsych. Cogn.*, 4, 140, 1997.
63. Johnson, M.K. et al., An age-related deficit in prefrontal cortical function associated with refreshing information, *Psychol. Sci.*, 15, 127, 2004.
64. Rajah, M.N. and D'Esposito, M., Region-specific changes in prefrontal function with age: a review of PET and fMRI studies of working and episodic memory, *Brain*, 128, 1964, 2005.
65. Rypma, B. et al., Dissociating age-related changes in cognitive strategy and neural efficiency using event-related fMRI, *Cortex*, 41, 582, 2005.
66. Hasher, L. and Zacks, R.T., Working memory, comprehension, and aging: a review and a new view, in *The Psychology of Learning and Motivation: Advances in Research and Theory I*, Bower, G.H., Editor Eds., Academic Press, San Diego, CA, 1988, 193.
67. Lustig, C., May, C.P., and Hasher, L., Working memory span and the role of proactive interference, *J. Exp. Psychol. Gen.*, 130, 199, 2001.
68. Gazzaley, A. et al., Top-down suppression deficit underlies working memory impairment in normal aging, *Nat. Neurosci.*, 8, 1298, 2005.
69. May, C.P., Hasher, L., and Kane, M.J., The role of interference in memory span, *Mem. Cognit.*, 27, 759, 1999.
70. Zacks, R.T., Radvansky, G., and Hasher, L., Studies of directed forgetting in older adults, *J. Exp. Psychol. Learn. Mem. Cogn.*, 22, 143, 1996.
71. Burke, D.M., Language, aging, and inhibitory deficits: evaluation of a theory, *J. Gerontol. B. Psychol. Sci. Soc. Sci.*, 52, 254, 1997.
72. Verhaeghen, P. and De Meersman, L., Aging and the Stroop effect: a meta-analysis, *Psychol. Aging*, 13, 120, 1998.
73. Aron, A.R., Robbins, T.W., and Poldrack, R.A., Inhibition and the right inferior frontal cortex, *Trends Cogn. Sci.*, 8, 170, 2004.
74. Stroop, J.R., Studies of interference in serial verbal reactions, *J. Exp. Psychol.*, 18, 643, 1935.
75. Langenecker, S.A., Nielson, K.A., and Rao, S.M., fMRI of healthy older adults during Stroop interference, *NeuroImage.*, 21, 192, 2004.
76. Milham, M.P. et al., Attentional control in the aging brain: insights from an fMRI study of the stroop task, *Brain Cogn.*, 49, 277, 2002.
77. Persson, J. et al., Selection requirements during verb generation: differential recruitment in older and younger adults, *Neuroimage*, 23, 1382, 2004.
78. Thompson-Schill, S.L. et al., Effects of frontal lobe damage on interference effects in working memory, *Cogn. Affect. Behav. Neurosci.*, 2, 109, 2002.
79. Jonides, J. et al., Age differences in behavior and PET activation reveal differences in interference resolution in verbal working memory, *J. Cogn. Neurosci.*, 12, 188, 2000.
80. Monsell, S., Task switching, *Trends Cogn. Sci.*, 7, 134, 2003.
81. Wager, T.D. et al., Toward a taxonomy of attention shifting: individual differences in fMRI during multiple shift types, *Cogn. Affect. Behav. Neurosc.*, 5, 127, 2005.
82. Kray, J. and Lindenberger, U., Adult age differences in task switching, *Psychol. Aging*, 15, 126, 2000.
83. Reimers, S. and Maylor, E.A., Task switching across the life span: effects of age on general and specific switch costs, *Dev. Psychol.*, 41, 661, 2005.

84. Verhaeghen, P. and Cerella, J., Aging, executive control, and attention: a review of meta-analyses, *Neurosci. Biobehav. Rev.*, 26, 849, 2002.
85. DiGirolamo, G.J. et al., General and task-specific frontal lobe recruitment in older adults during executive processes: a fMRI investigation of task-switching, *Neuroreport*, 12, 2065, 2001.
86. Smith, E.E. et al., The neural basis of task-switching in working memory: effects of performance and aging, *Proc. Natl. Acad. Sci. U.S.A.*, 98, 2095, 2001.
87. Chen, P.S. et al., Correlation between different memory systems and striatal dopamine D2/D3 receptor density: a single photon emission computed tomography study, *Psychol. Med.*, 35, 197, 2005.
88. Goldman-Rakic, P.S. and Brown, R.M., Regional changes of monoamines in cerebral cortex and subcortical structures of aging rhesus monkeys, *Neuroscience*, 6, 177, 1981.
89. Volkow, N.D. et al., Measuring age-related changes in dopamine D2 receptors with 11C-raclopride and 18F-N-methylspiroperidol, *Psychiatry Res.*, 67, 11, 1996.
90. Volkow, N.D. et al., Dopamine transporters decrease with age, *J. Nucl. Med.*, 37, 554, 1996.
91. Volkow, N.D. et al., Parallel loss of presynaptic and postsynaptic dopamine markers in normal aging, *Ann. Neurol.*, 44, 143, 1998.
92. Volkow, N.D. et al., Association between age-related decline in brain dopamine activity and impairment in frontal and cingulate metabolism, *Am. J. Psychiatry*, 157, 75, 2000.
93. Kumakura, Y. et al., PET studies of net blood-brain clearance of FDOPA to human brain: age-dependent decline of [^{18}F]fluorodopamine storage capacity, *J. Cereb. Blood Flow Metab.*, 25, 807, 2005.
94. Backman, L. et al., Age-related cognitive deficits mediated by changes in the striatal dopamine system, *Am. J. Psychiatry*, 157, 635, 2000.
95. Braver, T.S. and Barch, D.M., A theory of cognitive control, aging cognition, and neuromodulation, *Neurosci. Biobehav. Rev.*, 26, 809, 2002.
96. Li, S.C. and Sikstrom, S., Integrative neurocomputational perspectives on cognitive aging, neuromodulation, and representation, *Neurosci. Biobehav. Rev.*, 26, 795, 2002.
97. Cabeza, R., Cognitive neuroscience of aging: contributions of functional neuroimaging, *Scand. J..Psychol.*, 42, 277, 2001.
98. Cabeza, R., Hemispheric asymmetry reduction in older adults: the HAROLD model, *Psychol. Aging*, 17, 85, 2002.
99. Prull, M.W., Gabrieli, J.D.E., and Bunge, S.A., Age-related changes in memory: a cognitive neuroscience perspective, in *The Handbook of Aging and Cognition*, Craik, F.I.M. and Salthouse, T.A., Eds., Lawrence Erlbaum Associates, Mahwah, NJ, 2000, 91.
100. Erickson, C.A. and Barnes, C.A., The neurobiology of memory changes in normal aging, *Exp. Gerontol.*, 38, 61, 2003.
101. Sullivan, E.V., Marsh, L., and Pfefferbaum, A., Preservation of hippocampal volume throughout adulthood in healthy men and women, *Neurobiol. Aging*, 26, 1093, 2005.
102. Van Petten, C. et al., Memory and executive function in older adults: relationships with temporal and prefrontal gray matter volumes and white matter hyperintensities, *Neuropsychologia*, 42, 1313, 2004.
103. Raz, N. et al., Differential aging of the medial temporal lobe: a study of a five-year change, *Neurology*, 62, 433, 2004.
104. Small, S.A. et al., Imaging hippocampal function across the human life span: is memory decline normal or not? *Ann. Neurol.*, 51, 290, 2002.

105. Van Petten, C., Relationship between hippocampal volume and memory ability in healthy individuals across the lifespan: review and meta-analysis, *Neuropsychologia*, 42, 1394, 2004.
106. Rosen, A.C. et al., Differential associations between entorhinal and hippocampal volumes and memory performance in older adults., *Behav. Neurosci.*, 117, 1150, 2003.
107. Rodrigue, K.M. and Raz, N., Shrinkage of the entorhinal cortex over five years predicts memory performance in healthy adults, *J. Neurosci.*, 24, 956, 2004.
108. Daselaar, S.M. et al., Neuroanatomical correlates of episodic encoding and retrieval in young and elderly subjects, *Brain*, 126, 43, 2003.
109. Gutchess, A.H. et al., Aging and the neural correlates of successful picture encoding: frontal activations compensate for decreased medial-temporal activity, *J. Cogn. Neurosci.*, 17, 84, 2005.
110. Moffat, S.D., Elkins, W., and Resnick, S.M., Age differences in the neural systems supporting human allocentric spatial navigation., *Neurobiol. Aging*, 27, 965, 2006.
111. Mitchell, K.J. et al., fMRI evidence of age-related hippocampal dysfunction in feature binding in working memory, *Brain Res. Cogn. Brain Res.*, 10, 197, 2000.
112. Morcom, A.M. et al., Age effects on the neural correlates of successful memory encoding, *Brain*, 126, 213, 2003.
113. Rosen, A.C. et al., Relating medial temporal lobe volume to frontal fMRI activation for memory encoding in older adults, *Cortex*, 41, 595, 2005.
114. Rosen, A.C. et al., Variable effects of aging on frontal lobe contributions to memory, *Neuroreport*, 13, 2425, 2002.
115. deToledo-Morrell, L. et al., MRI-derived entorhinal volume is a good predictor of conversion from MCI to AD, *Neurobiol. Aging*, 25, 1197, 2004.
116. Stoub, T.R. et al., MRI predictors of risk of incident Alzheimer disease: a longitudinal study, *Neurology*, 64, 1520, 2005.
117. Jack, C.R., Jr. et al., Comparison of different MRI brain atrophy rate measures with clinical disease progression in AD, *Neurology*, 62, 591, 2004.
118. Pennanen, C. et al., Hippocampus and entorhinal cortex in mild cognitive impairment and early AD, *Neurobiol. Aging*, 25, 303, 2004.
119. Grundman, M. et al., Mild cognitive impairment can be distinguished from Alzheimer disease and normal aging for clinical trials, *Arch. Neurol.*, 61, 59, 2004.
120. Thompson, P.M. et al., Mapping hippocampal and ventricular change in Alzheimer disease, *Neuroimage*, 22, 1754, 2004.
121. Johnson, S.C. et al., Hippocampal adaptation to face repetition in healthy elderly and mild cognitive impairment, *Neuropsychologia*, 42, 980, 2004.
122. Golby, A. et al., Memory encoding in Alzheimer's disease: an fMRI study of explicit and implicit memory, *Brain*, 128, 773, 2005.
123. Remy, F. et al., Verbal episodic memory impairment in Alzheimer's disease: a combined structural and functional MRI study, *Neuroimage*, 25, 253, 2005.
124. Sperling, R.A. et al., fMRI studies of associative encoding in young and elderly controls and mild Alzheimer's disease, *J. Neurol. Neurosurg. Psychiatry*, 74, 44, 2003.
125. Johnson, M.K. et al., An age-related deficit in prefrontal cortical function associated with refreshing information, *Psychol. Sci.*, 15, 127, 2004.
126. Lamar, M., Yousem, D.M., and Resnick, S.M., Age differences in orbitofrontal activation: an fMRI investigation of delayed match and nonmatch to sample, *Neuroimage*, 21, 1368, 2004.
127. Grady, C.L. et al., Age-related changes in brain activity across the adult lifespan, *J. Cogn. Neurosci.*, 18, 227, 2006.

128. Madden, D.J. et al., Age-related changes in neural activity during visual target detection measured by fMRI, *Cereb. Cortex.*, 14, 143, 2004.

129. Reuter-Lorenz, P.A. et al., Age differences in the frontal lateralization of verbal and spatial working memory revealed by PET, *J. Cogn. Neurosci.*, 12, 174, 2000.

130. Reuter-Lorenz, P.A. and Lustig, C., Brain aging: reorganizing discoveries about the aging mind, *Curr. Opin. Neurobiol.*, 15, 245, 2005.

131. Cabeza, R. et al., Aging gracefully: compensatory brain activity in high-performing older adults, *Neuroimage*, 17, 1394, 2002.

132. Colcombe, S.J. et al., The implications of cortical recruitment and brain morphology for individual differences in inhibitory function in aging humans, *Psychol. Aging*, 20, 363, 2005.

133. Erickson, K.I. et al., Training-induced plasticity in older adults: effects of training on hemispheric asymmetry, *Neurobiol. Aging*, Epub, 2006.

134. Logan, J.M. et al., Under-recruitment and nonselective recruitment: dissociable neural mechanisms associated with aging, *Neuron*, 33, 827, 2002.

135. Persson, J. et al., Structure-function correlates of cognitive decline in aging, *Cereb. Cortex*, 16, 907, 2006.

136. Dannhauser, T.M. et al., The functional anatomy of divided attention in amnestic mild cognitive impairment, *Brain*, 128, 1418, 2005.

137. Remy, F. et al., Mental calculation impairment in Alzheimer's disease: a functional magnetic resonance imaging study, *Neurosci. Lett.*, 358, 25, 2004.

138. Trollor, J.N. et al., Regional cerebral blood flow deficits in mild Alzheimer's disease using high resolution single photon emission computerized tomography, *Psychiatry Clin. Neurosci.*, 59, 280, 2005.

139. Rosano, C. et al., Event-related functional magnetic resonance imaging investigation of executive control in very old individuals with mild cognitive impairment, *Biol. Psychiatry*, 57, 761, 2005.

140. Ylikoski, R. et al., Heterogeneity of cognitive profiles in aging: successful aging, normal aging, and individuals at risk for cognitive decline, *Eur. J. Neurol.*, 6, 645, 1999.

141. Small, S.A., Age-related memory decline: current concepts and future directions, *Arch. Neurol.*, 58, 360, 2001.

142. Glisky, E.L., Rubin, S.R., and Davidson, P.S.R., Source memory in older adults: an encoding or retrieval problem? *J. Exp. Psychol. Learn. Mem. Cogn.*, 27, 1131, 2001.

143. Hedden, T. and Park, D.C., Contributions of source and inhibitory mechanisms to age-related retroactive interference in verbal working memory, *J. Exp. Psychol. Gen.*, 132, 93, 2003.

144. Glisky, E.L., Polster, M.R., and Routhieaux, B.C., Double dissociation between item and source memory, *Neuropsychology*, 9, 229, 1995.

145. Aguirre, G.K., Zarahn, E., and D'Esposito, M., The variability of human BOLD hemodynamic responses, *Neuroimage*, 8, 360, 1998.

146. Aron, A.R., Gluck, M.A., and Poldrack, R.A., Long-term test-retest reliability of functional MRI in a classification learning task, *Neuroimage*, 29, 1000, 2006.

147. Miller, M.B. et al., Extensive individual differences in brain activations associated with episodic retrieval are reliable over time, *J. Cogn. Neurosci.*, 14, 1200, 2002.

148. Hedden, T., Race, E.A., and Gabrieli, J.D.E., Intra-individual and inter-group reliability of functional activation related to working memory in younger and older adults, in *Annual Meeting of the Cognitive Neuroscience Society,* San Francisco, CA, 2006.

149. Grossman, M., et al., Age-related changes in working memory during sentence comprehension: an fMRI study, *Neuroimage*, 15, 302, 2002.
150. Jonides, J. et al., Inhibition in verbal working memory revealed by brain activation, *Proc. Natl. Acad. Sci. U.S.A.*, 95, 8410, 1998.

Section IV

Mechanisms Contributing to Brain Aging

12 Regulation of Cerebrovascular Aging

*William E. Sonntag, Delrae M. Eckman,
Jeremy Ingraham, and David R. Riddle*

CONTENTS

I.   INTRODUCTION

Normal function of virtually all tissues depends on adequate blood flow. As one would expect, deficits in blood flow under basal or stimulated conditions result in diminished metabolic capacity and impairments in function. Importantly, functional deficits in organs and tissues are one of the hallmarks of biological aging but the etiology of these deficits and the potential relationship between alterations in blood flow and the deterioration of tissue function with age remain enigmatic. Empirical and rigorous scientific evidence demonstrates that functional deterioration of many tissues begins in early adulthood and progresses throughout life. Concurrently, there is an increase in tissue pathology, including deposition of insoluble collagen and tissue fibrosis. Despite the structural changes with age, which are generally considered permanent or irreversible, tissue function can be improved even in late ages by several disparate types of interventions, supporting the conclusion that age-related impairments in cellular and tissue function, and perhaps some aspects of aging itself, remain "plastic." Whether such "plastic" changes depend on increased basal blood flow or the capacity to increase blood flow in response to metabolic challenge remains unknown.

The strong relationship that exists between cellular metabolic capacity and regional blood flow leads to the conclusion that a clear understanding of age-related changes in the regulation of blood flow (including microvascular architecture, plasticity, and vessel reactivity) is essential for understanding the progressive decline in cellular metabolic activity and eventually tissue function with age. Nevertheless, there are a limited number of studies that have considered the potential interrelationships between these variables. The guiding principle of this chapter, and for which there remain insufficient data, is that alterations in the vasculature have the capacity to impact biological aging. These alterations may include, but are not limited to, changes in microvascular density (density of arterioles, arteriolar to arteriolar anastomoses, capillaries, and venules); ultrastructure (cellular components that comprise the vasculature); plasticity (e.g., elaboration, regression, or replacement of microvessels that may occur over days, weeks, or months); and the dynamic regulation of blood flow through the vasculature (e.g., vessel reactivity). Despite the importance of each of these components, historical and technical aspects of research in these areas isolate the scientific disciplines and they are rarely considered a functional unit. This chapter reviews the current state of information in each of these areas as it relates to functional changes within the central nervous system with age.

II. EXPERIMENTAL CAVEATS AND POTENTIAL CONFOUNDS IN AGING RESEARCH

A cursory review of age-related changes in blood flow and/or vascular density reveals marked variability in experimental results that raises broader issues within the context of gerontology. Studies that address the biological and cellular mechanisms of aging are extraordinarily complex and require attention to a number of experimental variables. However, even with rigorous attention to experimental details, issues considered generally benign in other scientific experiments have the potential to produce an immense impact on the outcome of gerontological studies. These issues include the effects of minor changes in a single variable that, over time, have the potential to impact a diverse array of experimental outcomes. For example, the presence of subclinical infections or exposure to pathogens within an animal facility clearly will produce differential effects between young and old animals. Unintended crowding of animals within cages, noise, or other non-specific stresses produce different effects in old compared to younger animals (including substantially greater losses of body weight in old compared to younger animals). Subtle changes in early husbandry experiences within a population represent a less-explored area. Within the same animal facility, the specific details of animal husbandry (room temperature, population density, handling characteristics) may be unique to a specific cohort of animals as they progress from birth to old age. Differential prenatal and early life experiences of animals have the potential to result in modifications in the development of specific tissues [1] and would likely impact the appearance of age-related pathologies and potentially unique aging trajectories and lifespan. Other issues, including specific diets, the presence of underlying pathology, and strain differences, are likely to be important sources of experimental variance. Experimental confounds related to methodology including, but not limited to, differential effects of anesthesia, fixation methods, tissue atrophy, the absence of rigorous stereological methods for counting blood vessels, and the consequences of poor categorization of cells and/or blood vessels by region, size, and function have received little attention. These and related experimental caveats undoubtedly have the potential to alter experimental outcomes and hence produce artificial, exaggerated, or attenuated effects that are labeled as "aging." Furthermore, comparison of three age groups (young, middle-aged, and old) has been the "gold standard" for gerontological studies but these multiple age comparisons are rarely completed due to availability of animals, costs, or technical limitations associated with the experimental design. Finally, the rationale for analysis of specific ages within an animal strain has received little attention and, as a result, one might be comparing animals at the end of their lifespan (when endogenous organ systems are poorly regulated and substantial tissue pathology is present) with animals of another strain at the same chronological age but in which homeostatic mechanisms are maintained and tissue pathology is limited. Unfortunately, there are no rigorous standards between laboratories for animal husbandry in aging research and, as a result, it is not surprising (indeed it should be expected) that results on the same dependent variable within the same tissue vary between laboratories. In fact, it is sometimes remarkable the amount of agreement that does exist.

III. FUNCTIONAL CHANGES WITHIN THE CENTRAL NERVOUS SYSTEM

Impairments in tissue function are common phenomena in the aging population; however, compared to other tissues, loss of function within the central nervous system (CNS) has the potential to have more profound social and psychological consequences and can be an important factor in loss of independence. Although marked variability exists between individuals, there are numerous reports demonstrating a decline in cognitive function with age unrelated to a specific disease process. In otherwise healthy individuals, perceptual-motor performance and information processing speed, visual and auditory attention, as well as fluid intelligence are generally compromised with age [2, 3]. In addition, impairments in synaptic efficacy, neurogenesis, glucose metabolism, neurotransmitter levels, and long-term potentiation (an electrophysiological correlate of memory) are evident. Also, risk for degenerative diseases (e.g., Alzheimer's disease, Parkinson's disease, among others) increases and recovery from stoke damage is impaired. Although a number of cellular and subcellular correlates of this decline have been identified to date, there is no single unifying hypothesis for the decline in function of the CNS and increased risk of disease with age.

A.   CEREBRAL BLOOD FLOW

Whether the decline in CNS function with age is the result of a decrease in cerebral blood flow (CBF) remains a topic of considerable debate in which no consensus has emerged [4]. In part, this lack of consensus is related to some of the issues discussed previously. However, equally important is the technical difficulty in associating functional defects that occur in highly specific brain regions with an accurate measurement of flow to these same regions. Generally, the vast majority of analyses provide a "snapshot" of alterations in CBF in a large region of brain obtained under static conditions. However, the regulation of CBF is not static, and localized brain regions have the ability to regulate blood flow in response to minute alterations in metabolic requirements of the surrounding tissues. As glial and neuronal metabolism increase, blood flow increases concomitantly to support the increased metabolic requirements. Thus, local cellular metabolism and blood flow are tightly coupled in the CNS. The extremely limited data assessing the dynamic processes of changes in cerebral blood flow represent an important missing link in our analyses of age-related changes in CBF.

Despite the limitations described above, investigators using a variety of imaging methods have reported that CBF is significantly reduced in aged humans compared to young adults (see, for example, [5–7]). Similar conclusions were reached when comparing average measures of blood flow in groups of young and old subjects [8] or correlating CBF and age in individuals [9, 10]. Significantly, age-related changes in CBF appear to be regionally distinct [5, 6, 11–13] and may begin as early as middle age [10]. In addition to studies of humans, regionally specific, aging-related declines in CBF are found in both rodents and nonhuman primates [14–18]. Of course, several mechanisms regulate flow into and through each capillary bed, including the density of precapillary arterioles and capillaries [19], the structure of the vessels, and the reactivity of the arterioles (discussed in [7, 20, 21]). All or some of these mechanisms may be compromised with age.

B.   MICROVASCULAR DENSITY

The absence of an appropriate vascular network (including arterioles, arteriolar-arteriolar anastomoses, pre-capillary arterioles, and capillaries) supplying a tissue has the potential to result in inadequate blood flow either under basal conditions or conditions that require an increase in blood flow to meet metabolic demand. There are, in fact, numerous reports of age-related rarefaction or loss of arterioles in many tissues throughout the body (including cardiac and skeletal muscle [22–24]); however, only a few investigators have studied the effects of aging on the density of cerebral arterioles. Knox and Oliveira [25] reported that the number of arterioles in a strip of cortex extending from the pia to the white matter was similar in rats at 3 and 24 months of age, and Bell and Ball [26] reported an increase in arteriolar density in the subiculum of the aging human hippocampus. More recently, a

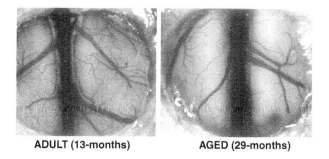

ADULT (13-months)   **AGED (29-months)**

FIGURE 12.1 (SEE COLOR INSERT FOLLOWING PAGE 204) Representative photographs of the cortical surface microvasculature in 13- and 29-month-old Brown-Norway rats, as seen through a cranial window. The entire parietal cranium has been removed. The cortex visible in this window extends from the frontal to the occipital cortex. Vascular measurements were made over the sensorimotor cortex. (*Source:* From [27]. With permission.)

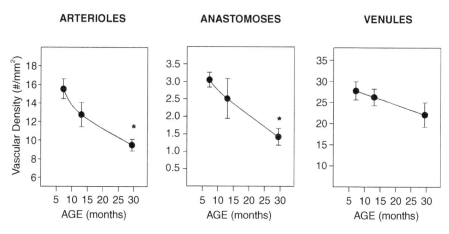

FIGURE 12.2 Summary of arteriolar (left), arteriole-to-arteriole anastomotic (center), and venular endpoint (right) density in male Brown-Norway rats. Data represent mean ± SEM for 18 young, 14 middle-age, and 13 old animals. (*Source:* From [27]. With permission.)

substantial age-related rarefaction of the surface arterioles that supply the parenchymal vessels of the cerebral cortex was reported [24, 27]. In otherwise healthy aging rats, the density of arterioles on the cortical surface was almost 40% lower in senescent animals than in young adults (29 vs. 13 months of age, Figure 12.1). Similar decreases were evident in arteriole-arteriole anastomoses and venules (Figure 12.2), suggesting that surface vessels and possibly vasculature in deeper layers of the cortex are affected by aging. Although it is difficult to reconcile the differences in these studies due to the specific ages, species, and brain regions compared, the substantial changes observed on the cortical surface and corresponding decreases in regional blood flow provide the first evidence that rarefaction of arterioles may be an important contributing factor to decreases in blood flow with resulting impairments in cortical function.

The putative decrease in afferent vessels raises the question of whether there is a corresponding decrease in cerebral capillaries supplied by the afferent arterioles. As in other tissues, the length of capillary per volume of tissue arguably represents the fundamental measure of microvascular status because it determines, at the simplest level, the surface area for exchange between tissue and blood and how far a given cell is from the source of oxygen and nutrients. Surprisingly, there is as yet no striking consensus for the effects of aging on capillary density within the brain. One recent review concluded that there is little, if any, decrease in capillary density [20], whereas others report compelling evidence for an aging-related decline in capillary density [7]. How such disparate conclusions can be drawn becomes clear when one reviews the literature from the past three decades (summarized in Table 12.1, from [28]), which includes reports of aging-related decreases in capillary density, stability of capillary density from adulthood through senescence, and of increased capillary density (presumably as a result of neural atrophy). Several possibilities exist for the different conclusions. First, although significant differences exist among species, these differences alone do not account for the disparate findings reported to date. All possible age-related changes in capillary density (decrease, increase, or no change) have been reported for both humans and rats, the subjects of virtually all available studies. Second, differential responses in localized regions of the brain most likely contribute to the disparity in the literature, but regional differences alone cannot explain the varied results. In some cases, the same neural region in the same species has been examined in different laboratories and conflicting conclusions have been drawn (e.g., rat frontal cortex: [29] vs. [30–32]; rat occipital cortex: [25] vs. [30]; human frontal cortex: [33] vs. [34]). Third, capillary changes with aging may be multiphasic. At least two studies suggest that capillary density increases during late adulthood and then declines during later senescence [35, 36]. If supported, the comparison of young and old animals without the appropriate middle-aged group may potentially bias interpretation of experimental results. Finally, previous studies indicate that the magnitude of age-related changes in capillary density, where they occur, do not exceed approximately 10 to 20%.

Taken together, the available literature suggests there is a substantial rarefaction of surface arterioles and limited but significant changes in capillary density in some regions of the brain, including the hippocampus and cerebral cortex. However, the evidence for capillary loss is tenuous and more extensive studies are required. In part, the disparate findings for capillary density changes with aging result from methodological differences among laboratories and improved stereological methods may resolve many of these issues [48–50]. To reliably reveal the regional and temporal patterns of microvascular changes, however, it will be necessary to analyze many neural areas in a single species at multiple ages using a consistent methodology. Such studies not only are required to establish the structural bases of aging-related changes in blood flow, but also are necessary to provide the critical baseline data for studies of microvascular plasticity.

TABLE 12.1
Capillary Changes in the CNS with Age

Species	Region(s)	Change	Ages Examined	Ref.
Report Aging-Related Decrease in Capillary Density				
Rat (Wistar, F)	Fr, Occ	↓[a]	8 vs. 27 mos	[30]
Human (F, M)	Precentral gyrus	↓ (17%)	74–94 years	[35][a]
Human (F, M)	Hipp	↓ (16%)	Avg 38 vs. avg 74 years	[26]
Rat (Wag/RIj x BN, F)	Fr	↑ followed by ↓	3 vs. 19 vs. 29 mos	[36]
Rat (Crl: CD(SD)BR, M)	Olfactory bulb	↓ (15%)	3–36 mos (27–36)	[37]
Rat (SD, M)	MTB	↓ (30%)	3–33 mos (3/6–27/33)	[38]
Human (F, M)	Calcarine cortex	↓ (16%)	Avg 38 vs. avg 74 years	[39]
Human (F, M)	Fr, Temp	↓ (Fr only)	26–96 years (correlation analysis)	[34]
Rat (Long Evans, M)	Multiple	↓ (10-30%)	8–10 vs. 28–33 mos	[40]
Rat (F344, M)	CA1, Par	↓	18 vs. 28 mos	[41, 42]
Human (F, M)	V1	↓ (16%)	Avg 31 vs. avg 79 years	[43]
Human (F, M)	Hypothalamus	↓ (16%)	30–76 years (correlation analysis)	[44]
Rat (Wistar, M)	Hipp, Fr, Occ	↓	12 vs. 27 mos	[31]
Rat (Wistar, M)	Hipp, Fr, Occ, Cb	↓	12 vs. 24 mos	[32]
Report No Aging-Related Decrease in Capillary Density				
Rat (SD, ns)	Occ	↑ (19%)	6 vs. 30 mos	[45]
Human (F, M)	PCG	↑ (17%)	19–74 years	[35][b]
Human (ns)	Fr, Occ, PCG, PsCG, Temp	No change	19–94 years	[33]
Rat (Wistar, F)	Occ	No change	3, 12, and 24 mos	[25]
Human	Cerebral Cortex	↑		[46]
Rat (SD, F)	Par	No Change	12 vs. 36 mos	[47]
Rat (Wistar, M)	Fr	↑[c]	3 vs. 20 mos	[29]

[a] Approximately 20% decrease, no statistics reported.

[b] Authors emphasize age-related increase in capillary density but data also reveal later decrease in density.

[c] Apparent increase restricted to superficial region of cortex.

Abbreviations: Cb: cerebellum; F: female; Fr: frontal cortex; Hipp: hippocampus; M: male; MTB: medial nucleus of the trapezoid body; NS: sex not specified; Occ: occipital cortex; Par: parietal cortex; PCG: precentral gyrus; PsCG: postcentral gyrus; Temp: temporal cortex; V1: primary visual cortex.

C.   MICROVASCULAR PLASTICITY

Capillary density is highest in regions rich in synapses, somewhat lower in regions containing primarily cells bodies, and lowest in fiber tracts [7]. Even within the gray matter of the cerebral cortex, sensory and association regions have higher densities of microvessels than motor regions; within a cortical region, layers and modules with greater cytochrome oxidase activity (indicative of greater synaptic activity) have higher capillary densities [72–74]. Thus, there must be developmentally regulated mechanisms by which the elaboration of the microvasculature is matched to the local level of neuronal signaling, presumably contributing to the differential growth of more active regions of the brain [73, 75, 76].

In principle, microvascular density in each region of the brain could be genetically programmed. The developmental mechanisms must be dynamic, however, because changes in neural activity during development result in predictable changes in microvascular density. Raising animals from the time of weaning in complex environments significantly increases synaptogenesis and the growth of neuropil in the cerebral cortex [77, 78]. Greenough and colleagues also demonstrated that the associated increase in metabolic demand from this paradigm produces significant growth of new capillaries [79, 80], even after the end of the normal period of developmental angiogenesis [81].

Conversely, decreased activity reduces vascular growth. Raising animals in complete darkness is commonly used to investigate the effects of activity deprivation on cortical development. Argandona and Lafuente [82, 83] demonstrated that dark-rearing rats from the time of birth significantly decreased the elaboration of the microvascular bed in the primary visual cortex. When examined as adults, the capillary density was 22% lower in dark-reared animals than in age-matched controls. Thus, the microvasculature within the CNS is actively modified during development to maintain a match between the local level of neural activity and the level of metabolic and vascular support necessary for that activity.

For many aspects of neural development, there are critical periods during which specific aspects of neural structure or function change in response to alterations in activity [84, 85]. Critical periods may be absolute, after which no significant change is possible, or they may be relative, such that change remains possible but only in response to greater perturbations than are required to elicit plasticity during earlier development. A variety of studies indicate that, for the cerebral microvasculature, plasticity is not limited to the developmental period; rather, the microvasculature in adult animals can be altered to maintain or improve function in response to changes in activity, damage, or other perturbations. The extent to which such plasticity is maintained during aging has not been clearly defined but undoubtedly depends on the specific factors eliciting the microvascular response.

Greenough and co-workers [86] have used the enriched environment paradigm to test whether microvascular plasticity in response to increased neural activity is limited to developing animals or is maintained in adults. These investigators demonstrated that housing adult rats (2 months of age) in complex environments resulted in microvascular growth within 10 days, just as in developing rats. Additional studies revealed, however, that the extent of the effect was reduced with age. The response in middle-aged rats was less than that in young adults, and no statistically significant change in microvascular density was elicited in old rats [87]. This age-related decrement in microvascular plasticity is consistent with reports that synaptic and dendritic plasticity also are reduced in old animals [79]. Thus, it is difficult to establish whether vascular plasticity decreases with age because neuronal plasticity declines, or whether neuronal plasticity is lost because there is insufficient vascular plasticity to support the generation and maintenance of new synapses [87]. Clearly, however, this type of microvascular plasticity is maintained into adulthood but sustained only poorly, if at all, during senescence [88].

Microvascular plasticity in the adult cerebellum was also investigated to assess the influence of learning vs. increased neural activity associated with simple motor activity. Microvascular growth was seen after motor learning, which also elicited synaptogenesis and growth of neuropil, and also after simple exercise, which had no effect on synapses and neuropil [89]. Voluntary exercise increased neural activity, as evidenced by increased glucose utilization [90], suggesting that microvascular growth occurs to meet the greater metabolic demands of increased neuronal signaling, even in adult animals. Consistent with this hypothesis, recent studies find that chronic exercise in adult animals, with no motor learning, promotes microvascular growth in the cerebral cortex [91, 92]. Unfortunately, to our knowledge there exists little or no data on the effect of exercise or motor learning on vascular plasticity in aged animals.

In addition to activity-induced angiogenesis, adult microvascular plasticity is important clinically. The success of strategies for treating neurodegenerative diseases by implanting stem cells or neurons critically depends on microvascular plasticity to establish metabolic support for the foreign cells [93, 94]. Thus, several laboratories have investigated the ability of the microvasculature to invade and support new tissue or cells after implantation in the adult CNS. Following transplantation, solid tissue allografts are infiltrated and supported primarily by host blood vessels [95, 96], although some donor vessels also are maintained within the graft [97]. Host blood vessels also elaborate to support grafts of dissociated cells [98–100], in which microvascular growth is more effective than in solid grafts [101]. Given that grafts can survive in aged brains [102–105], the necessary microvascular plasticity must be maintained during senescence.

Significant microvascular plasticity also occurs in response to chronic hypoperfusion or ischemia [7, 106, 107]. The restoration of blood flow after arterial occlusion relies in part on increased blood flow through collateral vessels supplying the ischemic region [108, 109], but significant new microvascular growth also occurs [110]. This includes both sprouting from preexisting capillaries and de novo vasculogenesis involving bone marrow-derived endothelial progenitor cells [107]. Similar to the microvascular changes that accompany changes in neural activity, post-ischemic microvascular plasticity appears to decrease in aged animals and humans [111, 112].

Several pharmacological agents promote microvascular growth and plasticity in the adult brain. Treatment of aging animals with a calcium channel blocker from 21 to 27 months of age, for example, significantly increased capillary density in the cerebral cortex and hippocampus [31, 32]. Similarly, 4 to 6 weeks of treatment with the plant alkaloid vincamine or its derivative increased capillary density in the cortex and hippocampus of adult rats [41, 47]. The extent of microvascular response appeared to be similar in 1-year-old and 3-year-old rats. Thus, at least for the responses to these pharmacological agents, there is no significant decline in plasticity during aging.

Clarifying the mechanisms that regulate microvascular growth and function in the developing and adult brain, and establishing how those mechanisms are affected by age, is critical for understanding the nature and functional consequences of age-related changes in the brain and for assessing prospects for preventing or reversing cognitive deficits. Recent studies by Sonntag et al. [27] demonstrate that, although microvascular plasticity may be reduced, growth of precapillary arterioles can be elicited even in aged animals. The studies also suggest a potential mechanism for age-related changes in the microvasculature and related plasticity. Microvascular density on the surface of the cerebral cortex was reported to decline with age [27]. Notably, the density of surface arterioles correlated with plasma insulin-like growth factor 1 (IGF-1) levels at the time of vascular mapping. That correlation suggested that microvascular rarefaction may be the consequence of the age-related decline in circulating growth hormone and IGF-1, particularly given evidence that growth hormone and IGF-1 are important anabolic growth factors that may influence many aspects of blood vessel growth and repair [113]. Consistent with that hypothesis, twice-daily injections of growth hormone to 30-month-old animals, sufficient to increase plasma IGF-1, dramatically increased the number of cortical arterioles. Thus, growth hormone and IGF-1 appear to mediate, at least in part, age-related changes in the microvasculature and potentially cerebral blood flow [113]. Moreover, although microvascular plasticity may decline in aged animals, it can be restored if appropriate trophic conditions are present.

In addition to growth hormone and IGF-1, other trophic factors profoundly influence the microvasculature. Although their potential roles in the etiology of age-related vascular changes have not been established, both basic fibroblast growth factor (bFGF) and vascular endothelial growth factor (VEGF) significantly influence angiogenesis and microvascular plasticity. Both factors exert a mitogenic effect on human microvascular endothelial cells in culture [114, 115]. VEGF prevents cultured microvascular endothelial cells from entering replicative senescence [116]. Additionally, VEGF is upregulated in spatial and temporal coincidence with angiogenesis associated with various CNS pathologies [117–119] and is involved in exercise-induced neovascularization [120]. Expression of bFGF is upregulated endogenously in response to focal cerebral infarction in rats, and exogenous administration of bFGF improves functional recovery, potentially via induction of angiogenesis in the damaged brain [121]. These factors do not appear always to benefit the microvasculature, however, because VEGF has been implicated in the breakdown of the blood-brain barrier associated with various CNS insults [122, 123]. Thus, the roles of these factors in modulating angiogenesis are complex and require further clarification.

In addition to trophic factors such as VEGF and BDNF, endocrine growth factors influence neuronal turnover in the adult brain. Plasma-derived IGF-1 reverses the decline in hippocampal neurogenesis that is produced by hypophysectomy [124] and also ameliorates the age-related decline in neuronal turnover [125]. These findings suggest that IGF-1 is an important regulator of neurogenesis, and that the decline in neuronal turnover during senescence is the result of decreased IGF-1 levels. The effects of aging on the multiple sources of IGF-1 within the CNS remain unclear, but the decline in plasma levels of IGF-1 may be exacerbated in many regions by decreased blood flow and by microvascular rarefaction, which also would reduce local production of IGF-1 and potentially other important growth factors by endothelial and smooth muscle cells.

Understanding the relationship between microvascular plasticity and neural activity, and how aging-related changes in the microvasculature affect metabolic support for neuronal signaling, is essential for clarifying the basis of cognitive changes during senescence. Accumulating evidence suggests that age-related changes in the microvasculature also may influence other critical aspects of neural function and plasticity. As noted previously, new neurons are continually produced in some regions of the adult brain [126–128] (see also Chapter 6), and the microvasculature is critically involved in regulating adult neurogenesis, both as a local source of factors that create an appropriate milieu for neurogenesis and as the source of blood-borne factors that influence proliferation. The production of new granule neurons in the subgranular zone of the adult dentate gyrus occurs within "neuroangiogenic foci" where neuronal, glial, and endothelial precursors divide in tight clusters [129, 130]. Proliferative precursors in other regions of the hippocampus are not found within such a vascular niche and do not give rise to neurons, only glia. Thus, the association between endothelial and neuronal proliferation in the subgranular zone suggests that either signals originating from somatic tissues or from the CNS act simultaneously to stimulate neurogenesis and angiogenesis, or that the initiating signal activates proliferation of one cell type, which then stimulates proliferation of the other. A recent demonstration that intracerebroventricular infusion of VEGF into the adult brain increases the genesis of both endothelial cells and granule neurons is consistent with a mechanistic link between angiogenesis and neurogenesis [131]. Also supporting this hypothesis is evidence that the reduction in neurogenesis that follows whole brain irradiation is due, in part, to alterations in the microenvironment, including disruption of microvascular angiogenesis [132]. More direct evidence that endothelial-produced factors regulate neurogenesis comes from the demonstration that culturing precursor cells from the adult rodent forebrain subependymal zone (SZ) on monolayers of endothelial cells, rather than on astrocytes or fibroblasts, increases neurogenesis and neuronal survival [133]. Thus, much remains to be determined concerning the complex interactions between vasculature and neurons.

D.   MICROVASCULAR ULTRASTRUCTURE

Alterations in microvessel ultrastructure potentially contribute to alterations in both blood flow and the transport of materials across the capillary wall, even where capillary density is unchanged. The effects of aging on arteriolar and capillary ultrastructure have been recently reviewed [7, 20].

In arterioles, aging appears to decrease the distensible components of the vessel wall (smooth muscle and elastin) and increase less distensible components (collagen and basement membrane; see [51]). Along with thickening of the endothelial basement membrane, cerebral arterioles in aged animals often contain flocculent material and intracellular inclusions that are not evident in the vessels of young animals [52, 53]. These alterations in arteriolar structure presumably contribute to age-related changes in arteriolar reactivity (see below).

Age-related alterations have been described in capillary endothelial cells, their basement membrane, in pericytes, and in the astrocytic endfeet that are opposed to the abluminal vascular surface (reviewed in [7]; see also [54]). The increase in thickness of the basement membrane and the abnormal inclusions reported for aging arterioles, including enlarged perivascular space, also are evident in capillaries [37, 38, 55–61]. The complete source and mechanisms of basement membrane changes remain to be established [7], but the flocculent deposits observed in aging capillaries have been attributed to the degeneration of pericytes [62]. The various age-related ultrastructural changes in the capillary wall must be regulated by several mechanisms, because chronic treatment with calcium channel blockers decreases the deposition of extracellular collagenous fibers but has no effect on the degeneration of pericytes [58, 59]. The functional impact of these age-related alterations in the capillary wall are numerous, and are likely to include both increased leakage of materials normally excluded by the blood brain barrier and reduced transport of substances (e.g., glucose, amino acids, growth factors) that are actively transported into the brain parenchyma. Recent studies suggest that the age-related increase in leakage may be less than previously suggested [63], but that the decrease in carrier function appears to be pronounced [7].

Reports of age-related changes in the shape of arterioles and capillaries were reported in the early 20th century [64]. Although the extent of such abnormalities during normal aging is still debated [21], there are sufficient descriptions of microvessel looping, tortuosity, and twisting to conclude that such changes occur in many neural regions [20, 52, 65–69]. Whether such alterations reflect primary changes in blood vessels or secondary effects of atrophy of surrounding neural tissue is not clear, but regardless of the specific mechanism, one would expect modification of vessel shape to produce profound hemodynamic and rheological changes within the microvascular bed [52, 68–71], contributing to decreased blood flow and reduced delivery of oxygen and nutrients to the brain parenchyma.

E.   SUMMARY

In many regions of the aging brain, metabolic support for neuronal signaling may be compromised by decreased blood flow. Rarefaction of arterioles and changes in vessel shape and structure most likely contribute to reduced flow although the possibility of capillary rarefaction and the regulation of capillary density with age remains an area for additional research. The metabolic impact of reduced blood flow may be exacerbated by altered transport across the capillary wall. In addition to influencing blood vessel structure and function, aging reduces microvascular plasticity such that capillaries respond less to increases in neural activity although responses to other factors that promote angiogenesis may be maintained. The age-related loss of plasticity certainly influences neural plasticity as well, because neuronal turnover in the adult brain is linked mechanistically to capillaries and their growth. Trophic factors produced by endothelial cells are additional important regulators of ongoing neurogenesis within the adult hippocampus, and impairments in secretion of these factors may have independent actions on the aging brain. Thus, aging-related changes in microvascular structure and plasticity potentially contribute in multiple ways to the decline in cognitive function that accompanies brain aging.

IV. VASCULAR REACTIVITY

A.   AGE-RELATED CHANGES IN VASCULAR REACTIVITY

Although decreases in vascular density and alterations in vessel ultrastructure have the ability to contribute to decreased blood flow and tissue dysfunction with age, alterations in vascular tone (basal vessel diameter) and vascular reactivity (dynamic changes in vessel diameter) are equally important because matching blood flow to tissue metabolic demand is critical for normal cellular function. Despite recent advances in the field, there are conflicting reports of age-related alterations in cerebrovascular tone and reactivity in the literature. For example, Thorin-Trescases [134] observed no effect of age on arterial tone in isolated human pial vessels with diameters ranging between 300–1200 microns, whereas Geary and Buchholz [135] reported increased middle cerebral artery tone in aged Fisher-344 rats. This inconsistency is potentially the result of a disparity in the size and location of the vessels examined, as well as species-based differences in vascular responses. However, recent studies in our laboratory indicate that there are age-related changes in vascular tone and reactivity, and that these alterations are secondary to changes in the balance between endothelium-derived relaxing and contracting factors released from either the micro- and/or macro-circulation (D.M. Eckman et al., unpublished data).

B.   ROLE OF THE ENDOTHELIUM IN AGING

Ultimately, blood flow through a vessel depends on the close interactions of several cell types that compose the vessel wall. Endothelial cells and smooth muscle cells form the basis of this interaction; the complex interactions between relaxing and constricting factors derived from endothelial cells result in a dynamic regulation of vascular smooth muscle cell activity, vessel dilation or constriction, and hence regulation of blood flow to tissue. Mechanistically, endothelium-dependent relaxing factors (EDRFs) result in hyperpolarization of smooth muscle cells and dilation, whereas endothelium-derived constriction factors (EDCFs) result in smooth muscle depolarization and vessel constriction. The roles of each of these factors are discussed below. Despite the recognized importance of these factors in the regulation of cerebral blood flow, there is generally little information available on age-related changes in vessel tone and reactivity in the cerebral circulation. Therefore, data from

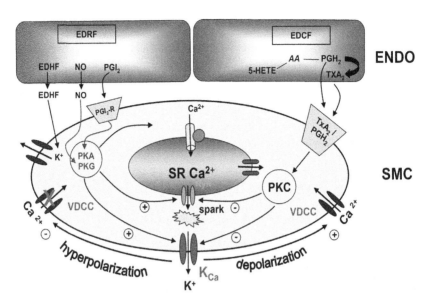

FIGURE 12.3 (SEE COLOR INSERT FOLLOWING PAGE 204) The degree of vascular constriction (vascular tone) regulates blood flow and depends on a close communication between endothelial cells (ENDO) and smooth muscle cells (SMC). Endothelium-dependent relaxing factors (EDRFs) include endothelium-dependent hyperpolarizing factor (EDHF), NO, and PGI_2. These compounds result in hyperpolarization of smooth muscle cells and dilation. Other factors such as endothelium-derived constriction factors (EDCFs), including PGH_2 and TXA_2 result in smooth muscle cell depolarization and vessel constriction. Many of the reported endothelium-dependent dilations depend on the actions of PKA/PKG and PKC. These kinases act on various intracellular targets that regulate/modulate $[Ca^{2+}]_i$ and/or directly influence ion channel activity. With aging, the contribution of endothelium-derived relaxing factors (EDRFs) decreases, whereas the contribution of endothelium-derived contracting factors (EDCFs) increases in many vascular beds. A decrease in endothelium-derived NO and PGI_2 leads to a relative decrease in the production of PKA/PKG, reducing membrane hyperpolarization, and increasing vascular tone. Furthermore, aging-associated elevation in PGH_2 and/or TxA_2 could increase PKC, thus decreasing K^+-channel activity and leading to greater increases in vascular tone. The additive effects of decreased PKA/PKG activity along with elevated PKC activity result in membrane depolarization, increasing $[Ca^{2+}]_i$ entry via voltage-dependent Ca^{2+} channels (VDCCs), leading to increased vascular tone/decreased blood flow in the cerebral circulation. (*Source:* Modified from [177]. With permission.)

other vascular beds are presented such that they might provide some insight into potential age-related changes in the cerebrovascular system.

1.   Endothelium-Derived Relaxing Factors (EDRFs)

a.   Nitric Oxide (NO)

The contribution of nitric oxide (NO) to the modulation of vascular tone has been the focus of multiple human and animal studies. The primary source of NO in the cerebral circulation is endothelial nitric oxide synthase (eNOS). As the name suggests, eNOS is located in the endothelial cells that line the lumen of the blood vessel. NO diffuses to vascular smooth muscle cells where it increases cGMP formation through the activation of cyclic guanylate cyclase (cGC). Activation of this pathway results in the dilation of vascular smooth muscle via multiple mechanisms. While the role of NO signaling in healthy aging-associated vascular dysfunction is not well understood, there are both human and animal studies that provide compelling data suggesting that altered vascular function associated with advancing age may be attributed, at least in part, to perturbations in NO signaling [136–144]. For example, in carotid arteries from aging mice [143], as well as forearm vessels of healthy elderly humans [142], vessel dilation following acetylcholine (ACh) administration (which stimulates endothelial NO production) is significantly reduced, suggesting a blunted production of NO occurs in endothelial cells with age. However, both of these studies also showed reduced vessel dilation in response to sodium nitroprusside (SNP), which directly donates NO to smooth muscle cells. Taken together, these data suggest both endothelial-dependent NO production and endothelial-independent NO sensitivity are altered with aging. In contrast, at least one study reported no age-related differences in coronary artery responses to ACh or nitroprusside have been observed in 24-month-old male F344 rats [145]. These inconsistent findings may reflect methodological differences but more importantly suggest that the mechanisms of age-related vascular dysfunction may be unique to each vascular bed and species.

The mechanisms underlying the disrupted NO signaling with aging identified thus far appear to be complex. In the systemic circulation, both an increase and a decrease in nitric oxide synthase (NOS) activity have been reported [146, 147], as well as an age-associated decrease in agonist-induced vascular cGMP levels [141, 148–150]. In middle cerebral arteries from Fisher-344 rats, Geary and Buchholz [135] demonstrated an increase in arterial tone with advancing age, a finding that appears to be, at least in part, secondary to the dysfunction of eNOS-sensitive mechanisms. Others report declines in the levels of the β subunit of soluble guanylate cyclase (sGC) and reduced sGC activity [141], reduced protein kinase G-1 (PKG-1) activation [151], and decreased eNOS mRNA expression [144, 147, 152] and phosphorylation [153]. Finally, either unchanged [145, 154] or increased eNOS protein expression has been reported in aged vasculature [138, 154–159].

b.   *Endothelium-Derived Hyperpolarizing Factors*
            (EDHFs)

It is well accepted that endothelium-derived hyperpolarizing factors (EDHFs) are important regulators of vascular tone in resistance-size arteries. However, the role of EDHFs in modulating vascular tone in the aging systemic circulation, especially in cerebral circulation, has received little attention. Interestingly, aging appears to significantly impair EDHF-mediated relaxations in isolated human gastroepiploic arteries, distal microvessels [160], and gracilis arterial segments [161]. In contrast, the magnitude of EDHF-mediated relaxation of renal arteries from WKY rats appears unaffected by increasing age [162].

2. Endothelium-Derived Contracting Factors (EDCFs)

a. Endothelin

There are limited data regarding the role of the potent vasoconstrictor, endothelin, in the modulation of vascular tone with age. Barton and colleagues [152] reported a rise in plasma endothelin-1 (ET-1) levels with increasing age in old female Ro-Ro Wistar rats (32 to 33 months). Furthermore, they have shown attenuated ET-1-induced constriction in the aorta but not the femoral artery of old female rats [152]. In contrast, the contractile response to ET-1 has been shown to increase in coronary arteries from aged Wistar-Kyoto [163] and Fisher-344 rats [145], as well as in basilar arteries from aged female rats [164]. Selective inhibition of endothelin-A receptors in young animals abolishes ET-1-induced coronary artery constriction, whereas inhibition of these receptors in aged animals has no effect on ET-1-induced constriction [145]. Thus, the role of endothelin in the modulation of vascular tone and reactivity in the aging vasculature appears complex and requires further investigation.

b. Prostanoids

The role of prostanoids, which include prostaglandins, prostacyclin, and thromboxane, in vascular regulation is well known. These molecules are created from arachidonic acid by cyclooxygenase (COX-1 and COX-2) and prostaglandin H synthase (PGHS-1 and PGHS-2) in most mammalian cells. In vasculature, prostanoids, especially thromboxane, stimulate vasoconstriction. Recent data suggest that aging results in a significant increase of thromboxane A_2 and the prostaglandins PGE_2, PGF_2alpha, and PGI_2 [165, 166]. Other studies have shown that the blunted vasodilatory response of aged vessels to administration of ACh or SNP, while partially attributable to dysregulation of NO, could be partially or completely reversed by inhibition of COX [138, 167] or PGHS2 [168]. Additionally, Davidge and colleagues [167] found that COX inhibition reversed an age-related hypersensitivity to administration of the vasoconstrictor phenylephrine [167]. Furthermore, age-related impairments in vasodilatory responses can be ameliorated by thromboxane A_2/PGH_2 receptor blockade [138, 167, 168]. Finally, age-associated endothelial dysfunction appears to occur as early as 12 months of age via inhibition of the synthesis of COX-2-derived constrictors as well as superoxide anions [169], suggesting an important role for prostanoids in the vascular dysfunction seen with aging.

c. Reactive Oxygen Species (ROS)

There are extensive data suggesting that oxidative stress plays an important role in the mechanisms of aging in multiple tissues [170] (see also Chapter 15). This concept is supported by data revealing a direct correlation between the activity of superoxide dismutase (SOD), an endogenous antioxidant, and lifespan in several species [171]. Although it is well recognized that changes in the antioxidant profile occur with advancing age, relatively little is known regarding the role of oxidative stress in aging-associated vascular dysfunction. In cultured aortic vascular smooth muscle cells from 16-month-old mice, reduced SOD activity has been shown to result in increased levels of reactive oxygen species (ROS) as well as increased lipid peroxidation and damage to mitochondrial DNA[172]. In aging rats and mice, increased

ROS production has been linked to decreased NO bioavailability [143, 173], with concomitant quenching of NO by the formation of peroxynitrite followed by nitration and inhibition of mitochondrial MnSOD [174]. These alterations have the potential to interfere with endothelial NO signaling, resulting in increased vasoconstrictive tone in aged vessels. Indeed, coronary arterioles from aging rats show significantly diminished flow-induced, NO-mediated dilation as a result of increased O_2^{-} anion and peroxynitrite production [144]. In contrast to the above data, at least one study reported that, despite increasing oxidative stress in both male and female Fisher-344 × Brown Norway rats with advancing age, vascular function appears to be preserved in mesenteric arteries [175]. Thus, specific vascular beds may be sensitive to increased oxidative stress associated with age, whereas others may be relatively insensitive to such effects.

C.   SUMMARY

Perturbations in multiple signaling pathways (NO, EDHF, ROS, prostanoids) have been described in different vascular beds in the healthy aging animal. The majority of the research to date suggests that endothelium-dependent responses are attenuated, primarily due to decreased NO production and/or impaired downstream signaling in the NO pathway. The apparent decrease in endothelium-dependent vasodilators coincides with an increase in endothelium-dependent vasoconstrictors in many vascular beds. Additionally, there is an evolving literature suggesting that both ROS and prostanoids may be responsible for elevated vasoconstrictor activity. As most of the aforementioned information is derived from peripheral vascular studies, the mechanism(s) underlying cerebral vascular dysfunction in the aging animal remain unknown. It is well accepted that the cerebral circulation is highly autoregulated. Small changes in arterial tone result in rapid adjustment of regional cerebral blood flow to meet neuronal and metabolic demands. Although it can be argued that the effects of aging on cerebral circulation are predictable based on other vascular beds, the diversity of changes observed in other vascular beds with age argue against this position [176]. In addition, the basic control mechanisms in the cerebral circulation are unique compared to other vascular beds and include, but are not limited to, features such as the blood-brain barrier, perivascular innervation, intracellular communication between neurons, perivascular glial cells, and smooth muscle cells, a high tissue metabolic rate, lack of anoxic tolerance, and the presence of collateral arteries in some species. Therefore, extrapolation of findings from other vascular beds to the cerebral circulation is difficult, and further studies of the altered regulation of the cerebrovasculature in aged animals are necessary.

V.   CONCLUSION

Cerebrovascular aging can be viewed from several perspectives, including alterations in vascular density (the number of capillaries and arterioles), vascular plasticity (the dynamic regulation of vessel density or structure), and vascular reactivity (the adjustment of vessels to acute metabolic changes that occur in tissues). There is evidence that in otherwise healthy humans and animals, age-related changes occur in each of these variables. Data on vascular changes in the brain with aging are limited by the absence of highly controlled studies, as well as by the complexities common to gerontological investigations. Nevertheless, there are substantial data that the density of some cerebral vessels, especially precapillary arterioles, decreases with age. However, the analysis of capillary density can be more challenging, and the introduction of stereological analyses may aid in the development of more precise analyses and resolve some of the current controversies. Certainly the growth of new vessels appears to be compromised with age, which has important implications for management of disease processes including stroke. Finally, matching acute metabolic changes to alterations in blood flow is critical for normal tissue function. Unfortunately, the majority of data on microvascular reactivity has been gathered from peripheral vascular beds. Whether changes in the cerebrovasculature are similar to those in the periphery remain to be established. However, each vascular bed appears to have unique regulatory properties and therefore additional direct studies will be required. The underlying basic question to be addressed is whether age-related alterations in blood flow or transport of nutrients from blood to brain limit tissue function in highly localized areas of the brain and directly or indirectly lead to impaired function. Obviously this is a complex question that will require non-invasive imaging techniques that are still in development. Once these studies are complete, the detailed studies of vascular density and vessel reactivity that are ongoing can be integrated to determine whether pharmacological interventions can be designed to improve function.

ACKNOWLEDGMENTS

This work was supported by National Institutes of Health Grants P01 AG11370 (WES and DRR) and R01 AG19886 (DRR).

REFERENCES

1. Figueroa, J.P. et al., Alterations in fetal kidney development and elevations in arterial blood pressure in young adult sheep after clinical doses of antenatal glucocorticoids, *Pediatr. Res.*, 58, 510, 2005.
2. Gallagher, M. and Nicolle, M.M., Animal models of normal aging: relationship between cognitive decline and markers in hippocampal circuitry, *Behav. Brain Res.*, 57, 155, 1993.
3. Ramsey, M.W. and Sonntag W.E, Growth hormone and insulin-like growth factor-1 and their interactions on brain circuits involved in cognitive function, in *The Somatotophic Axis in Brain Function*, Nyberg, F., Ed., Elsevier, New York, 2005, chap. 14, pp. 185–208.
4. Meltzer, C.C. et al., Does cerebral blood flow decline in healthy aging? A PET study with partial-volume correction, *J. Nucl. Med.*, 41, 1842, 2000.
5. Martin, A.J. et al., Decreases in regional cerebral blood flow with normal aging, *J. Cereb. Blood Flow Metab.*, 11, 684, 1991.

6. Moeller, J.R. et al., The metabolic topography of normal aging, *J. Cereb. Blood Flow Metab.*, 16, 385, 1996.
7. Farkas, E. and Luiten, P.G., Cerebral microvascular pathology in aging and Alzheimer's disease, *Prog. Neurobiol.*, 64, 575, 2001.
8. Kawamura, J. et al., Leuko-araiosis and cerebral perfusion in normal aging, *Exp. Aging Res.*, 19, 225, 1993.
9. Krejza, J. et al., Transcranial color Doppler sonography of basal cerebral arteries in 182 healthy subjects: age and sex variability and normal reference values for blood flow parameters, *AJR Am. J. Roentgenol.*, 172, 213, 1999.
10. Schultz, S.K. et al., Age-related changes in regional cerebral blood flow among young to mid-life adults, *Neuroreport,* 10, 2493, 1999.
11. Hagstadius, S. and Risberg, J., Regional cerebral blood flow characteristics and variations with age in resting normal subjects, *Brain Cogn.*, 10, 28, 1989.
12. Bentourkia, M. et al., Comparison of regional cerebral blood flow and glucose metabolism in the normal brain: effect of aging, *J. Neurol. Sci.*, 181, 19, 2000.
13. Pagani, M. et al., Regional cerebral blood flow as assessed by principal component analysis and (99m)Tc-HMPAO SPET in healthy subjects at rest: normal distribution and effect of age and gender, *Eur. J. Nucl. Med. Mol. Imaging,* 29, 67, 2002.
14. Ohata, M. et al., Regional cerebral blood flow during development and ageing of the rat brain, *Brain,* 104, 319, 1981.
15. Berman, R.F., Goldman, H., and Altman, H.J., Age-related changes in regional cerebral blood flow and behavior in Sprague-Dawley rats, *Neurobiol. Aging,* 9, 691, 1988.
16. Linville, D.G. and Arneric, S.P., Cortical cerebral blood flow governed by the basal forebrain: age-related impairments, *Neurobiol. Aging,* 12, 503, 1991.
17. Lartaud, I. et al., *In vivo* cerebrovascular reactivity in Wistar and Fischer 344 rat strains during aging, *Am. J. Physiol.*, 264, H851, 1993.
18. Noda, A. et al., Age-related changes in cerebral blood flow and glucose metabolism in conscious rhesus monkeys, *Brain Res.,* 936, 76, 2002.
19. Gjedde, A. and Diemer, N.H., Double-tracer study of the fine regional blood-brain glucose transfer in the rat by computer-assisted autoradiography, *J. Cereb. Blood Flow Metab.,* 5, 282, 1985.
20. Kalaria, R.N., Cerebral vessels in ageing and Alzheimer's disease, *Pharmacol. Ther.,* 72, 193, 1996.
21. De la Torre, J.C., Cerebromicrovascular pathology in Alzheimer's disease compared to normal aging, *Gerontology,* 43, 26, 1997.
22. Cook, J.J. et al., Age-related alterations in the arterial microvasculature of skeletal muscle, *J. Gerontol.*, 47, B83, 1992.
23. Rakusan, K. and Nagai, J., Morphometry of arterioles and capillaries in hearts of senescent mice, *Cardiovasc. Res.,* 28, 969, 1994.
24. Hutchins, P.M. et al., The microcirculation in experimental hypertension and aging, *Cardiovasc. Res.,* 32, 772, 1996.
25. Knox, C.A. and Oliveira, A., Brain aging in normotensive and hypertensive strains of rats. III. A quantitative study of cerebrovasculature, *Acta Neuropathol. (Berl),* 52, 17, 1980.
26. Bell, M.A. and Ball, M.J., Morphometric comparison of hippocampal microvasculature in ageing and demented people: diameters and densities, *Acta Neuropathol. (Berl.),* 53, 299, 1981.
27. Sonntag, W.E. et al., Decreases in cerebral microvasculature with age are associated with the decline in growth hormone and insulin-like growth factor 1, *Endocrinology,* 138, 3515, 1997.

28. Riddle, D.R., Sonntag, W.E., and Lichtenwalner, R.J., Microvascular plasticity in aging, *Ageing Res. Rev.,* 2, 149, 2003.
29. Hughes, C.C. and Lantos, P.L., A morphometric study of blood vessel, neuron and glial cell distribution in young and old rat brain, *J. Neurol. Sci.,* 79, 101, 1987.
30. Klein, A.W. and Michel, M.E., A morphometric study of the neocortex of young adult and old maze-differentiated rats, *Mech. Ageing Dev.,* 6, 441, 1977.
31. Amenta, F. et al., Effect of long-term treatment with the dihydropyridine-type calcium channel blocker darodipine (PY 108-068) on the cerebral capillary network in aged rats, *Mech. Ageing Dev.,* 78, 27, 1995.
32. Amenta, F. et al., Age-related changes in brain microanatomy: sensitivity to treatment with the dihydropyridine calcium channel blocker darodipine (PY 108-068), *Brain Res. Bull.,* 36, 453, 1995.
33. Meier-Ruge, W. et al., Stereological changes in the capillary network and nerve cells of the aging human brain, *Mech. Ageing Dev.,* 14, 233, 1980.
34. Mann, D.M. et al., Quantitative changes in cerebral cortical microvasculature in ageing and dementia, *Neurobiol. Aging,* 7, 321, 1986.
35. Hunziker, O., Abdel'Al, S., and Schulz, U., The aging human cerebral cortex: a stereological characterization of changes in the capillary net, *J. Gerontol.,* 34, 345, 1979.
36. Wilkinson, J.H., Hopewell, J.W., and Reinhold, H.S., A quantitative study of age-related changes in the vascular architecture of the rat cerebral cortex, *Neuropathol. Appl. Neurobiol.,* 7, 451, 1981.
37. Hinds, J.W. and McNelly, N.A., Capillaries in aging rat olfactory bulb: a quantitative light and electron microscopic analysis, *Neurobiol. Aging,* 3, 197, 1982.
38. Casey, M.A. and Feldman, M.L., Aging in the rat medial nucleus of the trapezoid body. III. Alterations in capillaries, *Neurobiol. Aging,* 6, 39, 1985.
39. Bell, M.A. and Ball, M.J., The correlation of vascular capacity with the parenchymal lesions of Alzheimer's disease, *Can. J. Neurol. Sci.,* 13, 456, 1986.
40. Buchweitz-Milton, E. and Weiss, H.R., Perfused capillary morphometry in the senescent brain, *Neurobiol. Aging,* 8, 271, 1987.
41. Jucker, M., Battig, K., and Meier-Ruge, W., Effects of aging and vincamine derivatives on pericapillary microenvironment: stereological characterization of the cerebral capillary network, *Neurobiol. Aging,* 11, 39, 1990.
42. Jucker, M. and Meier-Ruge, W., Effects of brovincamine on stereological capillary parameters in adult and old Fischer-344 rats, *Microvasc. Res.,* 37, 298, 1989.
43. Bell, M.A. and Ball, M.J., Neuritic plaques and vessels of visual cortex in aging and Alzheimer's dementia, *Neurobiol. Aging,* 11, 359, 1990.
44. Abernethy, W.B. et al., Microvascular density of the human paraventricular nucleus decreases with aging but not hypertension, *Exp. Neurol.,* 121, 270, 1993.
45. Bar, T., Morphometric evaluation of capillaries in different laminae of rat cerebral cortex by automatic image analysis: changes during development and aging, *Adv. Neurol.,* 20, 1, 1978.
46. Meier-Ruge, W., Ulrich, J., and Abdel-Al, S., Stereologic findings in normal brain aging and Alzheimer's disease, in Werthemimer, J. and Marios, M., Eds., *Senile Dementia: Outlook for the Future,* Alan R. Liss, New York, 1984, pp. 125–135.
47. Meier-Ruge, W. and Schulz-Dazzi, U., Effects of brovincamine on the stereological parameters of corticocerebral capillaries, *Life Sci.,* 40, 943, 1987.
48. Lokkegaard, A., Nyengaard, J.R., and West, M.J., Stereological estimates of number and length of capillaries in subdivisions of the human hippocampal region, *Hippocampus,* 11, 726, 2001.

49. Manoonkitiwongsa, P.S. et al., A simple stereologic method for analysis of cerebral cortical microvessels using image analysis, *Brain Res. Brain Res. Protoc.*, 8, 45, 2001.

50. Villena, A. et al., Stereological changes in the capillary network of the aging dorsal lateral geniculate nucleus, *Anat. Rec. A Discov. Mol. Cell Evol. Biol.*, 274, 857, 2003.

51. Hajdu, M.A. et al., Effects of aging on mechanics and composition of cerebral arterioles in rats, *Circ. Res.*, 66, 1747, 1990.

52. Ravens, J.R., Vascular changes in the human senile brain, *Adv. Neurol.*, 20, 487, 1978.

53. Knox, C.A. et al., Effects of aging on the structural and permeability characteristics of cerebrovasculature in normotensive and hypertensive strains of rats, *Acta Neuropathol. (Berl.)*, 51, 1, 1980.

54. Mooradian, A.D., Effect of aging on the blood-brain barrier, *Neurobiol. Aging*, 9, 31, 1988.

55. Burns, E.M., Kruckeberg, T.W., and Gaetano, P.K., Changes with age in cerebral capillary morphology, *Neurobiol. Aging*, 2, 283, 1981.

56. Hicks, P. et al., Age-related changes in rat brain capillaries, *Neurobiol. Aging*, 4, 69, 1983.

57. Stewart, P.A. et al., A quantitative analysis of blood-brain barrier ultrastructure in the aging human, *Microvasc. Res.*, 33, 270, 1987.

58. de Jong, G.I. et al., Nimodipine effects on cerebral microvessels and sciatic nerve in aging rats, *Neurobiol. Aging*, 13, 73, 1992.

59. De Jong, G.I., Traber, J., and Luiten, P.G., Formation of cerebrovascular anomalies in the ageing rat is delayed by chronic nimodipine application, *Mech. Ageing Dev.*, 64, 255, 1992.

60. Keuker, J.I., Luiten, P.G., and Fuchs, E., Capillary changes in hippocampal CA1 and CA3 areas of the aging rhesus monkey, *Acta Neuropathol. (Berl.)*, 100, 665, 2000.

61. Maclullich, A.M. et al., Enlarged perivascular spaces are associated with cognitive function in healthy elderly men, *J. Neurol. Neurosurg. Psychiatry*, 75, 1519, 2004.

62. Luiten, P.G., de Jong, G.I., and Schuurman, T., Cerebrovascular, neuronal, and behavioral effects of long-term Ca2+ channel blockade in aging normotensive and hypertensive rat strains, *Ann. N.Y. Acad. Sci.*, 747, 431, 1994.

63. Shah, G.N. and Mooradian, A.D., Age-related changes in the blood-brain barrier, *Exp. Gerontol.*, 32, 501, 1997.

64. Cerletti, U., Die Gefabvermehrung im Zentralnervensystem, *Nissls Hist. Histopathol. Arbeiten*, 11, 41, 1910.

65. Ferszt, R. and Cervos-Navarro, J., Cerebrovascular pathology-aging and brain failure, in *Brain Aging: Neuropathology and Neuropharmacology*, Cervos-Navarro, J. and Sarkander, H.I., Eds., Raven Press, New York, 1983, pp. 133–151.

66. Akima, M. et al., A study on the microvasculature of the cerebral cortex. Fundamental architecture and its senile change in the frontal cortex, *Lab. Invest.*, 55, 482, 1986.

67. Cervos-Navarro, J., Gertz, H.J., and Frydl, V., Cerebral blood vessel changes in old people, *Mech. Ageing Dev.*, 39, 223, 1987.

68. Moody, D.M., Santamore, W.P., and Bell, M.A., Does tortuosity in cerebral arterioles impair down autoregulation in hypertensives and elderly normotensives? A hypothesis and computer model, *Clin. Neurosurg.*, 37, 372, 1991.

69. Moody, D.M. et al., Cerebral microvascular alterations in aging, leukoaraiosis, and Alzheimer's disease, *Ann. N.Y. Acad. Sci.*, 826, 103, 1997.

70. De la Torre, J.C. and Mussivand, T., Can disturbed brain microcirculation cause Alzheimer's disease? *Neurol. Res.*, 15, 146, 1993.

71. De la Torre, J.C., Impaired brain microcirculation may trigger Alzheimer's disease, *Neurosci. Biobehav. Rev.*, 18, 397, 1994.

72. Bell, M.A. and Ball, M.J., Laminar variation in the microvascular architecture of normal human visual cortex (area 17), *Brain Res.*, 335, 139, 1985.
73. Riddle, D.R. et al., Differential metabolic and electrical activity in the somatic sensory cortex of juvenile and adult rats, *J. Neurosci.*, 13, 4193, 1993.
74. Zheng, D., LaMantia, A.S., and Purves, D., Specialized vascularization of the primate visual cortex, *J. Neurosci.*, 11, 2622, 1991.
75. Riddle, D. et al., Growth of the rat somatic sensory cortex and its constituent parts during postnatal development, *J. Neurosci.*, 12, 3509, 1992.
76. Purves, D. et al., Neural activity and the development of the somatic sensory system, *Curr. Opin. Neurobiol.*, 4, 120, 1994.
77. Diamond, M.C. et al., Differences in occipital cortical synapses from environmentally enriched, impoverished, and standard colony rats, *J. Neurosci. Res.*, 1, 109, 1975.
78. Sirevaag, A.M. and Greenough, W.T., Differential rearing effects on rat visual cortex synapses. III. Neuronal and glial nuclei, boutons, dendrites, and capillaries, *Brain Res.*, 424, 320, 1987.
79. Black, J.E., Sirevaag, A.M., and Greenough, W.T., Complex experience promotes capillary formation in young rat visual cortex, *Neurosci. Lett.*, 83, 351, 1987.
80. Sirevaag, A.M. et al., Direct evidence that complex experience increases capillary branching and surface area in visual cortex of young rats, *Brain Res.*, 471, 299, 1988.
81. Caley, D.W. and Maxwell, D.S., Development of the blood vessels and extracellular spaces during postnatal maturation of rat cerebral cortex, *J. Comp Neurol.*, 138, 31, 1970.
82. Argandona, E.G. and Lafuente, J.V., Effects of dark-rearing on the vascularization of the developmental rat visual cortex, *Brain Res.*, 732, 43, 1996.
83. Argandona, E.G. and Lafuente, J.V., Influence of visual experience deprivation on the postnatal development of the microvascular bed in layer IV of the rat visual cortex, *Brain Res.*, 855, 137, 2000.
84. Fox, K. and Zahs, K., Critical period control in sensory cortex, *Curr. Opin. Neurobiol.*, 4, 112, 1994.
85. Berardi, N., Pizzorusso, T., and Maffei, L., Critical periods during sensory development, *Curr. Opin. Neurobiol.*, 10, 138, 2000.
86. Black, J.E., Zelazny, A.M., and Greenough, W.T., Capillary and mitochondrial support of neural plasticity in adult rat visual cortex, *Exp. Neurol.*, 111, 204, 1991.
87. Black, J.E., Polinsky, M., and Greenough, W.T., Progressive failure of cerebral angiogenesis supporting neural plasticity in aging rats, *Neurobiol. Aging*, 10, 353, 1989.
88. Black, J.E., Isaacs, K.R., and Greenough, W.T., Usual vs. successful aging: some notes on experiential factors, *Neurobiol. Aging*, 12, 325, 1991.
89. Isaacs, K.R. et al., Exercise and the brain: angiogenesis in the adult rat cerebellum after vigorous physical activity and motor skill learning, *J. Cereb. Blood Flow Metab*, 12, 110, 1992.
90. Vissing, J., Andersen, M., and Diemer, N.H., Exercise-induced changes in local cerebral glucose utilization in the rat, *J. Cereb. Blood Flow Metab.*, 16, 729, 1996.
91. Kleim, J.A., Cooper, N.R., and VandenBerg, P.M., Exercise induces angiogenesis but does not alter movement representations within rat motor cortex, *Brain Res.*, 934, 1, 2002.
92. Swain, R.A. et al., Prolonged exercise induces angiogenesis and increases cerebral blood volume in primary motor cortex of the rat, *Neuroscience*, 117, 1037, 2003.
93. Rosenstein, J.M., Why do neural transplants survive? An examination of some metabolic and pathophysiological considerations in neural transplantation, *Exp. Neurol.*, 133, 1, 1995.

94. Redmond, D.E., Jr., Cellular replacement therapy for Parkinson's disease — where we are today? *Neuroscientist*, 8, 457, 2002.

95. Broadwell, R.D. et al., Allografts of CNS tissue possess a blood-brain barrier. II. Angiogenesis in solid tissue and cell suspension grafts, *Exp. Neurol.*, 112, 1, 1991.

96. Miyoshi, Y., Date, I., and Ohmoto, T., Three-dimensional morphological study of microvascular regeneration in cavity wall of the rat cerebral cortex using the scanning electron microscope: implications for delayed neural grafting into brain cavities, *Exp. Neurol.*, 131, 69, 1995.

97. Baker-Cairns, B.J. et al., Contributions of donor and host blood vessels in CNS allografts, *Exp. Neurol.*, 142, 36, 1996.

98. Dusart, I. et al., Vascularization of fetal cell suspension grafts in the excitotoxically lesioned adult rat thalamus, *Brain Res. Dev. Brain Res.*, 48, 215, 1989.

99. Finger, S. and Dunnett, S.B., Nimodipine enhances growth and vascularization of neural grafts, *Exp. Neurol.*, 104, 1, 1989.

100. Grabowski, M. et al., Vascularization of fetal neocortical grafts implanted in brain infarcts in spontaneously hypertensive rats, *Neuroscience*, 51, 673, 1992.

101. Leigh, K., Elisevich, K., and Rogers, K.A., Vascularization and microvascular permeability in solid versus cell-suspension embryonic neural grafts, *J. Neurosurg.*, 81, 272, 1994.

102. Gash, D.M., Collier, T.J., and Sladek, J.R., Jr., Neural transplantation: a review of recent developments and potential applications to the aged brain, *Neurobiol. Aging*, 6, 131, 1985.

103. Gage, F.H. and Bjorklund, A., Neural grafting in the aged rat brain, *Annu. Rev. Physiol*, 48, 447, 1986.

104. Matsumoto, A. et al., Ultrastructural and immunohistochemical analysis of fetal mediobasal hypothalamic tissue transplanted into the aged rat brain, *Ann. N.Y. Acad. Sci.*, 495, 404, 1987.

105. Zaman, V. and Shetty, A.K., Survival of fetal hippocampal CA3 cell grafts in the middle-aged and aged hippocampus: effect of host age and deafferentation, *J. Neurosci. Res.*, 70, 190, 2002.

106. Krupinski, J. et al., Some remarks on the growth-rate and angiogenesis of microvessels in ischemic stroke. Morphometric and immunocytochemical studies, *Patol. Pol.*, 44, 203, 1993.

107. Zhang, Z.G. et al., Bone marrow-derived endothelial progenitor cells participate in cerebral neovascularization after focal cerebral ischemia in the adult mouse, *Circ. Res.*, 90, 284, 2002.

108. Coyle, P. and Heistad, D.D., Blood flow through cerebral collateral vessels one month after middle cerebral artery occlusion, *Stroke*, 18, 407, 1987.

109. Garcia, J.H. et al., Brain microvessels: factors altering their patency after the occlusion of a middle cerebral artery (Wistar rat), *Am. J. Pathol.*, 145, 728, 1994.

110. Sbarbati, A. et al., The microvascular system in ischemic cortical lesions, *Acta Neuropathol. (Berl.)*, 92, 56, 1996.

111. Yamaguchi, S. et al., Effect of aging on collateral circulation via pial anastomoses in cats, *Gerontology*, 34, 157, 1988.

112. Szpak, G.M. et al., Border zone neovascularization in cerebral ischemic infarct, *Folia Neuropathol.*, 37, 264, 1999.

113. Sonntag, W.E. et al., The effects of growth hormone and IGF-1 deficiency on cerebrovascular and brain ageing, *J. Anat.*, 197 Pt 4, 575, 2000.

114. Kraling, B.M. and Bischoff, J., A simplified method for growth of human microvascular endothelial cells results in decreased senescence and continued responsiveness to cytokines and growth factors, *In Vitro Cell Dev. Biol. Anim.*, 34, 308, 1998.

115. Rosenstein, J.M. et al., Patterns of brain angiogenesis after vascular endothelial growth factor administration *in vitro* and *in vivo*, *Proc. Natl. Acad. Sci. U.S.A.*, 95, 7086, 1998.

116. Watanabe, Y. et al., Vascular permeability factor/vascular endothelial growth factor (VPF/VEGF) delays and induces escape from senescence in human dermal microvascular endothelial cells, *Oncogene*, 14, 2025, 1997.

117. Slevin, M. et al., Serial measurement of vascular endothelial growth factor and transforming growth factor-beta1 in serum of patients with acute ischemic stroke, *Stroke*, 31, 1863, 2000.

118. Ferrara, N., Vascular endothelial growth factor and the regulation of angiogenesis, *Recent Prog. Horm. Res.*, 55, 15, 2000.

119. Zagzag, D. and Capo, V., Angiogenesis in the central nervous system: a role for vascular endothelial growth factor/vascular permeability factor and tenascin-C. Common molecular effectors in cerebral neoplastic and non-neoplastic "angiogenic diseases," *Histol. Histopathol.*, 17, 301, 2002.

120. Gustafsson, T. and Kraus, W.E., Exercise-induced angiogenesis-related growth and transcription factors in skeletal muscle, and their modification in muscle pathology, *Front. Biosci.*, 6, D75-D89, 2001.

121. Kawamata, T., Speliotes, E.K., and Finklestein, S.P., The role of polypeptide growth factors in recovery from stroke, *Adv. Neurol.*, 73, 377, 1997.

122. Nag, S., The blood-brain barrier and cerebral angiogenesis: lessons from the cold-injury model, *Trends Mol. Med.*, 8, 38, 2002.

123. Zhang, Z. and Chopp, M., Vascular endothelial growth factor and angiopoietins in focal cerebral ischemia, *Trends Cardiovasc. Med.*, 12, 62, 2002.

124. Aberg, M.A. et al., Peripheral infusion of IGF-I selectively induces neurogenesis in the adult rat hippocampus, *J. Neurosci.*, 20, 2896, 2000.

125. Lichtenwalner, R.J. et al., Intracerebroventricular infusion of insulin-like growth factor-I ameliorates the age-related decline in hippocampal neurogenesis, *Neuroscience*, 107, 603, 2001.

126. Altman, J. and Das, G.D., Autoradiographic and histological evidence of postnatal hippocampal neurogenesis in rats, *J. Comp Neurol.*, 124, 319, 1965.

127. Eriksson, P.S. et al., Neurogenesis in the adult human hippocampus, *Nat. Med.*, 4, 1313, 1998.

128. Gould, E. et al., Neurogenesis in the neocortex of adult primates, *Science*, 286, 548, 1999.

129. Palmer, T.D., Adult neurogenesis and the vascular Nietzsche, *Neuron*, 34, 856, 2002.

130. Palmer, T.D., Willhoite, A.R., and Gage, F.H., Vascular niche for adult hippocampal neurogenesis, *J. Comp Neurol.*, 425, 479, 2000.

131. Jin, K. et al., Vascular endothelial growth factor (VEGF) stimulates neurogenesis *in vitro* and *in vivo*, *Proc. Natl. Acad. Sci. U.S.A.*, 99, 11946, 2002.

132. Monje, M.L. et al., Irradiation induces neural precursor-cell dysfunction, *Nat. Med.*, 8, 955, 2002.

133. Leventhal, C. et al., Endothelial trophic support of neuronal production and recruitment from the adult mammalian subependyma, *Mol. Cell Neurosci.*, 13, 450, 1999.

134. Thorin-Trescases, N. et al., Diameter dependence of myogenic tone of human pial arteries. Possible relation to distensibility, *Stroke*, 28, 2486, 1997.

135. Geary, G.G. and Buchholz, J.N., Selected contribution: effects of aging on cerebrovascular tone and [Ca^{2+}]i, *J. Appl. Physiol.*, 95, 1746, 2003.

136. Taddei, S. et al., Aging and endothelial function in normotensive subjects and patients with essential hypertension, *Circulation*, 91, 1981, 1995.

137. Egashira, K. et al., Effects of age on endothelium-dependent vasodilation of resistance coronary artery by acetylcholine in humans, *Circulation*, 88, 77, 1993.

138. Matz, R.L. et al., Vascular bed heterogeneity in age-related endothelial dysfunction with respect to NO and eicosanoids, *Br. J. Pharmacol.*, 131, 303, 2000.

139. Hinschen, A.K., Rose'Meyer, R.B., and Headrick, J.P., Age-related changes in adenosine-mediated relaxation of coronary and aortic smooth muscle, *Am. J. Physiol. Heart Circ. Physiol.*, 280, H2380, 2001.

140. Woodman, C.R., Price, E.M., and Laughlin, M.H., Selected contribution: aging impairs nitric oxide and prostacyclin mediation of endothelium-dependent dilation in soleus feed arteries, *J. Appl. Physiol.*, 95, 2164, 2003.

141. Moritoki, H. et al., Possible mechanisms of age-associated reduction of vascular relaxation caused by atrial natriuretic peptide, *Eur. J. Pharmacol.*, 210, 61, 1992.

142. Al-Shaer, M.H. et al., Effects of aging and atherosclerosis on endothelial and vascular smooth muscle function in humans, *Int. J Cardiol.*, 109, 201, 2006.

143. Blackwell, K.A. et al., Mechanisms of aging-induced impairment of endothelium-dependent relaxation: role of tetrahydrobiopterin, *Am. J. Physiol. Heart Circ. Physiol.*, 287, H2448, 2004.

144. Csiszar, A. et al., Aging-induced phenotypic changes and oxidative stress impair coronary arteriolar function, *Circ. Res.*, 90, 1159, 2002.

145. Korzick, D.H. et al., Exaggerated coronary vasoreactivity to endothelin-1 in aged rats: role of protein kinase C, *Cardiovasc. Res.*, 66, 384, 2005.

146. Cernadas, M.R. et al., Expression of constitutive and inducible nitric oxide synthases in the vascular wall of young and aging rats, *Circ. Res.*, 83, 279, 1998.

147. Challah, M. et al., Circulating and cellular markers of endothelial dysfunction with aging in rats, *Am. J. Physiol.*, 273, H1941, 1997.

148. Ueda, H. and Moritoki, H., Possible association of decrease of ATP-induced vascular relaxation with reduction of cyclic GMP during aging, *Arch. Int. Pharmacodyn. Ther.*, 310, 35, 1991.

149. Moritoki, H. et al., Age-associated decrease in histamine-induced vasodilation may be due to reduction of cyclic GMP formation, *Br. J. Pharmacol.*, 95, 1015, 1988.

150. Moritoki, H. et al., Evidence for the involvement of cyclic GMP in adenosine-induced, age-dependent vasodilatation, *Br. J. Pharmacol.*, 100, 569, 1990.

151. Lin, C.S. et al., Age-related decrease of protein kinase G activation in vascular smooth muscle cells, *Biochem. Biophys. Res. Commun.*, 287, 244, 2001.

152. Barton, M. et al., Anatomic heterogeneity of vascular aging: role of nitric oxide and endothelin, *Hypertension*, 30, 817, 1997.

153. Smith, A.R. and Hagen, T.M., Vascular endothelial dysfunction in aging: loss of Akt-dependent endothelial nitric oxide synthase phosphorylation and partial restoration by (R)-alpha-lipoic acid, *Biochem. Soc. Trans.*, 31, 1447, 2003.

154. Chou, T.C. et al., Alterations of nitric oxide synthase expression with aging and hypertension in rats, *Hypertension*, 31, 643, 1998.

155. van der, L.B. et al., Expression and activity patterns of nitric oxide synthases and antioxidant enzymes reveal a substantial heterogeneity between cardiac and vascular aging in the rat, *Biogerontology*, 6, 325, 2005.

156. Tschudi, M.R. et al., Effect of age on kinetics of nitric oxide release in rat aorta and pulmonary artery, *J. Clin. Invest.*, 98, 899, 1996.

reproductive function. Collectively, these functions enable "fight or flight" behaviors to remove the organism from immediate danger, while later restoring bodily homeostasis.

Although many hormones are released in response to stress, much research has focused on the role of glucocorticoids (GCs). It is important to note, however, that stress and elevated GC levels are not equivalent, though their effects on behavior, plasticity, and other measures may be similar. GCs are synthesized in the adrenal glands, released directly into the peripheral circulatory system, and readily cross the blood-brain barrier. Two forms of GC receptors, the mineralocorticoid receptor (MR) and glucocorticoid receptor (GR), are each widely distributed throughout the brain [7–10], enabling GCs to have tremendous influence on brain function. The primary GC in humans and other primates is cortisol, whereas the main GC in rodents is corticosterone.

Links between GCs and peripheral signs of aging were first proposed after clinicians observed that patients with Cushing's syndrome (also called hypercortisolemia; characterized by excessive secretion of GCs via the adrenal glands) exhibit pathologies often seen in aged individuals [11, 12]. These problems include heart disease, osteoporosis, hypertension, Type II diabetes, depression of the immune system, and loss of muscle. The idea that GCs might contribute to brain aging did not emerge until the early 1970s. At that time, studies had revealed that one particular region of the brain, the hippocampus, was especially enriched for GC receptors [13], and the contribution of the hippocampus to reducing activation of the HPA axis was beginning to be appreciated [14]. It was also known that the hippocampus was especially vulnerable to both normal and pathological changes observed with aging [15, 16]. These factors led scientists to propose a glucocorticoid hypothesis of aging [17–20]. This hypothesis predicted that life-long exposure to normal levels of GCs would cause deleterious effects of GCs to accumulate in GC-sensitive neurons, such as those of the hippocampus. Moreover, because hippocampal dysfunction could reduce hippocampus-mediated inhibition of the HPA axis [21], GC secretion was predicted to gradually increase over time, leading to an acceleration of both damage and dysfunction.

In accordance with the GC hypothesis of aging, basal plasma levels of GCs [22–24] and other hormones in the HPA axis [23, 25] increase in senescent rodents. Additionally, older rodents exhibit exaggerated endocrine stress responses; peak levels of stress hormones are unaffected with age, however GC levels take longer to return to basal levels [22, 26]. In contrast, the relationship between GC levels and aging is not as straightforward in primates. Generally, studies of nonhuman primates [27, 28] and humans [29, 30] reveal no increase in basal levels of GCs with aging until considering extremely aged cohorts. However, aged primates and humans do show some alterations in measures of HPA axis activity. For example, older primates exhibit higher cortisol levels and prolonged elevation of cortisol in response to some types of stimuli relative to younger primates [28, 32]. Some studies of aged humans have reported mild alterations in the diurnal cortisol rhythm [32–34]. Interestingly, several recent studies have suggested that age-related changes in HPA activity exhibit high levels of variability in primates, and identified sub-groups of rhesus monkeys [35] and humans [36–38] that have increasing and high basal cortisol levels with aging. These sub-groups were identified by tracking cortisol levels in individuals across a span of years, a time consuming approach that is rarely used. Because cortisol levels vary widely within a day, due both to an innate diurnal rhythm and to the recent experiences of the individual, repeated measures over time likely produce a more reliable indicator of cumulative GC exposure.

The nature of individual differences in HPA function in human populations is not well understood, but there are a variety of sources that may contribute to group differences in GC secretion, which could, in turn, drive differences in susceptibility to GC-accelerated aging. One factor that may contribute to sub-populations with increased GC release is the presence of neuropathological conditions in that sub-population. There are a number of conditions, including Alzheimer's disease [39] and depression [40], that result in high levels of cortisol, which have been speculated to contribute to accelerated brain aging [41]. A second factor that may contribute to individual differences in GC secretion is cumulative exposure to stress. Some chronic stressors in rodents [42, 43] and primates [44, 45] produce elevated basal GC levels. Similarly, in human populations, stressors such as caregiving or chronic illness can result in increased basal GC secretion [46, 47]. Another factor that may shape HPA axis activity is early life experiences. In rodents, unpredictable prenatal stress (produced by stressing the pregnant dam) causes life-long increases in HPA activity [48, 49]. In contrast, mild postnatal stress (short-term separation of the pups from the mother) is sufficient to reverse the effects of prenatal stress, and causes decreased activity of the HPA axis [50, 51]. Handling rodents during infancy causes long-lasting increases in GC receptors in the hippocampus, which enhances negative feedback of the HPA axis [51]. In these rat models of early experience, prenatal stress accelerates brain aging while mild postnatal stress of a form most readily construed as "stimulation" slows brain aging [52, 53]. A fourth modulator of HPA axis activity is genetic influences. It has been shown that people with genetically small hippocampi are more vulnerable to the pathological effects of stress [54]. It has also been shown that the human gene for GR has three single nucleotide polymorphisms, two of which produce a mild augmentation to psychosocial stress (reviewed in [55]).

Collectively, this evidence suggests that GC-mediated HPA activity is altered by aging, at least in a subset of the aged population. Whatever the underlying cause of age-related changes in GCs, many studies have now contributed to our understanding of the effects of GCs on neuronal function. These studies have revealed that stress and GCs have profound consequences for learning and memory and synaptic plasticity. Additional data have revealed that stress and GCs also contribute to neuronal atrophy, changes in rates of neuronal turnover, and perhaps to neuronal death. Subsequent work has provided evidence that these GC- and stress-induced changes are present in senescent animals, and have also demonstrated that interventions designed to reduce HPA activity can reduce signs of brain aging. By understanding the ways in which stress and GCs exacerbate brain aging, we also gain insight into ways to promote healthy brain aging.

II.   STRESS AND GLUCOCORTICOID EFFECTS ON LEARNING AND MEMORY

The ability of stress and GCs to affect learning and memory has been extensively documented, particularly in the hippocampus where GC receptors are highly expressed. It has been shown that the levels of GCs at the time of learning and testing, as well as the cumulative history of GC exposure prior to learning and testing, are each capable of influencing learning and memory. In rodents, transient alterations in GC levels produced by a single injection of exogenous corticosterone cause concentration-dependent, biphasic modulation of brain function. Both low and high physiological levels of circulating GCs impair multiple measures of brain function, including learning and memory, whereas middle levels facilitate these measures, giving a characteristic "inverted-U" shaped dose-response curve (see [56] for a review). Stressors given immediately prior to assessment of learning and memory may similarly impair [57, 58] or facilitate [59] memory. The effects of repeated stress or GC exposure appear more uniform. Chronic stress consistently impairs measures of brain function. For example, chronic stress has been shown to adversely affect hippocampus-dependent spatial learning [60–63]. Deficits in hippo-campus-dependent learning after chronic stress have also been noted for other organisms, including the tree shrew [64] and humans [65]. The effects of chronic stress on hippocampal function appear to be mediated by GCs, despite other stress-induced neuroendocrine changes. Removal of the adrenal glands prior to chronic stress is sufficient to prevent stress-induced memory problems [60]. Also, repeated injections of high physiological levels of exogenous GCs are sufficient to impair hippocampus-dependent task performance in rodents [60, 66].

Studies in humans also support a link between high circulating GC levels and poor learning and memory, although these impairments are not specific to hippo-campal function. However, two studies in nonhuman primates have indicated that GC receptors are expressed in the frontal and prefrontal cortices at levels similar to or greater than the hippocampus [10, 68], predicting that GC effects on memory may not be greatest in hippocampus-dependent tasks in the primate. Injection of synthetic cortisol in young adults during the peak (highest level) or trough (lowest level) of the diurnal rhythm of endogenous secretion produced an impairment or facilitation of memory, depending on the time of injection [68]. That is, at the highest levels (the combination of both exogenous and endogenous GCs), acutely elevated GCs impaired performance, while at the lowest levels, performance improved. Repeated injections of synthetic cortisol over ten days in healthy, young adult humans have been shown to produce deficits in tasks depending on the frontal cortex [69]. In humans with clinical depression, cortisol levels are elevated during the cicadian trough overall and levels are predictive of memory performance: high levels of cortisol correlate with poor task performance [70]. Finally, hypercortisolemic patients with Cushing's syndrome have been shown to have impaired performance on both cortical [71] and hippocampal [72] tasks. Thus, long-term exposure to high GC levels is capable of impairing learning and memory.

The effects of aging on learning and memory are similar to those produced by GCs and stress in younger animals. For example, rodents show age-related impair-ment of hippocampal function on a variety of hippocampus-dependent tasks such as spatial navigation [73, 74], the radial arm maze [75, 76], and contextual fear conditioning [77, 78]. Aged rats also show impairments on behavioral tasks that depend on frontal cortices, including medial frontal [79] and orbitofrontal [80, 81]. However, for all of these tasks, age-dependent impairment of learning and memory is quite variable, with subsets of animals exhibiting impairment and other cohorts showing little or no impairment [73–75, 81–86]; such variability can reflect important factors, such as strain or developmental history. Aged primates, including both monkeys [3, 87, 88] and humans [36, 38, 89, 90] show deficits in learning and memory, particularly in tasks that depend on the frontal cortices or hippocampus. In general, small sample sizes in these studies have precluded examining many of the factors that give rise to variability in these endpoints.

There is evidence to suggest that age-related impairments in learning and memory are related to GC levels. Increased HPA activity correlates with age-related cognitive impairment in rodents [4, 52, 91] and humans [5, 37], such that the greater the degree of cognitive impairment, the greater the measures of HPA activity. Adrenalectomy of rodents in mid-life, coupled with low-dose supplementation of exogenous GCs, retards age-related memory deficits [92]. In humans, elderly persons with subjective memory impairment have elevated basal cortisol levels [93]. Also, elderly humans with persistently high levels of basal cortisol measured across several years exhibited poorer performance on a hippocampus-dependent delayed memory task than elderly persons with lower cortisol levels [36, 38]. Finally, in humans with elevated basal cortisol levels, administration of metyrapone, a drug that maintains cortisol secretion at low basal rates, has been shown to reverse age-related memory impairments [94].

III. STRESS AND GLUCOCORTICOID EFFECTS ON PLASTICITY

Studies examining synaptic plasticity in animal models have demonstrated that putative cellular substrates for learning and memory are also regulated by stress and GCs. Acute administration of corticosterone to young adult rodents produces parallel effects on behavioral indicators of memory and synaptic plasticity; low to medium doses of corticosterone produce dose-dependent increases of hippocampal long-term potentiation (LTP, an increase in synaptic strength [95]),; whereas high doses impair LTP [96, 97]. High levels of exogenous corticosterone administered to young adult rats also reduce hippocampal prime burst potentiation (PBP, a form of LTP [98] in which stimulation patterns are designed to mimic stimulation of the hippocampus under natural conditions) [96, 99]. Similar reductions in PBP are observed after acute, intense psychological stress [100] or exposure to predator odor [101]. Repeated stress in young rats causes multiple changes in hippocampal electrophysiological measures, including reduction of stimulation thresholds, reduction of field EPSP amplitude, and a decrease in frequency potentiation (FP; a form of short-term plasticity in hippocampus [102] of the field EPSP) [103]. Intense, acute stress [104] and repeated stress [105] also impair LTP in young rats. Both acute and repeated stressors facilitate long-term depression (LTD [106], a reduction in synaptic strength) [107, 108].

Studies suggest that some of these effects on synaptic plasticity are mediated by GCs released during stress. For example, chronic injection of high physiological levels of GCs impairs hippocampal LTP in young rats [97]. Similar decrements in

LTP have been observed after 3 months of elevated corticosterone in middle-aged rats [60]. These studies demonstrate that GCs alone are capable of reducing plasticity in hippocampus. Adrenalectomy of adult rats reduces the ability of stress to diminish LTP [109]. Adrenalectomy also reduces afterhyperpolarizations in neurons of hippocampal slice preparations, enabling those neurons to fire action potentials in quicker succession; in contrast, bath application of GC agonists to hippocampal slice preparations from adrenalectomized rats enhances afterhyperpolarizations, indicating that GCs reduce the excitability of hippocampal neurons [110]. High levels of GCs also increase voltage-gated calcium currents in neurons [111, 112].

There are numerous studies that suggest that GC-induced changes in electrophysiological measures exist in aged animals. Paralleling the effects of stress and GCs, aging reduces both LTP, especially with lower intensity of stimulation [113, 114], and FP [115]. Aging rats also show increases in LTD [116]. Reductions in stimulation threshold and field EPSP amplitude, observed after stress in young rats, also are observed with normal aging [103]. Also, GC-sensitive afterhyperpolarizations in hippocampal neurons are greater in aged rats relative to young rats [117]. Finally, aged rats show increased calcium-dependent neuronal activity in hippocampus [118], and have large L-type calcium channel currents [119, 120], which contribute directly to impairment of synaptic plasticity [121].

IV. STRESS AND GLUCOCORTICOID CONTRIBUTIONS TO NEURONAL ATROPHY AND CELL DEATH

Some studies suggest that stress and GCs may lead to neuronal death, but this conclusion is not without controversy. In rodents, chronic injection of exogenous stress levels of corticosterone in young rats produced neuronal loss of CA3 comparable to that seen in aged rats [19], but it has also been shown that this effect is observed only if treatment begins when the rats are juveniles and does not happen if prolonged corticosterone exposure occurs only during adulthood [122]. Thus, high levels of corticosterone do not always cause neuron loss. Stress is even less likely to produce overt neuronal death than GC exposure [123]. Only truly exceptional levels of stress have ever been shown to cause neuron loss in the brain. Wild-born monkeys that died in captivity exhibiting multiple signs of severe social subordination stress (gastric ulcers, bite wounds, increased adrenal weight) have been shown to have stress-related changes in hippocampal neurons. These monkeys showed reduced numbers of hippocampal neurons and pronounced atrophy in those hippocampal neurons that remained [124].

Unlike stress or GCs, it is clear that senescence is accompanied by cell loss, and this cell loss is indirectly linked to GC exposure. In the rat, age-related neuronal loss in hippocampus is greatest in Ammon's horn pyramidal neurons, and minimal in the dentate gyrus [92, 125]. Because receptors for GCs are highest in Ammon's horn, and less dense in dentate gyrus [126, 127], this anatomical pattern of neuron loss implicates GC actions in age-related decline of hippocampal volume. Removal of endogenous corticosterone by adrenalectomy of rodents in middle-age attenuates this age-related loss of hippocampal neurons [92]. Both cognitive impairments and elevated corticosterone levels are correlated with hippocampal neuron loss in rats [4]. Finally, rats with low HPA activity as a result of postnatal handling as pups did not show age-related loss of hippocampal neurons, in contrast to their nonhandled littermates [51, 53]. Thus, GC levels clearly accelerate neuron loss in aged rodents.

One recent proposal [128] has suggested an interesting mechanism by which GCs, through GR-mediated signaling, may contribute to cell death. According to this hypothesis, high levels of GCs must first pass through the cell membrane and bind to the cytoplasmic GR. The activated GR acts through a combination of nongenomic (depolarization of the mitochondrial membrane [129]) and genomic mechanisms (increasing gene transcription of pro-apoptotic proteins such as Bax that further depolarize the mitochondria). Factors promoting apoptotic cell death, such as cytochrome c, are released from mitochondria upon sustained depolarization. Thus, GC-mediated apoptosis of neurons [130] is hypothesized to be mediated by direct and indirect actions of GR on mitochondria.

It is not clear whether healthy aging in humans is accompanied by neuron loss, nor is it clear whether high levels of cortisol in humans could lead to cell death. In the few studies to quantify hippocampal neuron numbers in postmortem human brains, the number of hippocampal neurons decreased with age in area CA1, the dentate gyrus, and the subiculum [131, 132]. Using MRI techniques to estimate volumetric changes in brain structures, volumetric loss in healthy subjects is particularly pronounced in various cortical regions, including frontal and parietal cortices, but there appears to be little volumetric loss in subcortical areas such as hippocampus, thalamus, and the amygdala [134]. Young and middle-aged humans with elevated cortisol due to Cushing's syndrome exhibit loss of hippocampal volume [134]; however, this effect is reversed when treatment is given to normalize corticosterone levels [135]. Although volumetric loss in human cases could be accounted for by cell death, the simple reversibility of volume loss in Cushing's patients with high cortisol suggests that at least some volumetric changes are more likely due to reversible dendritic atrophy.

An abundant literature illustrates strong links between stress, GCs, and neuronal atrophy. In rodents, chronic stress has been shown to cause neuronal atrophy in numerous brain regions, including the inferior colliculus [136], medial prefrontal cortex [137], and the hippocampus [138]. Administration of exogenous corticosterone [139–141] or a synthetic GC [141] to young rodents produces neuronal atrophy in the same regions showing atrophy after chronic stress. In primates, exposure to chronic and severe social stress caused atrophy in hippocampus, frontal and prefrontal cortices, and the cingulate cortex [124]. Implantation of a cortisol pellet directly into the hippocampus of adult monkeys caused extensive atrophy of local neurons after 1 year of cortisol exposure [142]. Administration of high levels of a synthetic GC to pregnant rhesus monkeys caused both hypercortisolemia (chronically elevated levels of cortisol) and marked hippocampal atrophy in the offspring [143].

If one accepts the premise that volumetric loss in humans is likely to reflect atrophy, then links can be made between stress, GCs, and atrophy in humans. For example, high levels of exogenous steroids administered to treat autoimmune disease in young and middle-aged humans caused brain atrophy, and the atrophy was reversed in several patients when steroids were no longer used [144]. As mentioned, patients with high cortisol levels due to Cushing's syndrome have small hippocampal volumes [134] but hippocampal volumes increase after treatment to reduce cortisol levels [135]. Smaller hippocampal volumes have been reported in patients with stress-related psychiatric disorders including PTSD [145], borderline personality disorder with abuse [146], and depression [147], and dissociative identity disorder [148].

Caution must be used, however, when correlating psychiatric disease with alterations in brain volumes, as it is possible that volumetric differences precede the disease. Such a finding was recently demonstrated for smaller hippocampal volumes in patients with PTSD [54]. Researchers identified monozygotic twin pairs, one of whom had combat exposure ("combat exposed") during military experience and the other without combat experience ("unexposed"). Of those pairs, a subset of the combat-exposed twins had developed PTSD after their combat experience, and the remainder did not; none of the "unexposed" subjects developed PTSD. By conducting volumetric MRI analysis of the hippocampus, the researchers were able to show that the combat veterans with PTSD had smaller right hippocampal volumes relative to individuals without PTSD. However, the identical twins of the combat-exposed veterans with PTSD also had smaller hippocampi relative to individuals without PTSD. This strongly suggests that small hippocampi constitute a risk factor for developing PTSD, and suggests that the "hippocampal atrophy" observed in some PTSD patients can reflect a preexisting condition and is not the result of trauma. Smaller hippocampi may reduce the ability of the hippocampus to inhibit the HPA axis during a stressor [21], thereby increasing the individual's exposure to cortisol and other stress hormones during a traumatic event.

There are several studies that indicate that neuronal atrophy accompanies aging but few studies quantify atrophy in animal models of aging. This is likely because the techniques (such as Golgi staining) are labor intensive and the analysis is time consuming. Studies in senescent rats show reduction in dendritic branching of the hippocampus [149] and the anterior cingulate cortex [150]. The largest age-related decline in human subjects is in the prefrontal lobes [151, 152] but volumetric reductions also are observed in other cortices and a small reduction has been reported for the hippocampus [152]. Interestingly, these areas that show atrophy in humans are also the areas that have been shown in nonhuman primates to contain high levels of GR. However, there is no direct evidence that altering GC levels in either human or nonhuman primates affects the aging process.

V. STRESS AND GLUCOCORTICOID REGULATION OF NEUROGENESIS

New neurons are generated in the adult brain via mitotic cell division, a phenomenon termed "neurogenesis." These new neurons have been shown to migrate from the subventricular zone and subgranular zone to the olfactory bulb and hippocampus respectively, and also to the neocortex, where they integrate with the local circuitry.

Neurogenesis has been shown in several species, including the rat [153, 154], nonhuman and human primates [154–156], and the tree shrew [157], but occurs in limited fashion. That is, even within the olfactory bulb and hippocampus, new neurons comprise only a very small portion of the total number of neurons in the structure. Although the functional purpose of neurogenesis is highly debated, the fact that these newborn neurons mature, form synapses, and integrate into neural networks suggests that they may play an important role in hippocampal function (see [158] for a review; see also Chapter 6).

Neurogenesis has been shown to be very sensitive to stress and GCs. A wide variety of acute stressors reduce proliferation of hippocampal cells [157–159]. Chronic stressors also produce similar effects on hippocampal proliferation [161–163]. Prolonged and high levels of corticosterone reduce neurogenesis in rats [164], as does transient elevation of circulating GCs via a single injection of a high dose of corticosterone [165]. Increased basal corticosterone levels in the offspring of a female rat stressed while pregnant is correlated with reduced hippocampal neurogenesis [166]. Adrenalectomy reverses the ability of acute stressors to impair neurogenesis in young rats [167]. Adrenalectomy of young rats also reverses corticosterone-induced impairment of neurogenesis [164].

Age-related changes in neurogenesis parallel those changes observed after stress and GC treatment in younger animals. In rodents, tremendous decreases in hippocampal cell proliferation accompany senescence [168–170]. Within a cohort of aged rats, significant correlations have been observed between basal corticosterone levels and levels of hippocampal neurogenesis; those aged rats with the highest levels of corticosterone also had the lowest levels of neurogenesis [171]. In mice, neuronal precursor cells in older animals express higher levels of both MR and GR than precursor cells of younger animals, suggesting that cell proliferation is likely more sensitive to corticosterone as aging progresses [172]. In agreement with this suggestion, increased sensitivity to GCs with age has been suggested in tree shrews; older animals exhibited greater inhibition of hippocampal cell proliferation in response to chronic stress than younger animals [173]. Rodents adrenalectomized in mid-life do not show age-related increases in corticosterone levels, nor do they show age-related decline of neurogenesis [171, but see 174]. Adrenalectomy of aged rats is also capable of increasing hippocampal cell proliferation to levels comparable to that of young rats, suggesting that high corticosterone levels in aged rats act to suppress neurogenesis [170]. No studies have examined the effects of stress on neurogenesis in aged animals; but because aged animals show such a large suppression of neurogenesis, it may be that neurogenesis is not capable of further suppression.

VI. CONCLUSIONS

An extensive body of work has substantiated the idea that repeated or prolonged exposure to GCs has a deleterious impact on brain function, and has also provided evidence that GCs likely contribute to age-related decline in brain function. These stress- and GC-mediated effects on age are evident across behavior, electrophysiological, and anatomical levels. Despite the sophistication of our knowledge of the effects of stress and GCs across many dimensions of brain function, future research will undoubtedly continue to expand our understanding of the ways by which this occurs and suggest new therapeutic targets for intervention within a subset of people whose brain function is disproportionately affected during senescence.

REFERENCES

1. Lehmann, H.E., Successful cerebral aging: clinical and pharmacological approaches to the aging brain, *J. Psychiatr. Pract.*, 6, 33, 2000.
2. Cabeza, R., et al., Aging gracefully: compensatory brain activity in high-performing older adults, *Neuroimage*, 17, 1394, 2002.
3. Rapp, P.R. and Amaral, D.G., Recognition memory deficits in a subpopulation of aged monkeys resemble the effects of medial temporal lobe damage, *Neurobiol. Aging*, 12, 481, 1991.
4. Issa, A.M. et al., Hypothalamic-pituitary-adrenal activity in aged, cognitively impaired and cognitively unimpaired rats, *J. Neurosci.*, 10, 3247, 1990.
5. Meaney, M.J. et al., Individual differences in hypothalamic-pituitary-adrenal activity in later life and hippocampal aging, *Exp. Gerontol.*, 30, 229, 1995.
6. Munck, A., Guyre, P., and Holbrook, N., Physiologial actions of glucocorticoids in stress and their relation to pharmacological actions, *Endoc. Rev.*, 5, 25, 1984.
7. Seckl, J.R. et al., Distribution of glucocorticoid and mineralocorticoid receptor messenger RNA expression in human postmortem hippocampus, *Brain Res.*, 561, 332, 1991.
8. Van Eekelen, J.A., Bohn, M.C., and de Kloet, E.R., Postnatal ontogeny of mineralocorticoid and glucocorticoid receptor gene expression in regions of the rat tel- and diencephalons, *Brain Res. Dev. Brain Res.*, 61, 33, 1991.
9. Meyer, U. et al., Cloning of glucocorticoid receptor and mineralocorticoid receptor cDNA and gene expression in the central nervous system of the tree shrew (*Tupaia belangeri*), *Brain Res. Mol. Brain Res.*, 55, 243, 1998.
10. Sanchez M.M. et al., Distribution of corticosteroid receptors in the rhesus brain: relative absence of glucocorticoid receptors in the hippocampal formation, *J. Neurosci.*, 20, 4657, 2000.
11. Findlay, T., Role of the neurohypophysis in the pathogenesis of hypertension and some allied disorders associated with aging, *Am. J. Med.*, 7, 70, 1949.
12. Wexler, B.C., Comparative aspects of hyperadrenocorticism and aging, in *Hypothalamus, Pituitary, and Aging*, Ereritt, V. and Burgess, J.A., Eds., Charles C. Thomas, Springfield, IL, 1976.
13. McEwen, B.S., Weiss, J.M., and Schwartz, L.S., Selective retention of corticosterone by limbic structures in rat brain, *Nature*, 220, 911, 1968.
14. Bohus, B., The hippocampus and the pituitary-adrenal system hormones, in *The Hippocampus*, Isaacson, R.L. and Pribram, K.H., Eds., Plenum Press, New York, 1975, 323.
15. Wisniewski, H.M. and Terry, R.D., Morphology of the aging brain, human and animal, in *Progress in Brain Research*, Ford, D.M., Ed., Elsevier, Amsterdam, 1973, 167.
16. Tomlinson, B.L. and Henderson, G., Some quantitative cerebral findings in normal and demented old people, in *Neurobiology of Aging,* Terry, R.D. and Gershon, S., Eds., Raven Press, New York, 1976, 183.

17. Landfield, P.W., Waymire, J.C., and Lynch, G., Hippocampal aging and adrenocorticoids: quantitative correlations, *Science,* 202, 1098, 1978.

18. Landfield, P.W., An endocrine hypothesis of brain aging and studies on brain-endocrine correlations and monosynaptic neurophysiology during aging, in *Parkinson's Disease, Vol. 2: Aging and Neuroendocrine Relationships,* Finch, C.E., Potter, D.E., and Kenny, A.D., Eds., Plenum Press, New York, 1978, 179.

19. Sapolsky, R.M., Krey, L.C., and McEwen, B.S., Prolonged glucocorticoid exposure reduces hippocampal neuron number: implications for aging, *J. Neurosci,* 5, 1222, 1985.

20. Sapolsky, R.M., Krey, L.C., and McEwen, B.S., The neuroendocrinology of stress and aging: the glucocorticoid cascade hypothesis, *Endocr. Rev.,* 7, 284, 1986.

21. Sapolsky, R.M., Krey, L.C., and McEwen, B.S., Glucocorticoid-sensitive hippocampal neurons are involved in terminating the adrenocortical stress response, *Proc. Natl. Acad. Sci. U.S.A.,* 81, 61, 1984.

22. Sapolsky, R.M., Krey, L.C., and McEwen, B.S., The adrenocortical stress-response in the aged male rat: impairment of recovery from stress, *Exp. Gerontol.,* 18, 55, 1983.

23. Meaney, M.J. et al., Basal ACTH, corticosterone and corticosterone-binding globulin levels over the diurnal cycle, and age-related changes in hippocampal type I and type II corticosteroid receptor binding capacity in young and aged, handled and nonhandled rats, *Neuroendocrinology,* 55, 204, 1992.

24. Sapolsky, R.M., Do glucocorticoid concentrations rise with age in the rat? *Neurobiol. Aging,* 13, 171, 1992.

25. Tang, F. and Phillips, J.G., Some age-related changes in pituitary-adrenal function in the male laboratory rat, *J. Gerontol.,* 33, 377, 1978.

26. Sapolsky, R.M., Krey, L.C., and McEwen, B.S., The adrenocortical axis in the aged rat: impaired sensitivity to both fast and delayed feedback inhibition, *Neurobiol. Aging,* 7, 331, 1986.

27. Goncharova, N.D. and Lapin, B.A., Changes of hormonal function of the adrenal and gonadal glands in baboons of different age groups, *J. Med. Primatol.,* 29, 26, 2000.

28. Goncharova, N.D. and Lapin, B.A., Effects of aging on hypothalamic-pituitary-adrenal system function in non-human primates, *Mech. Ageing Dev.,* 123, 1191, 2002.

29. Waltman, C. et al., Spontaneous and glucocorticoid-inhibited adrenocorticotropic hormone and cortisol secretion are similar in healthy young and old men, *J. Clin. Endocrinol. Metab.,* 73, 495, 1991.

30. Born J. et al., Effects of age and gender on pituitary-adrenocortical responsiveness in humans, *Eur. J. Endocrinol.,* 132, 705, 1995.

31. Lyons, D.M. et al., Cognitive correlates of white matter growth and stress hormones in female squirrel monkey adults, *J. Neurosci.,* 24, 3655, 2004.

32. Touitou, Y. et al., Adrenal circadian system in young and elderly human subjects: a comparative study, *J. Endocrinol.,* 93, 201, 1982.

33. Sherman, B., Wysham, C., and Pfohl, B., Age-related changes in the circadian rhythm of plasma cortisol in man, *J. Clin. Endocrinol. Metab.,* 61, 439, 1985.

34. Maes, M. et al., Effects of age on spontaneous cortisolaemia of normal volunteers and depressed patients, *Psychoneuroendocrinology,* 19, 79, 1994.

35. Erwin, J.M. et al., Age-related changes in fasting plasma cortisol in rhesus monkeys: implications of individual differences for pathological consequences, *J. Gerontol. A. Biol. Sci. Med. Sci.,* 59, 424, 2004.

36. Lupien, S.J. et al., Cortisol levels during human aging predict hippocampal atrophy and memory deficits, *Nat. Neurosci.,* 1, 69, 1998.

37. Lupien, S., Lecours, A.R., Lussier, I., Schwartz, G., Nair, N.P., Meaney, M.J., Basal cortisol levels and cognitive deficits in human aging. *J. Neurosci.*, 14, 2893, 1994.
38. Li, G. et al., Salivary cortisol and memory function in human aging, *Neurobiol. Aging*, 3, 27, 1705, 2006.
39. Armanini, D. et al., Alzheimer's disease: pathophysiological implications of measurement of plasma cortisol, plasma dehydroepiandrosterone sulfate, and lymphocytic corticosteroid receptors, *Endocrine*, 22, 113, 2003.
40. O'Brien, J.T. et al., A longitudinal study of hippocampal volume, cortisol levels, and cognition in older depressed subjects, *Am. J. Psychiatry*, 161, 2081, 2004.
41. Ferrari, E. et al., Cognitive and affective disorders in the elderly: a neuroendocrine study, *Arch. Gerontol. Geriatr. Suppl.*, 9, 171, 2004.
42. Du Ruisseau, P. et al., Effects of chronic stress on pituitary hormone release induced by combined hemi-extirpation of the thyroid, adrenal and ovary in rats, *Neuroendocrinology*, 24, 169, 1977.
43. Vernikos, J. et al., Pituitary-adrenal function in rats chronically exposed to cold, *Endocrinology*, 110, 413, 1982.
44. Abbott, D.H. et al., Are subordinates always stressed? A comparative analysis of rank differences in cortisol levels among primates, *Horm. Behav.*, 43, 67, 2003.
45. Suleman, M.A. et al., Physiologic manifestations of stress from capture and restraint of free-ranging male African green monkeys (*Cercopithecus aethiops*), *J. Zoo Wildl. Med.*, 35, 20, 2004.
46. Davis, L.L. et al., Biopsychological markers of distress in informal caregivers, *Biol. Res. Nurs.*, 6, 90, 2004.
47. Reiche, E.M., Morimoto, H.K., and Nunes, S.M., Stress and depression-induced immune dysfunction: implications for the development and progression of cancer, *Int. Rev. Psychiatry*, 17, 515, 2005.
48. Ader, R. and Plaut, S.M., Effects of prenatal maternal handling and differential housing on offspring emotionality, plasma corticosterone levels, and susceptibility to gastric erosions, *Psychosom. Med.*, 30, 277, 1968.
49. Maccari, S. et al., Prenatal stress and long-term consequences: implications of glucocorticoid hormones, *Neurosci. Biobehav. Rev.*, 27, 119, 2003.
50. Meaney, M.J. et al., Effect of neonatal handling on age-related impairments associated with the hippocampus, *Science*, 239, 766, 1988.
51. Meaney, M.J. et al., Postnatal handling attenuates certain neuroendocrine, anatomical, and cognitive dysfunctions associated with aging in female rats, *Neurobiol. Aging*, 12, 31, 1991.
52. Vallee, M. et al., Long-term effects of prenatal stress and postnatal handling on age-related glucocorticoid secretion and cognitive performance: a longitudinal study in the rat, *Eur. J. Neurosci.*, 11, 2906, 1999.
53. Lehmann, J. et al., Comparison of maternal separation and early handling in terms of their neurobehavioral effects in aged rats, *Neurobiol. Aging*, 23, 457, 2002.
54. Gilbertson, M.W. et al., Smaller hippocampal volume predicts pathologic vulnerability to psychological trauma, *Nat. Neurosci.*, 5, 1242, 2002.
55. DeRijk R. and de Kloet E.R., Corticosteroid receptor genetic polymorphisms and stress responsivity, *Endocrine*, 28, 263, 2005.
56. Lupien, S.J and McEwen, B.S., The acute effects of corticosteroids on cognition: integration of animal and human model studies, *Brain Res. Brain Res. Rev.*, 24, 1, 1997.
57. de Quervain, D.J., Roozendaal, B., and McGaugh, J.L., Stress and glucocorticoids impair retrieval of long-term spatial memory, *Nature*, 394, 787, 1998.

58. Kim, J.J. et al., Amygdalar inactivation blocks stress-induced impairments in hippocampal long-term potentiation and spatial memory, *J. Neurosci.*, 25, 1532, 2005.
59. Shors, T.J., Acute stress rapidly and persistently enhances memory formation in the male rat, *Neurobiol. Learn. Mem.*, 75, 10, 2001.
60. Bodnoff, S.R. et al., Enduring effects of chronic corticosterone treatment on spatial learning, synaptic plasticity, and hippocampal neuropathology in young and mid-aged rats, *J. Neurosci.*, 15, 61, 1995.
61. Conrad, C.D. et al., Chronic stress impairs rat spatial memory on the Y maze, and this effect is blocked by tianeptine pretreatment, *Behav. Neurosci.*, 110, 1321, 1996.
62. Pawlak, R. et al., Tissue plasminogen activator and plasminogen mediate stress-induced decline of neuronal and cognitive functions in the mouse hippocampus, *Proc. Natl. Acad. Sci. U.S.A.*, 102, 18201, 2005.
63. Song, L. et al., Impairment of the spatial learning and memory induced by learned helplessness and chronic mild stress, *Pharmacol. Biochem. Behav.*, 83, 186, 2006.
64. Ohl, F. and Fuchs, E., Differential effects of chronic stress on memory processes in the tree shrew, *Brain Res. Cogn. Brain Res.*, 7, 379, 1999.
65. Bergdahl, J. et al., Treatment of chronic stress in employees: subjective, cognitive and neural correlates, *Scand. J. Psychol.*, 46, 395, 2005.
66. McLay, R.N., Freeman, S.M., and Zadina, J.E. Chronic corticosterone impairs memory performance in the Barnes maze, *Physiol. Behav.*, 63, 933, 1998.
67. Patel, P.D. et al., Glucocorticoid and mineralocorticoid receptor mRNA expression in squirrel monkey brain, *J. Psychiatr. Res.*, 34, 383, 2000.
68. Lupien, S.J. et al., The modulatory effects of corticosteroids on cognition: studies in young human populations, *Psychoneuroendocrinology*, 27, 401, 2002.
69. Young, A.H. et al., The effects of chronic administration of hydrocortisone on cognitive function in normal male volunteers, *Psychopharmacology (Berl.)*, 145, 260, 1999.
70. Egeland, J. et al., Cortisol level predicts executive and memory function in depression, symptom level predicts psychomotor speed, *Acta Psychiatr. Scand.*, 112, 434, 2005.
71. Starkman, M.N. et al., Elevated cortisol levels in Cushing's disease are associated with cognitive decrements, *Psychosom. Med.*, 63, 985, 2001.
72. Grillon, C. et al., Deficits in hippocampus-mediated Pavlovian conditioning in endogenous hypercortisolism, *Biol. Psychiatry*, 56, 837, 2004.
73. Drapeau, E. et al., Spatial memory performances of aged rats in the water maze predict levels of hippocampal neurogenesis, *Proc. Natl. Acad. Sci. U.S.A.*, 100, 14385, 2003.
74. Meijer, O.C. et al., Correlations between hypothalamus-pituitary-adrenal axis parameters depend on age and learning capacity, *Endocrinology*, 146, 1372, 2005.
75. Ingram, D.K., London, E.D., and Goodrick, C.L., Age and neurochemical correlates of radial maze performance in rats, *Neurobiol. Aging*, 2, 41, 1981.
76. Kadar, T. et al., Age-related structural changes in the rat hippocampus: correlation with working memory deficiency, *Brain Res.*, 512, 113, 1990.
77. Moyer, J.R., Jr. and Brown, T.H., Impaired trace and contextual fear conditioning in aged rats, *Behav. Neurosci.*, 120, 612, 2006.
78. Wati, H. et al., A decreased survival of proliferated cells in the hippocampus is associated with a decline in spatial memory in aged rats, *Neurosci. Lett.*, 399, 171, 2006.
79. Barense, M.D., Fox, M.T., and Baxter, M.G., Aged rats are impaired on an attentional set-shifting task sensitive to medial frontal cortex damage in young rats, *Learn. Mem.*, 9, 191, 2002.

80. Schoenbaum, G. et al., Teaching old rats new tricks: age-related impairments in olfactory reversal learning, *Neurobiol. Aging*, 23, 555, 2002.
81. Schoenbaum, G. et al., Encoding changes in orbitofrontal cortex in reversal-impaired aged rats, *J. Neurophysiol.*, 95, 1509, 2006.
82. Gage, F.H., Dunnett, S.B., and Bjorklund, A., Spatial learning and motor deficits in aged rats, *Neurobiol. Aging*, 5, 43, 1984.
83. Gage, F.H., Kelly, P.A., and Bjorklund, A., Regional changes in brain glucose metabolism reflect cognitive impairments in aged rats, *J. Neurosci.*, 4, 2856, 1984.
84. Gallagher, M. and Pelleymounter, M.A., An age-related spatial learning deficit: choline uptake distinguishes "impaired" and "unimpaired" rats, *Neurobiol. Aging*, 9, 363, 1988.
85. Burger, C. et al., Changes in transcription within the CA1 field of the hippocampus are associated with age-related spatial learning impairments, *Neurobiol. Learn. Mem.*, 87, 21, 2007.
86. Sandi, C. and Touyarot, K., Mid-life stress and cognitive deficits during early aging in rats: individual differences and hippocampal correlates, *Neurobiol. Aging*, 27, 128, 2006.
87. O'Donnell, K.A., Rapp, P.R., and Hof, P.R., Preservation of prefrontal cortical volume in behaviorally characterized aged macaque monkeys, *Exp. Neurol.*, 160, 300, 1999.
88. Rapp, P.R., Kansky, M.T., and Roberts, J.A., Impaired spatial information processing in aged monkeys with preserved recognition memory, *Neuroreport*, 8, 1923, 1997.
89. Moffat, S.D., Zonderman, A.B., and Resnick, S.M., Age differences in spatial memory in a virtual environment navigation task, *Neurobiol. Aging.*, 22, 787, 2001.
90. Nordahl, C.W. et al., White matter changes compromise prefrontal cortex function in healthy elderly individuals, *J. Cogn. Neurosci.*, 18, 418, 2006.
91. Rowe, W. et al., Antidepressants restore hypothalamic-pituitary-adrenal feedback function in aged, cognitively-impaired rats, *Neurobiol. Aging*, 18, 527, 1997.
92. Landfield, P.W., Baskin, R.K., and Pitler, T.A., Brain aging correlates: retardation by hormonal-pharmacological treatments, *Science*, 214, 581, 1981.
93. Wolf, O.T. et al., Subjective memory complaints in aging are associated with elevated cortisol levels, *Neurobiol. Aging*, 26, 1357, 2005.
94. Lupien, S.J. et al., Acute modulation of aged human memory by pharmacological manipulation of glucocorticoids, *J. Clin. Endocrinol. Metab.,* 87, 3798, 2002.
95. Bliss, T.V. and Lomo T., Long-lasting potentiation of synaptic transmission in the dentate area of the anaesthetized rabbit following stimulation of the perforant path, *J. Physiol.*, 232, 331, 1973.
96. Diamond, D.M. et al., Inverted-U relationship between the level of peripheral corticosterone and the magnitude of hippocampal primed burst potentiation, *Hippocampus*, 2, 421, 1992.
97. Pavlides, C., Watanabe, Y., and McEwen, B.S., Effects of glucocorticoids on hippocampal long-term potentiation, *Hippocampus*, 3, 183, 1993.
98. Diamond, D.M., Dunwiddie, T.V., and Rose, G.M., Characteristics of hippocampal primed burst potentiation in vitro and in the awake rat, *J. Neurosci.*, 8, 4079, 1988.
99. Bennett, M.C. et al., Serum corticosterone level predicts the magnitude of hippocampal primed burst potentiation and depression in urethane-anaesthetized rats, *Psychobiology*, 19, 301, 1991.
100. Diamond, D.M., Fleshner, M., and Rose, G.M., Psychological stress repeatedly blocks hippocampal primed burst potentiation in behaving rats, *Behav. Brain Res.*, 62, 1, 1994.

101. Mesches, M.H. et al., Exposing rats to a predator blocks primed burst potentiation in the hippocampus *in vitro, J. Neurosci.*, 19, RC18, 1999.

102. Anderson, P. and Lomo, T., Control of hippocampal output by afferent volley frequency, in *Structure and Function of the Limbic System: Progress in Brain Research*, Vol. 27, Adey, W.R. and Tokizane, T., Eds., Elsevier, Amsterdam, 1967, 400.

103. Kerr, D.S. et al., Chronic stress-induced acceleration of electrophysiologic and morphometric biomarkers of hippocampal aging, *J. Neurosci.*, 11, 1316, 1991.

104. Foy, M.R. et al., Behavioral stress impairs long term potentiation in rodent hippocampus, *Behav. Neural Biol.*, 48, 138, 1987.

105. Pavlides, C., Nivon, L.G., and McEwen, B.S., Effects of chronic stress on hippocampal long-term potentiation, *Hippocampus*, 12, 245, 2002.

106. Dunwiddie, T. and Lynch, G., Long-term potentiation and depression of synaptic responses in the rat hippocampus: localization and frequency dependency, *J. Physiol.*, 276, 353, 1978.

107. Artola, A. et al., Long-lasting modulation of the induction of LTD and LTP in rat hippocampal CA1 by behavioural stress and environmental enrichment, *Eur. J. Neurosci.*, 23, 261, 2006.

108. Yang, J. et al., Acute behavioural stress facilitates long-term depression in temporoammonic-CA1 pathway, *Neuroreport*, 17, 753, 2006.

109. Shors, T.J., Levine, S., and Thompson, R.F., Effect of adrenalectomy and demedulation on the stress-induced impairment of long-term potentiation, *Neuroendocrinology*, 51, 70, 1990.

110. Joels, M. and de Kloet, E.R., Effects of glucocorticoids and norepinephrine on the excitability in the hippocampus, *Science*, 245, 1502, 1989.

111. Karst, H. et al., Glucocorticoids alter calcium conductances and calcium channel subunit expression in basolateral amygdala neurons, *Eur. J. Neurosci.*, 16, 1083, 2002.

112. Kole, M.H. et al., High-voltage-activated Ca^{2+} currents and the excitability of pyramidal neurons in the hippocampal CA3 subfield in rats depend on corticosterone and time of day, *Neurosci. Lett.*, 307, 53, 2001.

113. Deupree, D.L., Bradley, J., and Turner, D.A., Age-related alterations in potentiation in the CA1 region in F344 rats, *Neurobiol. Aging*, 14, 249, 1993.

114. Rosenzweig, E.S. et al., Role of temporal summation in age-related long-term potentiation-induction deficits, *Hippocampus*, 7, 549, 1997.

115. Landfield, P.W., McGaugh, J.L., and Lynch, G., Impaired synaptic potentiation processes in the hippocampus of aged, memory-deficient rats, *Brain Res.*, 150, 85, 1978.

116. Norris, C.M., Korol, D.L., and Foster, T.C., Increased susceptibility to induction of long-term depression and long-term potentiation reversal during aging, *J. Neurosci.*, 16, 5382, 1996.

117. Kerr, D.S. et al., Corticosteroid modulation of hippocampal potentials: increased effect with aging, *Science*, 245, 1505, 1989.

118. Landfield, P.W. and Pitler, T.A., Prolonged Ca^{2+}-dependent afterhyperpolarizations in hippocampal neurons of aged rats, *Science*, 226, 1089, 1984.

119. Moyer, J.R., Jr. et al., Nimodipine increases excitability of rabbit CA1 pyramidal neurons in an age- and concentration-dependent manner, *J. Neurophysiol.*, 68, 2100, 1992.

120. Davare, M.A. and Hell, J.W., Increased phosphorylation of the neuronal L-type Ca(2+) channel Ca(v)1.2 during aging, *Proc. Natl. Acad. Sci. U.S.A.*, 100, 16018, 2003.

121. Thibault, O., Hadley, R., and Landfield, P.W., Elevated postsynaptic [Ca²⁺]i and L-type calcium channel activity in aged hippocampal neurons: relationship to impaired synaptic plasticity, *J. Neurosci.*, 21, 9744, 2001.

122. Sousa, N., Madeira, M.D., and Paula-Barbosa, M.M., Effects of corticosterone treatment and rehabilitation on the hippocampal formation of neonatal and adult rats. An unbiased stereological study, *Brain Res.*, 794, 199, 1998.

123. Sousa, N. et al., Maintenance of hippocampal cell numbers in young and aged rats submitted to chronic unpredictable stress. Comparison with the effects of corticosterone treatment, *Stress*, 2, 237, 1998.

124. Uno, H. et al., Hippocampal damage associated with prolonged and fatal stress in primates, *J. Neurosci.*, 9, 1705, 1989.

125. Coleman, P.D. and Flood, D.G., Neuron numbers and dendritic extent in normal aging and Alzheimer's disease, *Neurobiol. Aging*, 8, 521, 1987.

126. Sousa, R.J., Tannery, N.H., Lafer, E.M., *In situ* hybridization mapping of glucocorticoid receptor messenger ribonucleic acid in rat brain, *Mol. Endocrinol.*, 3, 481, 1989.

127. Van Eekelen, J.A. and De Kloet, E.R., Co-localization of brain corticosteroid receptors in the rat hippocampus, *Prog. Histochem. Cytochem.*, 26, 250, 1992.

128. Zhang, L. et al., Stress-induced change of mitochondria membrane potential regulated by genomic and non-genomic GR signaling: a possible mechanism for hippocampus atrophy in PTSD, *Med. Hypotheses*, 66, 1205, 2006.

129. Moutsatsou, P. et al., Localization of the glucocorticoid receptor in rat brain mitochondria, *Arch. Biochem. Biophys.*, 386, 69, 2001.

130. Crochemore, C. et al., Direct targeting of hippocampal neurons for apoptosis by glucocorticoids is reversible by mineralocorticoid receptor activation, *Mol. Psychiatry*, 10, 790, 2005.

131. West, M.J. and Gundersen, H.J., Unbiased stereological estimation of the number of neurons in the human hippocampus, *J. Comp. Neurol.*, 296, 1, 1990.

132. West, M.J., Regionally specific loss of neurons in the aging human hippocampus, *Neurobiol. Aging*, 14, 287, 1993.

133. Grieve, S.M. et al., Preservation of limbic and paralimbic structures in aging, *Hum. Brain Mapp.*, 25, 391, 2005.

134. Starkman, M.N. et al., Hippocampal formation volume, memory dysfunction, and cortisol levels in patients with Cushing's syndrome, *Biol. Psychiatry*, 32, 756, 1992.

135. Starkman, M.N. et al., Decrease in cortisol reverses human hippocampal atrophy following treatment of Cushing's disease, *Biol. Psychiatry*, 46, 1595, 1999.

136. Dagnino-Subiabre, A. et al., Chronic stress impairs acoustic conditioning more than visual conditioning in rats: morphological and behavioural evidence, *Neuroscience*, 135, 1067, 2005.

137. Radley, J.J. et al., Repeated stress induces dendritic spine loss in the rat medial prefrontal cortex, *Cereb. Cortex*, 16, 313, 2006.

138. Watanabe, Y., Gould, E., and McEwen, B.S., Stress induces atrophy of apical dendrites of hippocampal CA3 pyramidal neurons, *Brain Res.*, 588, 341, 1992.

139. Woolley, C., Gould, E., and McEwen, B.S., Exposure to excess glucocorticoids alters dendritic morphology of adult hippocampal pyramidal neurons, *Brain Res.*, 531, 225, 1990.

140. Wellman, C.L., Dendritic reorganization in pyramidal neurons in medial prefrontal cortex after chronic corticosterone administration, *J. Neurobiol.*, 49, 245, 2001.

141. Cerqueira, J.J. et al., Morphological correlates of corticosteroid-induced changes in prefrontal cortex-dependent behaviors, *J. Neurosci.*, 25, 7792, 2005.

142. Sapolsky, R.M. et al., Hippocampal damage associated with prolonged glucocorticoid exposure in primates, *J. Neurosci.*, 10, 2897, 1990.

143. Uno, H., et al., Neurotoxicity of glucocorticoids in the primate brain, *Horm. Behav.*, 28, 336, 1994.

144. Bentson, J. et al., Steroids and apparent cerebral atrophy on computed tomography scans, *J. Comput. Assist. Tomogr.*, 2, 16, 1978.

145. Smith, M.E., Bilateral hippocampal volume reduction in adults with post-traumatic stress disorder: a meta-analysis of structural MRI studies, *Hippocampus*, 15, 798, 2005.

146. Brambilla, P. et al. Anatomical MRI study of borderline personality disorder patients, *Psychiatry Res.*, 131, 125, 2004.

147. Hickie, I. et al., Reduced hippocampal volumes and memory loss in patients with early- and late-onset depression, *Br. J. Psychiatry*, 186, 197, 2005.

148. Vermetten, E., Schmahl, C., Lindner, S., Loewenstein, R.J., and Bremner, J.D., Hippocampal and amygdalar volumes in dissociative identity disorder. *Am. J. Psychiatry*, 163, 630, 2006.

149. Markham, J.A. et al., Sexually dimorphic aging of dendritic morphology in CA1 of hippocampus, *Hippocampus*, 15, 97, 2005.

150. Markham, J.A. and Juraska, J.M., Aging and sex influence the anatomy of the rat anterior cingulate cortex, *Neurobiol. Aging*, 23, 579, 2002.

151. Cowell, P.E., et al., Sex differences in aging of the human frontal and temporal lobes, *J. Neurosci.*, 14, 4748, 1994.

152. Raz, N. et al., Selective aging of the human cerebral cortex observed *in vivo:* differential vulnerability of the prefrontal gray matter, *Cereb. Cortex*, 7, 268, 1997.

153. Kaplan, M.S. and Hinds, J.W., Neurogenesis in the adult rat: electron microscopic analysis of light radioautographs, *Science*, 197, 1092, 1977.

154. Gould, E. et al., Adult-generated hippocampal and neocortical neurons in macaques have a transient existence, *Proc. Natl. Acad. Sci. U.S.A.*, 98, 10910, 2001.

155. Gould, E. et al., Neurogenesis in the neocortex of adult primates, *Science*, 286, 548, 1999.

156. Eriksson, P.S., Perfilieva, E., Bjork-Eriksson, T., Alborn, A.M., Nordborg, C., Peterson, D.A., and Gage, F.H., Neurogenesis in the adult human hippocampus, *Nat. Med.*, 1313, 1998.

157. Gould, E. et al., Neurogenesis in the dentate gyrus of the adult tree shrew is regulated by psychosocial stress and NMDA receptor activation, *J. Neurosci.*, 17, 2492, 1997.

158. Lledo, P.M., Alonso, M., and Grubb, M.S., Adult neurogenesis and functional plasticity in neuronal circuits, *Nat. Rev. Neurosci.*, 7, 179, 2006.

159. Tanapat, P., Galea, L.A., and Gould, E., Stress inhibits the proliferation of granule cell precursors in the developing dentate gyrus, *Int. J. Dev. Neurosci.*, 16, 235, 1998.

160. Mitra, R. et al., Social stress-related behavior affects hippocampal cell proliferation in mice, *Physiol. Behav.*, 89, 123, 2006.

161. Czeh, B. et al., Chronic psychosocial stress and concomitant repetitive transcranial magnetic stimulation: effects on stress hormone levels and adult hippocampal neurogenesis, *Biol. Psychiatry*, 52, 1057, 2002.

162. Dong, H. et al., Modulation of hippocampal cell proliferation, memory, and amyloid plaque deposition in APPsw (Tg2576) mutant mice by isolation stress, *Neuroscience*, 127, 601, 2004.

163. Lee, K.J. et al., Chronic mild stress decreases survival, but not proliferation, of newborn cells in adult rat hippocampus, *Exp. Mol. Med.*, 38, 44, 2006.

164. Wong, E.Y. and Herbert, J., Raised circulating corticosterone inhibits neuronal differentiation of progenitor cells in the adult hippocampus, *Neuroscience*, 137, 83, 2006.

165. Cameron, H.A. and Gould, E., Adult neurogenesis is regulated by adrenal steroids in the dentate gyrus, *Neuroscience*, 61, 203, 1994.

166. Lemaire, V. et al., Postnatal stimulation of the pups counteracts prenatal stress-induced deficits in hippocampal neurogenesis, *Biol. Psychiatry*, 59, 786, 2006.

167. Tanapat, P. et al., Exposure to fox odor inhibits cell proliferation in the hippocampus of adult rats via an adrenal hormone-dependent mechanism, *J. Comp. Neurol.*, 437, 496, 2001.

168. Seki, T. and Arai, Y., Age-related production of new granule cells in the adult dentate gyrus, *Neuroreport*, 6, 2479, 1995.

169. Kuhn, H.G., Dickinson-Anson, H., and Gage, F.H., Neurogenesis in the dentate gyrus of the adult rat: age-related decrease of neuronal progenitor proliferation, *J. Neurosci.*, 16, 2027, 1996.

170. Cameron, H.A. and McKay, R.D., Restoring production of hippocampal neurons in old age, *Nat. Neurosci.*, 2, 894, 1999.

171. Montaron, M.F. et al., Lifelong corticosterone level determines age-related decline in neurogenesis and memory, *Neurobiol. Aging*, 27, 645, 2006.

172. Garcia, A. et al.,. Age-dependent expression of glucocorticoid- and mineralocorticoid receptors on neural precursor cell populations in the adult murine hippocampus, *Aging Cell*, 3, 363, 2004.

173. Simon, M., Czeh, B., and Fuchs, E., Age-dependent susceptibility of adult hippocampal cell proliferation to chronic psychosocial stress, *Brain Res.*, 1049, 244, 2005.

174. Brunson, K.L., Baram, T. Z., and Bender, R.A., Hippocampal neurogenesis is not enhanced by lifelong reduction of glucocorticoid levels, *Hippocampus*, 15, 491, 2005.

14 Altered Calcium Homeostasis in Old Neurons

Emil C. Toescu

CONTENTS

I.   Ca^{2+} HYPOTHESIS OF AGING

It is now more than two decades since the first proposal of a "Ca^{2+} hypothesis of aging" [1]. In its mature formulation, the hypothesis aimed to provide a working hypothesis for explaining not only the aging process but also Alzheimer's disease (AD). Drawing on many neurophysiological processes and mechanisms, the hypothesis contained six interrelated key elements [2], providing an extremely wide explanatory blanket. The exposition of these elements is worth repeating not only for historical reasons and to illustrate the breath of the proposal, but also because it still represents the source of some misunderstandings.

The first element of Khachaturian's construct was simply that the cellular mechanisms that participate in Ca^{2+} homeostasis also play an important role in the process of aging and neurodegeneration. Consequently, altered Ca^{2+} homeostasis can account for a number of age-related changes associated with either aging or AD. The second element was that normal aging and the process of neurodegeneration, as in AD, must be seen as part of a continuum of processes associated with development and restructuring of the nervous system throughout life. Thus, the morphological changes in AD, such as dendritic pruning and loss of synapses and neurons, involve the same mechanisms that are responsible for neuroplasticity in the developing or mature brain. As an extension of the previous point, the third element of the hypothesis concentrated on the plasticity of the nervous system architecture seen, at any time point, as a balance between growth/regeneration and decaying/degeneration processes. In many of these processes the intracellular Ca^{2+} ($[Ca^{2+}]_i$) plays a crucial role and, from this perspective, the neuronal dysfunction of the aged or the AD brain results from an imbalance between the two types of opposing processes, an imbalance that can result from a breakdown of the homeostatic mechanisms regulating $[Ca^{2+}]_i$. The next, rather contentious element dealt with the temporal dimension of the aging/neurodegenerative processes and proposed that the functional product of the perturbation in $[Ca^{2+}]_i$ homeostasis and time is a constant. Thus, small changes in $[Ca^{2+}]_i$ (as those resulting, for example, from a less efficient Ca^{2+} extrusion pump, or an enhanced Ca^{2+} channel activity) exerted over a long period of time would have the same functional or morphological effects as a massive, but acute insult. It is clear now that the actions of Ca^{2+} in different temporal domains (i.e., over milliseconds, seconds, minutes, or days) generate very different types of responses and functional outcomes. A fifth element took into account the cellular effects of Ca^{2+} signaling and proposed that Ca^{2+}-mediated processes are an important part of the final common pathway that leads to neuronal dysfunction and cell death. The model presented at this point an extremely broad and flexible perspective, and almost any element along the path leading from the triggers of Ca^{2+} dysregulation to various Ca^{2+} homeostatic mechanisms to, eventually, any of the Ca^{2+}-dependent processes could fit the bill of explaining the involvement of Ca^{2+} in the process of aging and neurodegeneration. This point was even further expanded by the sixth element, which proposed that both the age-related and the AD-associated changes are not single factorial events but could be initiated by a wide variety of instances, acting single or in combination, simultaneous or sequentially, over a long period of time.

Underlying this hypothesis were two powerful ideas that reflected the predominant views of the time. One was that the difference between aging and neurodegeneration is just a matter of degree, both existing along a continuous path. The other idea was that intracellular Ca^{2+} signaling is one of the most important transducing processes involved in a wide range of cellular processes [3, 4]. Linking the two was the concept of Ca^{2+} regulation of neuronal death through the process of excitotoxicity. The term "excitotoxicity" was first coined by Olney in 1970 to describe the excessive activation of glutamate receptors that follows neuronal deprivation of oxygen and/or nutrients and resulting in neuronal death [5]. The subsequent demonstration in 1987 of the involvement of Ca^{2+} in mediating the excitotoxic outcome [6] strengthened the "Ca^{2+} hypothesis of aging."

Today, of the two central ideas discussed above, only the latter remains unchallenged; the issue of understanding the aging as a neurodegenerative process is very much disputed. From animal studies it is clear that the age-related changes in functional and biochemical characteristics of the cortical circuitry that might underlie the moderate cognitive decline do not involve frank neuronal death but a significant amount of synaptic restructuring [7]. Some of the reasons why, from the late 1960s to the mid-to-late 1980s the dogma of aging centered on the idea of associated significant neuronal loss were technological (the modern unbiased, dissector method for counting neurons was introduced only in 1984 [8] and helped demonstrate significant differences between neuronal numbers in normal aging and in neurodegenerative diseases [9]; see also Chapter 4) and methodological, involving the possible inclusion in some studies of material coming from subjects already affected by neurodegenerative diseases, (cf. [10]). Thus, in its initial formulation that links dysregulation of Ca^{2+} homeostasis to neuronal loss, the "Ca^{2+} hypothesis" is not directly applicable anymore to the process of normal aging, but retains much of its explanatory power in the context of Alzheimer's disease (see [11] for a recent review). What is undisputed, however, is the fact that intracellular Ca^{2+} signaling and its regulation are central to neuronal physiology, linking with a variety of other processes (Figure 14.1).

II. Ca^{2+} HOMEOSTASIS

A. Ca^{2+} ENTRY AND Ca^{2+} EXTRUSION PATHWAYS

At any time point, the values of intracellular free Ca^{2+}, as measured routinely by Ca^{2+}-sensitive fluorescent dyes with different affinities, represent the functional balance between processes that increase and those that decrease $[Ca^{2+}]_i$ (Figure 14.2). Neuronal activation usually is associated with increases in $[Ca^{2+}]_i$. For neurons, the source for these activation-induced Ca^{2+} responses is the extracellular medium, with Ca^{2+} ions flowing along a very steep (10,000-fold) concentration gradient (at rest $[Ca]_i$ is around 50 to 100 nM, whereas the extracellular Ca^{2+} is around 1.5 to 2 mM). This process involves a number of different types of ion channels; some are activated by the depolarization of the plasma membrane and have exclusive selectivity for Ca^{2+} ions (the voltage-operated Ca^{2+} channels, VOCCs). These channels exist as several types and are functionally divided into two categories: (1) the low voltage-activated (LVA) channels (prototype, the former T-type VOCC and current Cav3 family — for new VOCC nomenclature, see [12]), activated by smaller depolarizations of the plasma membrane; and (2) the high voltage-activated (HVA) channels. Of these HVAs, the best known functionally is the L-type Ca^{2+} channel (current Cav1 family), but the family also comprises the N-, P-, Q-, and R-types (all part of the Cav2 family) [13]. Additional types of channels involved in generating Ca^{2+} signals in neuronal cytosol are the ones activated by specific ligands (ligand operated Ca^{2+} channels, LOCs), such as NMDA, AMPA (or, in vivo, glutamate) or ATP (purinergic P2X receptors). These are nonspecific cationic channels, with a Ca^{2+} permeability that is usually lower than that for Na^+ (the latter ion having, nevertheless, a much lower electrochemical gradient). Another type of neuronal plasma

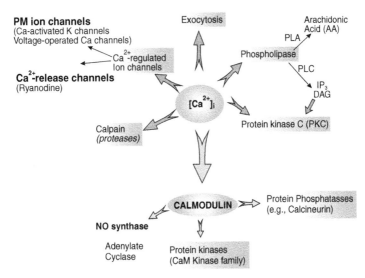

FIGURE 14.1 (SEE COLOR INSERT FOLLOWING PAGE 204) Scope of Ca^{2+} signaling. The figure illustrates some of the main targets of Ca^{2+} signaling, through which Ca^{2+} exerts its huge range of functional effects on cellular (neuronal) physiology [168]. For some of these interactions, Ca^{2+} has a direct interaction with the targets, whereas for many other function, calmodulin, the classical Ca^{2+} binding protein, is a mediator, so that the Ca^{2+}-calmodulin complex becomes the target activator [169]. Such targets, regulating a plethora of downstream physiological responses, include nitric oxide synthase (NOS [170]), adenylate cyclase [171], the family of CaM kinases [172], and the important family of Ca^{2+}-dependent protein phosphatases, such as calcineurin [173]. Of the direct targets, Ca^{2+} is an essential regulator of the exocytotic process [174]. Ca^{2+} also is an important regulator of a variety of channels, either on the plasma membrane, such as the VOCCs [175] and the Ca^{2+}-dependent K^+ channels [176], or on the ER membrane, such as the rynanodine receptor/channel [16, 177]. Through the activation of the PLA2 [178], Ca^{2+} regulates the generation of arachidonic acid and the prostaglandins signaling pathways. Finally, through the binding and activation of a series of proteases (e.g., calpain), Ca^{2+} is an important regulator and executioner of neuronal death [179].

membrane channel with Ca^{2+} permeability is represented by the second messenger-operated Ca^{2+} channels (SMOCs), with cyclic nucleotides or arachidonate as activators. Finally, a ubiquitous and ever-expanding family of nonselective plasma membrane channels is that of the transient receptor potential (TRP) channels, initially described during the study of the photoreceptor transduction process.

Recovery of resting $[Ca]_i$ values following such activation-evoked Ca^{2+} signals, which can generate increases of $[Ca]_i$ well in excess of 10 μM, taking into account the confined small volumes where these signals appear (synaptic boutons, dendritic spines), is an energy-dependent process involving either pumps (ATPases) or specific transporters. The pumps remove cytosolic Ca^{2+} either to the extracellular medium (the plasma membrane Ca^{2+} ATPase, PMCA) or into the endoplasmic reticulum, which is a very important Ca^{2+} storing organelle (through the sarco(endo)plasmic Ca^{2+} ATPase, SERCA). A specific transporter is the Na^+/Ca^{2+} exchanger (NCX), which harnesses the electrochemical gradient of Na^+. These transport systems have different thresholds for activity. While the pumps have lower transport rates, they have a higher affinity for Ca^{2+} and thus are able to respond to smaller changes in $[Ca]_i$ and ultimately to set the basal Ca^{2+} levels.

B.   INTRACELLULAR ORGANELLES

Many intracellular organelles participate in Ca^{2+} homeostasis and, as discussed in more detail below, another important mechanism for removal of cytosolic Ca^{2+} is the Ca^{2+} uniporter of the mitochondria. This system has a huge transport capacity (depending on conditions, mitochondria can accumulate millimolar Ca^{2+}) with an optimal affinity in the micromolar range, levels easily reached at the peak of Ca^{2+} responses during activation. The system is also able, in a sub-mode of action or through a separate uptake system (the rapid uptake mode, RaM), to take up cytosolic Ca^{2+} following smaller, submicromolar $[Ca]_i$ increases [14].

Endoplasmic reticulum (ER) is a multifunctional organelle, intimately involved in Ca^{2+} homeostasis, acting both as a direct source of Ca^{2+} signaling (e.g., metabotropic glutamate stimulation, mediating release of Ca^{2+} from the ER through the generation of $InsP_3$ and activation of the specific $InsP_3$ receptors) or as an important amplifier of the Ca^{2+} signal generated at the plasma membrane, through the process commonly known as the Ca^{2+}-induced Ca^{2+} release (CICR) [15]. As mentioned above, through the action of the SERCA pumps, the ER also can participate in the recovery of the resting $[Ca^{2+}]_i$ values following neuronal activation. While this role of the ER is very well established in nonexcitable cells and in some neurons of the peripheral nervous system, its participation in the intense Ca^{2+} signaling of central nervous system neurons is more restricted [16]. Irrespective of the cell type under consideration, the ER is always the site of protein synthesis and maturation, and many of these processes are controlled by proteins sensitive to Ca^{2+} [17].

C. CA^{2+} BUFFERS

All the mechanisms briefly described above involve transporting proteins, embedded in membranes, which are able to bind Ca^{2+} with various affinities and mediate the transmembrane movement of ions. Another set of proteins with an important role in cellular Ca^{2+} homeostasis is known under the general name of Ca^{2+}-binding proteins (CaBP). Many of these proteins are soluble, and this higher degree of mobility allows them to interact with Ca^{2+} with different affinities at various locations, and consequently shape the Ca^{2+} signal (either by transporting Ca^{2+} away from or by significant Ca^{2+} buffering at the site of generation). One of the largest families of CaBP is characterized by the EF-hand Ca^{2+}-binding domain, consisting of two perpendicular 10- to 12-residue, alpha-helix regions separated by a 12-residue loop region; EF-hand domains are often found in single or multiple pairs, giving rise to a huge variety of structural/functional variations in the proteins that form a family comprising more than 600 members [18]. The CaBP are divided into two functional, well-established categories. One, having calmodulin as the reference member, acts as a Ca^{2+} sensing mechanism that translates graded changes in $[Ca^{2+}]_i$ that follow cell stimulation into a graded response initiated by the binding of these CaBP to various Ca^{2+}-sensitive target enzymes. Within this category, a group of proteins, called the neuronal calcium-sensor (NCS) proteins, has recently acquired prominence due to the relatively specific localization and/or set of functions they perform [19]. One of these proteins, calsenilin, could be very relevant to the processes of neurodegeneration because, among other things, it can modify the processing of presenilins and regulate the processing of the amyloid precursor protein (APP), both intimately involved in the pathophysiological processes of Alzheimer's disease [20].

The other functional category, represented by proteins such as parvalbumin, calbindin, and calretinin (PB, CB, and CR, respectively), is that of the Ca^{2+} buffers. These proteins are widely expressed in the central nervous system, less in principal neurons, and more in the inhibitory GABAergic interneurons, each type being characterized by a predominant form of CaBP, and associated with a specific

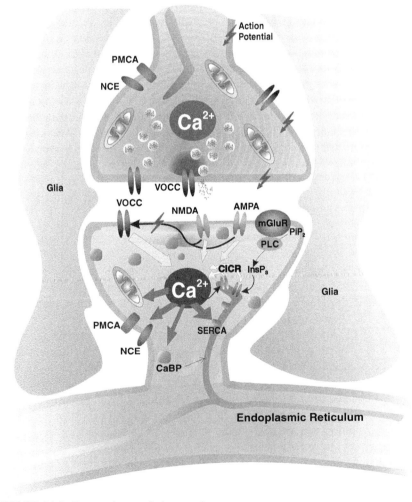

FIGURE 14.2 (See caption on facing page)

constellation of associated neurotransmitters, cell surface markers, and receptors [21]. Furthermore, experimental data and theoretical modeling, coupled with infor-mation on the biochemical properties of these CaBP buffers, show that they could exert profound effects on neuronal activity, from shaping the Ca^{2+} signal at local levels in the presynaptic active zone or postsynaptic densities, thus initiating the transfer of information in the neuronal networks [22] to modulate neuronal vulner-ability. Many studies have shown the neuroprotective effects of CaBP. For example, in hippocampal primary cultures, neurons expressing CB are more effective at recovering $[Ca^{2+}]_i$ levels after stimulation [23]; whereas for cortical neurons, expres-sion of CR appears to play this protective role [24]. Calbindin can protect neurons from both oxidative stress and reduce apoptosis [25]. Significantly more motor neurons survived a standard severe peripheral injury in parvalbumin-overexpressing transgenic mice than in control, wild-type littermates [26].

At the other end of the functional spectrum, the distribution and types of intra-cellular Ca^{2+} buffers can affect significantly the electrical activity of neurons. For example, a strong correlation has been found between the expression of parvalbumin and the firing pattern of neurons: the PV-positive GABAergic interneurons are capable of maintaining a higher rate of repetitive activity, an observation explained by the fact that PV is a "slow" Ca^{2+} buffer and thus able to decrease more effectively the $[Ca^{2+}]_i$ during higher frequency discharges [27]. Overall, it is important to mention in this discussion that a more general parameter, the Ca^{2+}-binding ratio (Ks), is used to measure and compare the overall capacity of various cells to buffer Ca^{2+}, independent of the type of Ca^{2+} buffer proteins involved. Experimental

FIGURE 14.2 (SEE COLOR INSERT FOLLOWING PAGE 204) Diagrammatic presenta-tion of the roles of Ca^{2+} in the synaptic transmission of information. At the presynaptic site, the major pathway of Ca^{2+} increase is the activation of the VOCCs that follows the depolar-ization of the presynaptic bouton by incoming action potentials. The entry of Ca^{2+} from the extracellular medium (either intra- or para-synaptic) activates the exocytotic process [174], with consequent release of neurotransmitters in the synaptic cleft. The entry of Ca^{2+} at the postsynaptic density is mediated by a wider range of channels: either the VOCCs (particularly the Cav1.2. and 1.3 L-type [13, 180]) or the glutamatergic ionotropic channels with Ca^{2+} permeability (NMDA- and AMPA-type). It is well established that the postsynaptic types of Ca^{2+}-permeable channels are integrated in elaborated protein complexes, with important signaling function, generating the so-called "signalosomes" [181, 182]. In addition, a Ca^{2+} signal with important modulator functions can be generated through the activation of the metabotropic glutamate receptors (mGluR) [183], which can trigger an $InsP_3$-mediated Ca^{2+} response [181]. Either this release of Ca^{2+} from the intracellular stores or the entry of Ca^{2+} from the extracellular medium can by amplified by the process of Ca^{2+}-induced Ca^{2+} release (CICR) [15]. The initial increase in $[Ca^{2+}]_i$ is immediately buffered by the soluble Ca^{2+}-binding proteins (CaBP). During the recovery phase, the free Ca^{2+} is either taken up by the mitochon-dria or into the ER, through the activity of the sarco(endo)plasmic reticulum Ca^{2+} ATPase (SERCA). The majority of the Ca^{2+} is extruded to the extracellular medium, through the activity of the plasma membrane Ca^{2+}ATPase (PMCA) or the operation of a membrane Na^+/Ca^{2+} exchanger (NCE). For a more "realistic" representation, the glial component of the synaptic complex also is shown, because glia act as an important sheath, with morphological, functional, and metabolic functions [184].

measurements of this important parameter show significant heterogeneity between different neuronal types — in hippocampus, the inhibitory interneurons have a two to three times larger buffering power (i.e., higher Ks) than the excitatory interneurons, and thus are able to withstand larger Ca^{2+} challenges [28]. In the spinal cord, the Ks of motor neurons is only about 50 (indicating that 1 in 50 Ca^{2+} ions entering the cells or 2% of the Ca^{2+} challenge remains free, unbound by the cytosolic buffers) [29], whereas the Ks of the sympathetic superior cervical ganglia (SCG) varies between 250 and 500, depending on the value of $[Ca^{2+}]_i$ at a given time [30]. Interestingly, the value of Ks appears to be developmentally regulated [31].

III. EFFECTS OF AGING ON Ca^{2+} HOMEOSTATIC SYSTEMS

There are relatively few direct experimental data analyzing and describing the putative age-related changes of the various Ca^{2+} homeostatic mechanisms. Overall, they tend to show dysfunction but, as discussed at length elsewhere, the interpretation is rendered difficult by the use of a variety of cellular preparations and by the heterogeneity of neuronal composition and ratio of glia to neurons in various regions of the brain [32].

A.   AGE-DEPENDENT EFFECTS ON CA^{2+} ENTRY PATHWAYS

The age-dependent changes in the activity of various Ca^{2+} entry systems illustrate the problems in interpretation. Some of the complications are intrinsic to the model; there are several pathways allowing Ca^{2+} entry, each of them composed of various subunits with different Ca^{2+} permeabilities and regulating different sets of neuronal activities and functions. The other source of complication is the regional heterogeneity.

1. Ca^{2+} Channels

With respect to the effect of aging on the voltage-operated Ca^{2+} channels, two regions have been studied more intensely: (1) the hippocampus, in particular the pyramidal neurons of CA1 region; and (2) the cortical neurons of the basal forebrain.

In the hippocampus, one of the most consistent findings is that of an age-dependent increase in Ca^{2+}-dependent afterhyperpolarization (AHP) [33–35], due to a demonstrated increase in the number of L-type VOCCs [34–36]. A somewhat similar conclusion was reached for the neurons of the basal forebrain, although the mechanisms mediating an increased Ca^{2+} load within aging appear different. In these latter neurons, the two large families of VOCCs — that is, the LVA and HVA — appear to respond differently to aging. While the LVA show an increased current density (i.e., larger current values per unit of surface area) with similar activation/inactivation kinetics [37], the HVA show the opposite — the same current density but with decreased inactivation [38]. While most of this electrophysiological evidence would indicate that in the CNS, aging might be associated with an increase in Ca^{2+} uptake through VOCCs, once again the peripheral neurons seem different; and for the dorsal root ganglia neurons, both LVA and HVA currents are decreased by aging [39]. Other lines of evidence, based on older biochemical studies, suggest an opposite functional outcome. An assessment of the binding sites for a typical, very specific VOCC antagonist (i.e., dihyropiridine) showed an age-dependent decrease in the binding affinity and sensitivity [40]. Work on another type of nervous system preparation, synaptosomes, also showed conflicting results in response to depolarization (the assumption being that depolarization by KCl will activate the VOCC present in the nerve terminals); some reported an increased Ca^{2+} uptake [41], whereas others showed an inhibition [42] or no effect [43]. Expanding the panoply of methods used for assessing the effects of aging on VOCC, one study [44] looked at the age-dependent changes in the α subunit composition of the VOCCs, using the cerebellum as a study model (for which, however, not much electrophysiology of the aging brain exists) and showed a consistent decrease in the $α_D$ subunit (encoding the L-type VOCC) in the Purkinje neurons. While the details of such investigations appear rather confusing, in general it appears that there is no unique effect of aging on VOCCs; and that for each type of VOCC, conclusions need to be drawn by direct experimentation on multiple neuronal types.

2.   Glutamate-Operated Channels

The other path of Ca^{2+} entry during neuronal activation is through one or another of the various ionotropic glutamatergic receptor/channels; both the NMDA and AMPA receptors have a sizable Ca^{2+} permeability [45]. The main receptor subunit of the NMDA receptor is the NR1 subunit, which has three alternative splicing regions [46] and its presence is required in all expressed NMDA receptors, as being essential in establishing the functional homo- or heteromeric complexes [47]. Two other subunits have been described: (1) the NR2 (A-D forms) and (2) the NR3 (A and B) [46]. The NMDA receptors also have a special set of properties that give the receptor important functional characteristics at rest; the NMDA channel pore is blocked in a voltage-dependent manner by Mg^+ ions [48]. This block is relieved by depolarization, but this induces a slight delay in the activation of the channel, generating a slower kinetic response [48]. There is an overwhelming body of evidence implicating the NMDA receptors in two functions that are affected by the aging process: (1) synaptic plasticity and memory, particularly in the hippocampus, and (2) excitotoxicity phenomena across the CNS. The overall view of the literature describing the changes in NMDA activity with aging is that of a decrease in effectiveness of NMDA signaling. As reviewed by Magnusson [49], the majority of studies have found an age-related decline in the number of NMDA receptor sites (as measured by a reduced B_{max} value), associated, in some of these studies, with no change in the affinity of the receptor for glutamate. In addition, the subunit composition of the expressed NMDA receptors appears to have an important developmental component. At embryonic stages, the NR2B subunit is present across the brain, with NR2D present only in the diencephalon and brain stem. After birth, the mRNA for NR2A becomes evident and prominent and, in the specific case of the cerebellum, prenatal expression of NR2B on the granule cell is changed to the NR2C subunit type [50]. At the other extreme of the lifespan, a decrease in the expression of the NR2B mRNA and protein has been reported as an age-related phenomenon, while the expression of NR2A was not affected [51]. These data are corroborated by electrophysiological evidence for an age-related decrease in NMDA responsive-ness in neostriatal slices of both aged rats (24 months old) and cats (16 years old) [52]. Others, however, have reported that the age-related decrease in the overall NMDA-mediated response is due to a reduction in the input to the NMDA receptor, rather than to the change in the electrophysiological NMDA response (rat CA1 region of the hippocampus, [53]). Experiments using short-term cell cultures derived from aged rats (25 to 26 months old) showed increased NMDA peak current when compared to middle-aged (9 to 10 months old) animals, associated with an increased Ca^{2+} signal [54]. Probably quite relevant in the attempt to systematize the results in the literature, in this last study, the NMDA response in the aged animals was larger than the one obtained in the middle-aged, but dramatically smaller (both NMDA and Ca^{2+} signal) than the signal recorded from cells derived from embryonic tissues [54].

AMPA receptor channels exist as homo- or, more common in their native form, as heteromers of the four possible subunits GluR1-GluR4 (or GluR-A to GluR-D). The AMPA channels are cation selective and are mainly permeable to the monovalent ions Na^+ and K^+. The permeability to Ca^{2+} depends on the inclusion and properties of the GluR2 subunit in the channel structure, such that AMPA-Rs assembled from combinations of GluR1, GluR2, and/or GluR4 are permeable to Ca^{2+} (and Zn^{2+}) and show a voltage-dependent block by intracellular polyamines [55]. The permeability properties of the GluR2 subunit have been traced to a single amino acid residue located in the pore-forming domain [56]. A positively charged arginine residue at this position prevents Ca^{2+} passage, whereas the presence of the neutral amino acid residue glutamine results in significant Ca^{2+} permeability [57]. Arginine is not encoded by the GluR2 genomic DNA and is introduced at this site by subsequent RNA editing, which in adult brains is very efficient [58]. As a result, the majority of AMPA receptors in the CNS have a low Ca^{2+} permeability, although some neurons displaying AMPA receptors with high Ca^{2+} permeability were reported in both the hippocampus [59] and neocortex [60]. AMPA binding does not appear to show significant changes with aging [61], although in many regions there are possible subtler age-associated changes, as shown for C57Bl/6 mice [62]. Despite this seem-ingly minor effect of age on AMPA binding, there are several brain regions for which a significant correlation between cognitive tests and AMPA binding densities was reported [63]. The lack of significant effect of aging on AMPA binding is consistent with the electrophysiological studies of the AMPA response showing no age-related changes in either the mean quantal sizes or the unitary synaptic response [64]. Another important issue, with relevance for $[Ca^{2+}]_i$ homeostasis, is that of the effect of age on GluR2 expression. The efficiency and fidelity of the RNA editing process-ing, ultimately conferring the Ca^{2+} resistance, is well conserved with aging in all the major regions of the brain [65]. In one of the few studies that analyzed specifically the distribution of GluR2 in the aged brain, analyzing primarily the short and long corticocortical projections, a notable downregulation in the expression of GluR2, as well as NMDA-R1, was demonstrated [66].

B. AGE-DEPENDENT EFFECTS ON CA²⁺ EXTRUSION PATHWAYS

A number of studies have indicated that both the activity and the expression levels of the PMCA in synaptosomal preparations are significantly reduced as a function of aging both in the Fisher-344 and in the longer-lived Fisher344/BNF1 rats [67, 68]. The functional decrease in activity could be explained by the inhibitory effects of free radicals (reactive oxygen species, ROS) on the PMCA, either as a direct effect on the pump activity [69] or on calmodulin, the essential CaBP that activates, in its Ca^{2+}-bound form, the PMCA [70]. Nevertheless, other studies using peripheral neurons (rat adrenergic neurons from the superior cervical ganglia) showed PMCA activity maintained with age and even a capacity to upregulate function (in conjunction with the other extrusion system — the Na^+/Ca^{2+} exchanger) in order to meet higher extrusion demands [71]. This probably is an important feature, because the PMCA has been reported as the major Ca^{2+} clearing system in this neuronal cell type [30]. In these types of neurons, it was the SERCA pumps, which mediate the re-uptake of Ca^{2+} into the endoplasmic reticulum, that appear to be affected by the process of aging, as shown in experiments using either specific SERCA inhibitors (e.g., thapsigargin) or inhibitors of other extrusion pathways, thus isolating the SERCA activity for inspection [72]. It is interesting to note that it is in these peripheral neurons that the intracellular Ca^{2+} stores, such as the ER, appear to play a more important role in Ca^{2+} homeostasis [16].

C. AGE-DEPENDENT EFFECTS ON CA²⁺ BUFFERS

Immunocytochemical determinations of calbindin (CB) and parvalbumin (PV) expression in animal models showed that age decreases the number of CB-positive neurons in the rabbit hippocampus without affecting the PV-positive neurons, although for the latter CaBP there were some subtler differences in subcellular distribution, with a proposed decrease in PV expression in the neurites [73]. A similar picture came from studies of human cortex, which showed a consistent trend for age-related decreases in the calbindin- and calretinin (CR)-positive neurons that attained a level of statistical significance only in few regions, while no change was recorded for parvalbumin (PV)-positive neurons [74]. These studies expanded on the previous one from the same group that showed a dramatic 60% loss of CB from the basal forebrain cholinergic neurons (BFCN) [75]. It is entirely possible, however, that the changes in CaBP expression are region specific and influenced by levels of activity. Thus, when assessing the number of PV- and CB-expressing neurons in the dorsal cochlear nucleus of mice, an age-related increase has been reported [76] This was consistent with the observation that excessive stimulation of neurons in the cochlear nucleus by noise exposure resulted in increased expression of the CaBP [77]. Similarly in human specimens, it was found that the number of CB-positive neurons in the temporal cortex increased with age, in contrast to the situation for the AD-afflicted specimens [78].

Functionally, intracellular Ca^{2+} buffering was reported to decline with aging in adrenergic nerves [79], based on the observation that norepinephrine release increased with age and that this effect was reversed by an increase of intracellular

Ca^{2+} buffering (with BAPTA-AM). Yet again, as for many others Ca^{2+} homeostasis parameters, the effect of aging on Ca^{2+} buffering is not simple, and other groups have described an increased Ca^{2+} buffering with aging, as in the case of the basal forebrain neurons [80]. When discussing Ca^{2+} buffering and the effects of this parameter on the values of $[Ca^{2+}]_i$, one should take into account not only the specific proteins that bind Ca^{2+}, the CaBPs discussed above, but also the participation of the internal organelles (e.g., the endoplasmic reticulum and mitochondria) with a Ca^{2+} uptake potential in shaping the Ca^{2+} signal. Thus, in assessing the dynamics of the $[Ca^{2+}]_i$ increase following stimulation (i.e., the shape of the Ca^{2+} signal), two phases normally are described — a rapid phase that limits the amplitude of the $[Ca^{2+}]_i$ response, followed by a second, slower phase that involves the Ca^{2+} extrusion systems, either Ca^{2+} removal or Ca^{2+} uptake into the intracellular compartments [81]. If the stimulus persists, then during this second phase, a new steady state (the Ca^{2+} plateau) is achieved, reflecting the balance between Ca^{2+} entry and Ca^{2+} removal from the cytosol. If the stimulation ceases, then this second, slower phase reflects the process of recovery of the resting $[Ca^{2+}]_i$ values. The surprising observation in the case of the basal forebrain neurons is that the reported increased Ca^{2+} buffering is manifest only during the rapid phase, and is not determined by changes in the function of either ER or the mitochondrial fraction (the latter being, in fact, reduced in the aged neurons [82]) and takes place in neurons with a decreased expression of CaBP [83].

D.   EFFECTS OF AGING ON INTRACELLULAR CA^{2+} COMPARTMENTS

1.   Endoplasmic Reticulum

The endoplasmic reticulum (ER) is an important intracellular Ca^{2+} store and, depending on its refill status, can act either as a "Ca^{2+} sink," buffering through SERCA pump-mediated Ca^{2+} reuptake into the ER, or as a "Ca^{2+} source," through a process that involves Ca^{2+}-induced Ca^{2+} release (CICR; [15]). When discussing the role of ER Ca^{2+} stores in neuronal physiology, a number of issues must be addressed, including:

- The morphology of the ER and its distribution is not uniform throughout the neuron. It is particularly patchy in the dendritic territory and is influenced by the morphology of the spine and the age of the preparation [84]. Thus, in adult animals, less than 25% of the thin spines contain SER, whereas almost 90% of the larger mushroom spines have SER. When all types of spines are analyzed, SER is present only in 50% of the spines (slightly more in the young preparations: 58% in immature brains vs. 48% in the adult spines). The important implication of these observations is that in about half of the spines, where synaptic activity presumably is still taking place, the entry of Ca^{2+} is buffered through mechanisms that do not involve ER Ca^{2+} reuptake. Where present, however, the ER is ideally adapted for Ca^{2+} uptake as its surface-to-ratio area is very large, with the

SER occupying only about 3% of the volume but up to 40% of the surface of the spine territory.

- In addressing the issue of the participation of the CICR in the control and modulation of the Ca^{2+} synaptic response, there appear to be differences between the various types of CNS neurons, particularly the cerebellar Purkinje neurons and the hippocampal pyramidal neurons, in respect to the mechanisms of release of Ca^{2+} from intracellular ER stores. In Purkinje neurons, the main ER Ca^{2+} release pathway is the InsP$_3$ receptor. As demonstrated in 1998 by two independent, but almost simultaneous, studies [85, 86], parallel fiber stimulation activates postsynaptically, even in the absence of membrane depolarization, a Ca^{2+} signal mediated by the activation of the mGluR1 receptors and which is able to trigger LTD. For the hippocampal neurons, the picture is more complex. For a start, the distribution of the Ca^{2+} release channels on the ER varies with the localization for the CA1 neurons; there are no InsP$_3$ receptors, only RynR, in the spines, whereas in the dendritic shaft both receptors are present [87]. Furthermore, whereas some studies asserted a significant role for the Ca^{2+}-induced Ca^{2+} release (CICR) process in postsynaptic Ca^{2+} signaling [88], others failed to detect a significant contribution [89].

- Intracellular Ca^{2+} stores can serve as "sinks" or "sources," and the role played by the ER Ca^{2+} stores depends to a significant degree on their filling status. It was shown in earlier studies that Ca^{2+} responses that involve mobilization from intracellular stores were significantly enhanced by depolarization protocols that allowed their filling [90, 91], indicating that the stores are functionally deplete and require constant uptake, and that the ER can play a dominant role as a Ca^{2+} buffering organelle following a Ca^{2+} challenge, acting on a much longer time-scale than the mitochondria [92]. This action explains why inhibition of the ER Ca^{2+} reuptake system can result in amplification of the Ca^{2+} signals [93].

Information about age-related changes in the function and activity of the ER Ca^{2+} stores is rather limited, with an overall view that the size of the caffeine-releasable ER Ca^{2+} store is reduced by aging, as shown both in granule neurons of the cerebellar slices [94] and in aged acutely dissociated basal forebrain neurons [80], but not in cultured hippocampal neurons [95]. There are several mechanisms that can explain a decrease in the size of the caffeine-sensitive Ca^{2+} stores, including a decreased efficiency of the reuptake mechanisms through the SERCA pumps or an increased Ca^{2+} leakage. When investigated directly, in acutely dissociated basal forebrain neurons, aging did not affect the rate of spontaneous depletion (i.e., leakage) but decreased the efficiency of the ER loading [96]. In contrast, in long-term (30 days *in vitro*) cultured hippocampal neurons, glutamate stimulation activated a sustained Ca^{2+} response that was inhibited by rynanodine, a blocker of CICR, thus indicating an increased ER Ca^{2+} leak [95]. It is not clear yet if this increased Ca^{2+} leak, in effect a sustained CICR, was due to an alteration in the function of the rynanodine receptors or was related to a possible coupling between the L-type VOCCs and the rynanodine Ca^{2+}-release channels [97], similar to the coupling between these types of Ca^{2+} channels in the muscle and which is known to be affected by the aging process [98]. An interesting observation on the role of intracellular Ca^{2+} stores in alterations in the normal Ca^{2+} homeostasis in the aged neurons has been recently reported with respect to the process of hippocampal LTP induction. Release of Ca^{2+} from the intracellular stores is an important participant in LTP induction for ranges of stimulation near the threshold of induction [99, 100]; but in the aged slices, inhibition of the Ca^{2+} release from the stores by either SERCA inhibitors or by rynanodine activated, rather than inhibited, LTP [101]. The explanation proposed for this paradoxical effect takes into account another well-established effect of Ca^{2+} in the aged neurons: activation of a slow afterhyperpolarization (AHP) current [102, 103], which in turn will affect the level of synaptic depolarization required for NMDA receptor and consequent LTP induction. The fact that aging is associated with a decline in LTP and synaptic plasticity [104, 105] might indicate an increase with age of the functional release of Ca^{2+} from the intracellular stores in these hippocampal neurons.

This area of discussion, the regulation of ER Ca^{2+} stores, is probably the most important one for appreciating the functional differences between normal physiological aging and the process of neurodegeneration, particularly AD, for which significant alterations in the ER Ca^{2+} handling were described [11]. Both bulwarks of pathology in AD (i.e., the $A\beta$ protein fragments and the presenilins) are associated with or induce alterations in Ca^{2+} homeostasis [106, 107], although is not yet clear whether the changes in Ca^{2+} homeostasis precede the protein alterations in AD or vice versa [108]. One of the best-established mechanisms through which $A\beta$ affects $[Ca^{2+}]_i$ regulation is by the formation by the $A\beta$ fragment of a cation-selective ion channel [109] with Ca^{2+} permeability. One effect of aggregated $A\beta$ is the increase of the oxidative stress, a mechanisms that has been linked with increases in the resting $[Ca^{2+}]_i$ [110]. The other culprits in AD pathogenesis are the presenilins (PS), which act as essential constituents of the β-secretase complex that cleaves a number of membrane proteins, including the amyloid precursor protein (APP), the latter generating the $A\beta$ fragments [111]. Experimental manipulations of expression of either of the two genes controlling PS (PS1 and PS2) in various animal models resulted in phenotypes with disrupted Ca^{2+} homeostasis characterized, in the main, by an ER Ca^{2+} store overload [11]. As a result, neurons expressing such mutations show increased vulnerability to glutamatergic stimulation as shown, for example, in the case of hippocampal neurons, both in slices [112] and in primary cell cultures [107]. The overloading of the internal stores appear to affect the release of Ca^{2+} mediated either by the rynanodine receptor [113] or by the $InsP_3$ receptor [114]. However, such drastic effects of presenilin mutations on ER Ca^{2+} homeostasis might indicate a possible physiological role, and it has been shown recently that PS-1 deficiency ($-/-$ homozygotes) can impair the glutamate-evoked Ca^{2+} signals, although the resting $[Ca^{2+}]_i$ levels were not affected [115]. Overall, these data illustrate the differences between normal aging and AD. In the former case, ER Ca^{2+} homeostasis is largely normal, with some tendency toward a reduction in the size of the Ca^{2+} store. In contrast, in the AD models, the ER stores are overfilled and the major dysfunctional proteins in AD are interfering with cellular Ca^{2+} homeostasis.

2.   Mitochondria

On the back of the "free radicals" theory of aging [116], and involving the effects of free radicals on mitochondrial DNA, Miquel [117] proposed the "mitochondrial theory" of aging more than two decades ago. In the intervening years, the role and participation of mitochondria in cellular Ca^{2+} homeostasis became clearer, and this relationship came to be included among the important processes that underlie the functional changes of normal brain aging [35, 118]. The role of mitochondria as regulators of the cell death mode, dictating the progression toward necrosis or apoptosis, has been well established for some time now [119] but, as discussed above, normal neuronal aging is not about cellular death and the role of apoptosis in brain aging is relatively small in contrast to the situation in neurodegenerative diseases [119–121]. Instead, the role of mitochondria as the primary site of neuronal energy production and major source of metabolically linked release of reactive oxygen and nitrogen species (ROS and RNS) is much more important for the process of cellular aging [122] (Figure 14.3). Also, it should be noted that mitochondria, through their capacity of taking up or releasing Ca^{2+}, can have a dramatic sculpting effect on the cytosolic Ca^{2+} signal.

The main drive for Ca^{2+} uptake is the steep mitochondrial membrane potential (−180 mV) generated by the activity of the electron transporters in the respiratory chain that couple electron transfer to proton extrusion (Figure 14.3). The transport of Ca^{2+} is implemented by a Ca^{2+} uniporter, which has only very recently been identified as a channel protein [123], that has a high affinity for Ca^{2+} (nanomolar range); is impermeable to K^+ and Mg^{2+}, ions that are abundant in the cytosol, and is inhibited by ruthenium red. The issue of Ca^{2+} affinity is problematic because functional studies have shown this mitochondrial Ca^{2+} uptake pathway as a low-affinity, high-capacity Ca^{2+} removal system [124]. It might then be more useful to talk about a Ca^{2+} uptake set point, at which the uptake and efflux of Ca^{2+} from the mitochondrial matrix are balanced, and above which net uptake of Ca^{2+} takes place [125]. One of the very important features of mitochondrial Ca^{2+} uptake is the potentially huge capacity of this Ca^{2+} store, a property that is based on the co-accumulation of phosphate together with Ca^{2+} to form a salt complex that is both rapidly dissociable and also osmotically inactive. In isolated mitochondria incubated in physiological buffers that mimic intracellular solutions, Ca^{2+} can reach concentrations of around 100 mM (i.e., 50 times larger than the extracellular Ca^{2+} concentrations), while maintaining a normal metabolic state [126]. More recent measurements of Ca^{2+} changes in intact cellular systems (lizard motor nerve terminals) confirmed the earlier data and showed that the accumulation of mitochondrial Ca^{2+} takes place while the concentration of free Ca^{2+} in the mitochondrial matrix ($[Ca^{2+}]_{mito}$) is maintained at stable levels [127].

This maintenance of a tight control on $[Ca^{2+}]_{mito}$ is essential as this parameter is a sword with two edges. Moderate increases in $[Ca^{2+}]_{mito}$ activate three important mitochondrial enzymes (pyruvate-, isocitrate-, and 2-oxoglutarate-dehydorgenases) that are involved in the Krebs (citric acid) cycle. The consequent increase in the reduction state of the NADH/NAD system will induce an increased electron transport and thus couple a cytosolic event that generated a Ca^{2+} response to a temporary

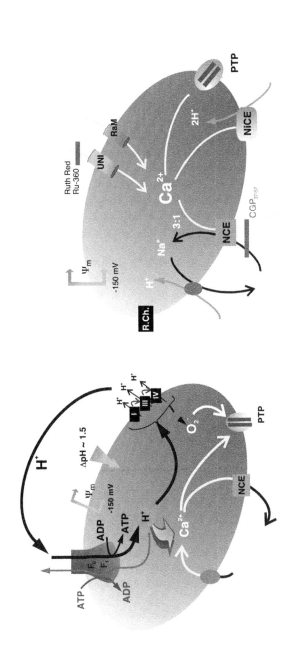

FIGURE 14.3 (SEE COLOR INSERT FOLLOWING PAGE 204) Mitochondrial physiology and mitochondrial Ca²⁺ handling. (Left panel): Central to the mitochondrial state is the electrochemical gradient established across the inner membrane. The gradient is established by the activity of the mitochondrial respiratory chain (or electron transport chain), composed of various multi-protein complexes (I, III, and IV, as the main proton pumps, with complex II acting as an alternative source of electrons). The energy required for proton transport is derived from the free energy of the electrons generated in the Krebs cycle that reduce initially the NAD and FAD pools. The proton gradient (generating both a mitochondrial membrane potential and a pH gradient) is coupled, according to the oxidative phosphorylation theory, to the activity of the ATP synthase (Complex V), which uses the energy of the proton gradient to phosphorylate ADP to ATP. (Right panel): The main pathway for Ca²⁺ uptake is represented by the Ca²⁺ uniporter (UNI), which only recently has been functionally characterized as a Ca²⁺ channel (see text for details). In addition, a rapid mode (RaM) transporter, with a higher Ca²⁺ affinity and rapid activation/inactivation kinetics, has been discussed [185]. Extrusion of Ca²⁺ takes two major routes, one driven by the Na⁺ gradient, a Na⁺/Ca²⁺ exchanger (NCE), and another pathway that is Na⁺-independent — the Na⁺-independent Ca²⁺ exchanger (NICE) — which couples Ca²⁺ extrusion with the proton gradient.

increase in ATP supply, a process called "metabolic coupling" [128]. At the other extreme, significant increases in $[Ca^{2+}]_{mito}$ will activate, together with other factors, the permeability transition pore (mPTP) and result in catastrophic consequences for the mitochondria [129], among which mitochondrial swelling is an early indicator. It is important to note that there is a likely tissue-specific heterogeneity in the activation of the mPTP, with liver mitochondria appearing to be more susceptible to Ca^{2+}-dependent activation than brain mitochondria, at least in isolated mitochondria preparations [130].

While the opening of the mPTP would lead to a rapid, unregulated redistribution of the Ca^{2+} accumulated in the matrix back to the cytosol, mitochondria have other transport systems that effect mitochondrial Ca^{2+} release. Two main pathways have been described, with a certain tissue specificity: an Na^+/Ca^{2+} exchange system that is predominant in the brain, heart, and skeletal muscle, whereas in the liver, kidney, and smooth muscles, Ca^{2+} efflux is predominantly Na^+ independent [131].

In discussing the effects of mitochondria on cellular Ca^{2+} homeostasis, the spatial dimension also must be take into account because, as demonstrated mainly in non-excitable cells, mitochondria, acting on limited spatial domains (functional "micro-domains"), can have significant effects on the Ca^{2+} release from the ER. This effect also takes into account the fact that cytosolic Ca^{2+} has a biphasic effect on ER Ca^{2+} release, both at the $InsP_3$ and the rynanodine receptors [16, 132]. Removal of Ca^{2+} from the immediate vicinity of the ER Ca^{2+} release channels should enhance the release and amplify the signal, and indeed, in *Xenopus* oocytes, enhancement of mitochondrial respiration increases the amplitude and velocity of the $InsP_3$-generated cytosolic Ca^{2+} waves [133]. In a similar fashion, the mitochondrial Ca^{2+} uptake could influence the entry of Ca^{2+} from the extracellular medium. One path responsible for Ca^{2+} entry and sensitive to the energetic status of the mitochondria, strategically placed in the submembranar space, is the capacitative Ca^{2+} entry pathway [134], activated by the depletion of the intracellular Ca^{2+} stores and inhibited either by ER store refilling or by permeating Ca^{2+} ions. To date, the evidence for such a pathway effective in the central nervous system's neurons is rather thin [135]. Although not yet investigated in detail, the same subplasmalemmal mitochondria also could modulate the activity of other Ca^{2+} channels that are inhibited by cytosolic Ca^{2+} increases, such as the voltage-operated Ca^{2+} channels [136]. Not only can Ca^{2+} uptake modulate neuronal function, but the mitochondrial release of Ca^{2+} can also affect neuronal physiology. Thus, tetanic stimulation of *Xenopus* motorneurons induces a potentiation of neurotransmitter release that is sensitive to the Ca^{2+} release from the mitochondria, but not from the ER [137].

To date, there is almost no information about the effects of aging on the biochemical properties of the mitochondrial Ca^{2+} transporters, either for uptake or for release, and this should be an important area of future research, both in the field of normal aging and for various neurodegenerative instances. However, other well-documented changes in mitochondrial status with age are affecting mitochondrial Ca^{2+} homeostasis. Of these, a chronic change in the mitochondrial membrane potential that progresses with age is one of the better-established features. Using a fluorescent dye (rhodamine 123) that equilibrates across cellular compartments as a function of the electrical potential across these membranes (Nerstian distribution), and thus accumulates preferentially in the mitochondria [138], it has been shown that in the aged preparations of isolated mitochondria, there is a population of mitochondria that is significantly depolarized [139]. Because the use of rhodamine has a number of important limitations — in particular, overloading of the mitochondrial compartment with a consequent quenching [138, 140] — other methods are available, including the use of a recording electrode sensitive to an ion with Nerstian distribution, tetraphenylphosphonium [141]. Use of such more precise techniques confirmed the chronic depolarization of aged mitochondria [142]. Because these experiments used preparations of isolated mitochondria that are susceptible to selective enrichment in viable mitochondria, and thus a potential underestimating bias, particularly for the more fragile aged cells [143], it was important to assess the situation in intact cellular preparations. Using the properties of protonophores to collapse the mitochondrial membrane potential and thus release the rhodamine accumulated in the mitochondria, it has been shown that in the aged neurons there is a significant age-dependent decrease in the amount of dye accumulated [143], in line with the idea of mitochondria in the aged cells being more depolarized. Metabolic control analysis showed, consistent with these ideas, that aged mitochondria have an increased mitochondrial proton leak, but it is difficult to assess if this observation is a cause or effect of reported mitochondrial depolarization, because in these experiments the aged mitochondria did not show a decreased membrane potential [144].

Clearly, a decrease in the mitochondrial potential would result in a decrease in the electrochemical force driving the mitochondrial Ca^{2+} uptake. Using simultaneous measurements of both cytosolic Ca^{2+} and mitochondrial depolarization response, it was estimated that in the aged cerebellar neurons there was an increase in the $[Ca^{2+}]_i$ threshold required for triggering mitochondrial uptake [14, 145]. Associated with this question of the threshold for mitochondrial uptake is the issue of the size and dynamics of the mitochondrial Ca^{2+} pool. It has been shown previously that Ca^{2+} mitochondrial loading (as assessed by a protonophore-induced Ca^{2+} release) depends on the level and duration of stimulation and that this loading is dynamic, with a spontaneous discharge over a period of minutes [146]. Also, the extent of mitochondrial depolarization resulting from mitochondrial loading depends on the type of stimulus, with significant differences between KCl and glutamate [147], or even among the various types of glutamatergic agonists [148]. The existence of possible changes with age in these parameters of mitochondrial Ca^{2+} storage currently is under investigation. Some early results show, for the cerebellar granule neurons, that following glutamatergic stimulation the major determinant of the size of the mitochondrial Ca^{2+} accumulation is the cytoplasmic Ca^{2+} levels irrespective of the age of the preparations, and thus, by extension, of the level of chronic mitochondrial depolarization [149].

Neuronal stimulation means mitochondrial depolarization but our understanding of the effects of this mitochondrial depolarization on the state of the cell is evolving. In some studies, mitochondrial depolarization that follows glutamate stimulation appears to be the early event that initiates excitotoxic death [150–152]. However, other studies have reported an opposite effect, and mitochondrial depolarization preceding the glutamatergic stimulation proved a very effective neuroprotective protocol [153, 154]. Rather than being exclusive, these data, taken together, indicate that the mitochondrial Ca^{2+} — either as amount of Ca^{2+} loading or as level of free matrix Ca^{2+} — is a dynamic parameter that controls the physiological state of the cell. One target of mitochondrial Ca^{2+} is the regulation of the mPTP opening, mentioned above, and not surprisingly inhibition of the mPTP proved an effective neuroprotective strategy, effective in a variety of pathological instances but also improving the status of aged mitochondria [155].

Another potential target for increased mitochondrial Ca^{2+} is the production of ROS, which has been demonstrated to follow NMDA stimulation [156], in a manner sensitive to removal of Ca^{2+} [157]. However, the interpretation of studies reporting measurements of ROS production is problematic, because the acute, real-time detection of free radicals (mainly through the use of fluorescent dyes) is notoriously difficult because of (1) the selectivity of various dyes for different ROS species, (2) the different sites at which the ROS are produced and their lifetime, and (3) the fact that the fluorescence of the dyes could be influenced by other enzymatic and non-enzymatic processes [158]. In addition, the bioenergetic process that leads from increased matrix Ca^{2+} to increased free radicals is not well established. Electron leak, generating free radicals, occurs predominantly within complex III in the respiratory chain, during the so-called "Q cycle," although complex I can also participate in the ROS generation process [159]. The crucial feature of this process is that it requires high mitochondrial membrane potential [160], and thus the Ca^{2+} uptake should inhibit rather than evoke an increase of ROS. One proposed explanation invokes (1) the stimulatory effect of Ca^{2+} on the citric acid cycle, mentioned above and that should accelerate the electron transfer rate; and (2) an effect of Ca^{2+} on nitric oxide (NO) generation, which in turn would inhibit the activity at the complex IV in the respiratory chain creating further favorable conditions for electron leak at complex III [161]. However, with respect to the effect of the respiration rate on the generation of ROS, a point of subtlety was made in a recent review by Nicholls [162]. The cytosolic environment is well hypoxic with respect to the values of the partial pressure of oxygen in the circulation or in the tissues, due to the increased diffusion pat, but even in these conditions oxygen, as a substrate for the final four-electron reduction to water, is in excess, and in sufficient supply. Under these conditions, the single electron reduction that generates free radicals is not simply a proportional slippage of the main electron carrier path, but rather the contrary. The generation of free radicals is inversely proportional to the rate of respiration, such that the higher the respiration rate and the lower the membrane potential, the less time will the electrons spend at the sites of leakage [162].

IV. AGING AND NEURODEGENERATION

Many times, "aging" and "neurodegeneration" are mentioned in the same breath, as if they are two state-points along a continuum, leading from the normality of old age to the state of confusion of senile dementia. Indeed, Terry and Katzman made this explicit prediction: they started from the observation that dementia occurs when there is a loss of about 40% of neocortical synapses and combined this with their estimations of the rate of age-dependent synaptic loss, as assessed by their analyses in human postmortem samples, extrapolating the data to the current estimations of human lifespan [163]. Apart from the anecdotal evidence of many centenarians that age successfully [164], including the *Guinness Book of Records'* oldest certified human being, Madame Calment, who died in 1997 at the age of over 122 years without showing any signs of clinical dementia, the set of data that underlies the provocative hypothesis mentioned above might have been corrupted, unknowingly, by the inclusion in the analysis of subclinical instances of neurodegenerative pathology. Indeed, a similar error crept in the early sets of data that led to the conclusion that normal aging is associated with significant neuronal loss in all regions of the brain, a conclusion that only recently has been disproved [10]. Even the term "neurodegeneration" is problematic, despite the obvious etymology, because the term has been used in reference to a large group of neurological diseases, with heterogeneous clinical and pathological manifestations, affecting specific, but different regions of the nervous system [165]. Another experimental observation that complicates the issues is that the pathological markers associated with various neurodegenerative diseases, such as Lewy bodies, neurofibrillary tangles (NFTs), senile plaques, or other protein depositions, can be detected in the brain of aged asymptomatic individuals [166]. These observations obviously raise the question of whether such individuals were just aging normally or were sampled at a presymptomatic stage of a neurodegenerative disease — there are, as yet, no definite answers to these issues. The study of the relationship between normal aging and neurodegeneration can be significantly helped by studies on animal models, because none of the human neurodegenerative diseases appear naturally in the animals. Through genetic manipulations, various animal models have been constructed that mimic one or another of the neurodegenerative phenotypes [167]. At the same time, behavioral studies allow a more and more detailed assessment of the cognitive status of the animals, leading to the generation of sophisticated models of learning and memory and the study of the effects of aging on such processes [105].

The animal studies also allowed a very detailed analysis of the metabolic changes associated with the process of normal aging, as reviewed in this chapter. What these studies indicate is that normal neuronal aging is a physiological process, characterized primarily by a decrease in the neuronal homeostatic reserve, where this homeostatic reserve is defined as the capacity of the cells to oppose the destabilizing effects of various metabolic stressors (Figure 14.4). A detailed discussion of the evidence was presented in earlier articles [122, 149]. Briefly, this hypothesis is based on the view that central to the changes in the cellular physiology of the aged neurons is a dysfunction of the metabolic triad: Ca^{2+} – mitochondria – ROS. It also states that the functional deficits of the aged neurons become evident only in a use-dependent manner, when the metabolic demands become excessive. This view accounts also for the lack of significant levels of neuronal loss with aging. On this weakened homeostatic reserve, any significant pathological instance that requires a strong metabolic response, be it trauma, stroke, or any idiopathic neurodegenerative process, would result in a significant level of neuronal death. In this model, it is the decreased homeostatic reserve that explains the increased neuronal vulnerability with age, an increased vulnerability that manifests itself in a variety of pathological scenarios.

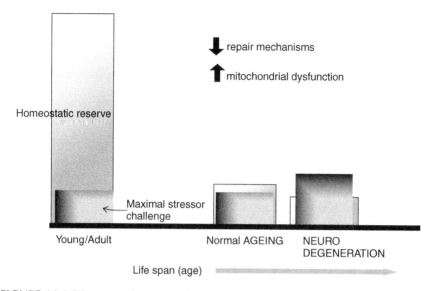

FIGURE 14.4 Diagrammatic presentation of the effects of changes in homeostatic reserve on the processes of aging and neurodegeneration. Cells, tissues, and organisms have an intrinsic property of fighting off the effects of various stressors, defined as the homeostatic reserve. In young/adult organisms, the homeostatic reserve is well in excess of the levels of maximal metabolic stressors still compatible with life. With the passage of time and increasing age, the combined effects of a decrease in the efficiency of the repair mechanisms, changes in mitochondrial status, and an increased accumulation of the ROS-induced damage drastically reduce the level of homeostatic reserve to levels that are still compatible with normal levels of activity. On this background, the neurodegenerative processes act either through an increase in the levels of metabolic stress or through a further decrease in the homeostatic reserve, such that in various regions of the brain where these changes take place, the homeostatic reserve becomes insufficient and neuronal loss ensues.

The fact that aging is "just" a functional state should be very encouraging. We might not be in a position to bring on immortality through engineering negligible senescence, but a better understanding of the metabolism of the aged neuron could open important avenues for therapeutic intervention that will impede or delay the possible cognitive decline of the aged.

ACKNOWLEDGMENTS

The author wishes to acknowledge the BBSRC, which provided, through the SAGE Initiative, a significant part of the financial support for the work performed in this laboratory. The author is also grateful to Professor A. Verkhratsky for discussions on various aspects of the work reported here. Siddhartha helped by providing a new perspective.

REFERENCES

1. Khachaturian, Z.S., Towards theories of brain aging, in *Handbook of Studies on Psychiatry and Old Age*, Kay, D. and Burrows, G., Eds., Elsevier, Amsterdam, 1984, 7.
2. Khachaturian, Z.S., Calcium hypothesis of Alzheimer's disease and brain aging, *Ann. N.Y. Acad. Sci.*, 747, 1, 1994.
3. Campbell, A.K., *Intracellular Calcium — Its Universal Role as Regulator*, John Wiley & Sons, New York, 1983.
4. Berridge, M.J. and Galione, A., Cytosolic calcium oscillators, *FASEB J.*, 2, 3074, 1988.
5. Olney, J.W. and Ho, O.L., Brain damage in infant mice following oral intake of glutamate, aspartate or cysteine, *Nature*, 227, 609, 1970.
6. Choi, D. W., Maulucci-Gedde, M., and Kriegstein, A.R., Glutamate neurotoxicity in cortical cell culture, *J. Neurosci.*, 7, 357, 1987.
7. Hof, P.R. and Morrison, J.H., The aging brain: morphomolecular senescence of cortical circuits, *Trends Neurosci.*, 27, 607, 2004.
8. Sterio, D.C., The unbiased estimation of number and sizes of arbitrary particles using the disector, *J. Microsci.*, 134, 127, 1984.
9. Gómez-Isla, T. et al., Profound loss of layer II entorhinal cortex neurons occurs in very mild Alzheimer's disease., *J. Neurosci.*, 16, 4491, 1996.
10. Morrison, J. and Hof, P., Life and death of neurons in the aging brain, *Science*, 278, 412, 1997.
11. LaFerla, F.M., Calcium dyshomeostasis and intracellular signaling in Alzheimer disease, *Nat. Rev. Neurosci.*, 3, 862, 2002.
12. Catterall, W.A. et al., International Union of Pharmacology. XL. Compendium of voltage-gated ion channels: calcium channels, *Pharmacol. Rev.*, 55, 579, 2003.
13. Trimmer, J.S. and Rhodes, K.J., Localization of voltage-gated ion channels in mammalian brain, *Annu. Rev. Physiol.*, 66, 477, 2004.
14. Xiong, J. et al., Mitochondrial polarisation status and $[Ca^{2+}]_i$ signaling in rat cerebellar granule neurons aged *in vitro*, *Neurobiol. Aging*, 25, 349, 2004.
15. Solovyova, N. et al., Ca^{2+} dynamics in the lumen of the endoplasmic reticulum in sensory neurons: direct visualization of Ca^{2+}-induced Ca^{2+} release triggered by physiological Ca(2+) entry, *Embo. J.*, 21, 622, 2002.
16. Verkhratsky, A., Physiology and pathophysiology of the calcium store in the endoplasmic reticulum of neurons, *Physiol. Rev.*, 85, 201, 2005.
17. Paschen, W., Endoplasmic reticulum: a primary target in various acute disorders and degenerative diseases of the brain, *Cell Calcium*, 34, 365, 2003.
18. Carafoli, E., Calcium signaling: a tale for all seasons, *Proc. Natl. Acad. Sci. U.S.A.*, 99, 1115, 2002.
19. Burgoyne, R.D. et al., Neuronal Ca^{2+}-sensor proteins: multitalented regulators of neuronal function, *Trends Neurosci.*, 27, 203, 2004.
20. Buxbaum, J.D., A role for calsenilin and related proteins in multiple aspects of neuronal function, *Biochem. Biophys. Res. Commun.*, 322, 1140, 2004.
21. Baimbridge, K.G., Celio, M.R., and Rogers, J.H., Calcium-binding proteins in the nervous system, *Trends Neurosci.*, 15, 303, 1992.
22. Augustine, G.J., Santamaria, F., and Tanaka, K., Local calcium signaling in neurons, *Neuron*, 40, 331, 2003.
23. Mattson, M.P. et al., Evidence for calcium-reducing and excito-protective roles for the calcium-binding protein calbindin-D28k in cultured hippocampal neurons, *Neuron*, 6, 41, 1991.

24. Lukas, W. and Jones, K.A., Cortical neurons containing calretinin are selectively resistant to calcium overload and excitotoxicity *in vitro, Neuroscience,* 61, 307, 1994.

25. Dowd, D.R., Calcium regulation of apoptosis, *Adv. Second Messenger Phosphoprotein Res.,* 30, 255, 1995.

26. Dekkers, J. et al., Over-expression of parvalbumin in transgenic mice rescues motoneurons from injury-induced cell death, *Neuroscience,* 123, 459, 2004.

27. Lee, S.H., Schwaller, B., and Neher, E., Kinetics of Ca^{2+} binding to parvalbumin in bovine chromaffin cells: implications for $[Ca^{2+}]$ transients of neuronal dendrites, *J. Physiol.,* 525(Pt. 2), 419, 2000.

28. Lee, S.H. et al., Differences in Ca^{2+} buffering properties between excitatory and inhibitory hippocampal neurons from the rat, *J. Physiol.,* 525(Pt. 2), 405, 2000.

29. Palecek, J., Lips, M.B., and Keller, B.U., Calcium dynamics and buffering in motoneurons of the mouse spinal cord, *J. Physiol.,* 520(Pt. 2), 485, 1999.

30. Wanaverbecq, N. et al., The plasma membrane calcium-ATPase as a major mechanism for intracellular calcium regulation in neurons from the rat superior cervical ganglion, *J. Physiol.,* 550, 83, 2003.

31. Fierro, L. and Llano, I., High endogenous calcium buffering in Purkinje cells from rat cerebellar slices, *J. Physiol.,* 496(Pt. 3), 617, 1996.

32. Verkhratsky, A. and Toescu, E., Calcium and neuronal aging, *Trends Neurosci.,* 21, 2, 1998.

33. Pitler, T.A. and Landfield, P.W., Aging-related prolongation of calcium spike duration in rat hippocampal slice neurons, *Brain Res.,* 508, 1, 1990.

34. Thibault, O. et al., Calcium dysregulation in neuronal aging and Alzheimer's disease: history and new directions, *Cell Calcium,* 24, 417, 1998.

35. Toescu, E.C. and Verkhratsky, A., Ca^{2+} and mitochondria as substrates for deficits in synaptic plasticity in normal brain aging, *J. Cell. Mol. Med.,* 8, 181, 2004.

36. Thibault, O. and Landfield, P.W., Increase in single L-type calcium channels in hippocampal neurons during aging, *Science,* 272, 1017, 1996.

37. Murchison, D. and Griffith, W.H., Low-voltage activated calcium currents increase in basal forebrain neurons from aged rats, *J. Neurophysiol.,* 74, 876, 1995.

38. Murchison, D. and Griffith, W.H., High-voltage-activated calcium currents in basal forebrain neurons during aging, *J. Neurophysiol.,* 76, 158, 1996.

39. Kostyuk, P. et al., Calcium currents in aged rat dorsal root ganglion neurons, *J. Physiol. Lond.,* 461, 467, 1993.

40. Govoni, S. et al., Age-related reduced affinity in ^{3}H nitrendipine labeling of brain voltage-dependent calcium channels, *Brain Res.,* 333, 374, 1985.

41. Alshuaib, W.B. and Fahim, M.A., Aging increases calcium influx at motor nerve terminal, *Int. J. Dev. Neurosci.,* 8, 655, 1990.

42. Martinez-Serrano, A. et al., Reduction of K^+-stimulated $^{45}Ca^{2+}$ influx in synaptosomes with age involves inactivating and noninactivating calcium channels and is correlated with temporal modifications in protein dephosphorylation, *J. Neurochem.,* 52, 576, 1989.

43. Farrar, R.P. et al., Aging does not alter cytosolic calcium levels of cortical synaptosomes in Fischer 344 rats, *Neurosci. Lett.,* 100, 319, 1989.

44. Chung, Y.H. et al., Differential alterations in the distribution of voltage-gated calcium channels in aged rat cerebellum, *Brain Res.,* 903, 247, 2001.

45. Burnashev, N., Calcium permeability of ligand-gated channels, *Cell Calcium,* 24, 325, 1998.

46. Dingledine, R. et al., The glutamate receptor ion channels, *Pharmacol. Rev.,* 51, 7, 1999.

47. Perez-Otano, I. et al., Assembly with the NR1 subunit is required for surface expression of NR3A-containing NMDA receptors, *J. Neurosci.,* 21, 1228, 2001.

48. Nowak, L. et al., Magnesium gates glutamate-activated channels in mouse central neurons, *Nature,* 307, 462, 1984.

49. Magnusson, K.R., The aging of the NMDA receptor complex, *Front. Biosci.,* 3, e70, 1998.

50. Monyer, H. et al., Developmental and regional expression in the rat brain and functional properties of four NMDA receptors, *Neuron,* 12, 529, 1994.

51. Clayton, D.A. and Browning, M.D., Deficits in the expression of the NR2B subunit in the hippocampus of aged Fisher 344 rats, *Neurobiol. Aging,* 22, 165, 2001.

52. Cepeda, C., Li, Z., and Levine, M.S., Aging reduces neostriatal responsiveness to N-methyl-D-aspartate and dopamine: an *in vitro* electrophysiological study, *Neuroscience,* 73, 733, 1996.

53. Barnes, C.A., Rao, G., and Shen, J., Age-related decrease in the N-methyl-D-aspartate-mediated excitatory postsynaptic potential in hippocampal region CA1, *Neurobiol. Aging,* 18, 445, 1997.

54. Cady, C., Evans, M.S., and Brewer, G.J., Age-related differences in NMDA responses in cultured rat hippocampal neurons, *Brain Res.,* 921, 1, 2001.

55. Verdoorn, T.A. et al., Structural determinants of ion flow through recombinant glutamate receptor channels, *Science,* 252, 1715, 1991.

56. Mishina, M. et al., A single amino acid residue determines the Ca^{2+} permeability of AMPA-selective glutamate receptor channels, *Biochem. Biophys. Res. Commun.,* 180, 813, 1991.

57. Seeburg, P.H., The TINS/TiPS Lecture. The molecular biology of mammalian glutamate receptor channels, *Trends Neurosci.,* 16, 359, 1993.

58. Lomeli, H. et al., Control of kinetic properties of AMPA receptor channels by nuclear RNA editing, *Science,* 266, 1709, 1994.

59. Isa, T. et al., Distribution of neurons expressing inwardly rectifying and Ca^{2+}-permeable AMPA receptors in rat hippocampal slices, *J. Physiol.,* 491, 719, 1996.

60. Itazawa, S. I., Isa, T., and Ozawa, S., Inwardly rectifying and Ca^{2+}-permeable AMPA-type glutamate receptor channels in rat neocortical neurons, *J. Neurophysiol.,* 78, 2592, 1997.

61. Magnusson, K.R., Influence of dietary restriction on ionotropic glutamate receptors during aging in C57B1 mice, *Mech. Aging. Dev.,* 95, 187, 1997.

62. Magnusson, K.R. and Cotman, C.W., Age-related changes in excitatory amino acid receptors in two mouse strains, *Neurobiol. Aging,* 14, 197, 1993.

63. Magnusson, K.R., Aging of glutamate receptors: correlations between binding and spatial memory performance in mice, *Mech. Aging Dev.,* 104, 227, 1998.

64. Barnes, C.A. et al., Region-specific age effects on AMPA sensitivity: electrophysiological evidence for loss of synaptic contacts in hippocampal field CA1, *Hippocampus,* 2, 457, 1992.

65. Carlson, N.G. et al., RNA editing (Q/R site) and flop/flip splicing of AMPA receptor transcripts in young and old brains, *Neurobiol. Aging,* 21, 599, 2000.

66. Tanaka, H. et al., The AMPAR subunit GluR2: still front and center-stage, *Brain Res.,* 886, 190, 2000.

67. Michaelis, M. et al., Decreased plasma membrane calcium transport activity in aging brain, *Life Sci.,* 59, 405, 1996.

68. Zaidi, A. et al., Age-related decrease in brain synaptic membrane Ca^{2+}-ATPase in F344/BNF1 rats, *Neurobiol. Aging,* 19, 487, 1998.

69. Zaidi, A. and Michaelis, M.L., Effects of reactive oxygen species on brain synaptic plasma membrane Ca^{2+}-ATPase, *Free Radic. Biol. Med.,* 27, 810, 1999.

70. Michaelis, M.L. et al., Decreased plasma membrane calcium transport activity in aging brain, *Life Sci.,* 59, 405, 1996.

71. Tsai, H. et al., Adrenergic nerve smooth endoplasmic reticulum calcium buffering declines with age, *Neurobiol. Aging,* 19, 89, 1998.

72. Pottorf, W.J., Duckles, S.P., and Buchholz, J.N., Aging and calcium buffering in adrenergic neurons, *Auton. Neurosci.,* 96, 2, 2002.

73. De Jong, G.I. et al., Age-related loss of calcium binding proteins in rabbit hippocampus, *Neurobiol. Aging,* 17, 459, 1996.

74. Bu, J. et al., Age-related changes in calbindin-D28k, calretinin, and parvalbumin-immunoreactive neurons in the human cerebral cortex, *Exp. Neurol.,* 182, 220, 2003.

75. Geula, C. et al., Loss of calbindin-D28k from aging human cholinergic basal forebrain: relation to neuronal loss, *J. Comp. Neurol.,* 455, 249, 2003.

76. Idrizbegovic, E. et al., The total number of neurons and calcium binding protein positive neurons during aging in the cochlear nucleus of CBA/CaJ mice: a quantitative study, *Hear. Res.,* 158, 102, 2001.

77. Idrizbegovic, E., Bogdanovic, N., and Canlon, B., Modulating calbindin and parvalbumin immunoreactivity in the cochlear nucleus by moderate noise exposure in mice. A quantitative study on the dorsal and posteroventral cochlear nucleus, *Brain Res.,* 800, 86, 1998.

78. Greene, J.R. et al., Accumulation of calbindin in cortical pyramidal cells with aging; a putative protective mechanism which fails in Alzheimer's disease, *Neuropathol. Appl. Neurobiol.,* 27, 339, 2001.

79. Tsai, H. et al., Intracellular calcium buffering declines in aging adrenergic nerves, *Neurobiol. Aging,* 18, 229, 1997.

80. Murchison, D. and Griffith, W., Increased calcium buffering in basal forebrain neurons during aging, *J. Neurophysiol.,* 80, 350, 1998.

81. Griffith, W.H. et al., Modification of ion channels and calcium homeostasis of basal forebrain neurons during aging, *Behav. Brain Res.,* 115, 219, 2000.

82. Murchison, D., Zawieja, D.C., and Griffith, W.H., Reduced mitochondrial buffering of voltage-gated calcium influx in aged rat basal forebrain neurons, *Cell Calcium,* 36, 61, 2004.

83. Wu, C.K. and Geula, C., Selective loss of calbindin D-28k from cholinergic neurons of the human basal forebrain in aging and Alzheimer's disease, in *Alzheimer's Disease Biology Diagnosis and Therapeutics,* Igbal, K., Winblad, B., Nishimura, T., Takeda, M., and Wisniewski, H.M., Eds., John Wiley & Sons, New York, 1997, 297.

84. Spacek, J. and Harris, K.M., Three-dimensional organization of smooth endoplasmic reticulum in hippocampal CA1 dendrites and dendritic spines of the immature and mature rat, *J. Neurosci.,* 17, 190, 1997.

85. Finch, E.A. and Augustine, G.J., Local calcium signaling by inositol-1,4,5-trisphosphate in Purkinje cell dendrites, *Nature,* 396, 753, 1998.

86. Takechi, H., Eilers, J., and Konnerth, A., A new class of synaptic response involving calcium release in dendritic spines, *Nature,* 396, 757, 1998.

87. Svoboda, K. and Mainen, Z.F., Synaptic [Ca^{2+}]: intracellular stores spill their guts, *Neuron,* 22, 427, 1999.

88. Emptage, N., Bliss, T.V.P., and Fine, A., Single synaptic events evoke NMDA receptor-mediated release of calcium from internal stores in hippocampal dendritic spines, *Neuron,* 22, 115, 1999.

89. Kovalchuk, Y. et al., NMDA receptor-mediated subthreshold Ca^{2+} signals in spines of hippocampal neurons, *J. Neurosci.*, 20, 1791, 2000.

90. Garaschuk, O., Yaari, Y., and Konnerth, A., Release and sequestration of calcium by ryanodine-sensitive stores in rat hippocampal neurons, *J. Physiol.*, 502, 13, 1997.

91. Irving, A.J. and Collingridge, G.L., A characterization of muscarinic receptor-mediated intracellular Ca^{2+} mobilization in cultured rat hippocampal neurons, *J. Physiol.*, 511(Pt. 3), 747, 1998.

92. Pozzo-Miller, L.D., Connor, J.A., and Andrews, S.B., Microheterogeneity of calcium signaling in dendrites, *J. Physiol.*, 525(Pt. 1), 53, 2000.

93. Toescu, E., Intraneuronal Ca^{2+} stores act mainly as a 'Ca^{2+} sink' in cerebellar granule neurons, *Neuroreport*, 9, 1227, 1998.

94. Kirischuk, S. and Verkhratsky, A., Calcium homeostasis in aged neurons, *Life Sci.*, 59, 451, 1996.

95. Clodfelter, G.V. et al., Sustained Ca^{2+}-induced Ca^{2+}-release underlies the post-glutamate lethal Ca^{2+} plateau in older cultured hippocampal neurons, *Eur. J. Pharmacol.*, 447, 189, 2002.

96. Murchison, D. and Griffith, W.H., Age-related alterations in caffeine-sensitive calcium stores and mitochondrial buffering in rat basal forebrain, *Cell Calcium*, 25, 439, 1999.

97. Chavis, P. et al., Functional coupling between ryanodine receptors and L-type calcium channels in neurons, *Nature*, 382, 719, 1996.

98. Renganathan, M., Messi, M.L., and Delbono, O., Dihydropyridine receptor-ryanodine receptor uncoupling in aged skeletal muscle, *J. Membr. Biol.*, 157, 247, 1997.

99. Harvey, J. and Collingridge, G.L., Thapsigargin blocks the induction of long-term potentiation in rat hippocampal slices, *Neurosci. Lett.*, 139, 197, 1992.

100. Raymond, C.R. and Redman, S.J., Different calcium sources are narrowly tuned to the induction of different forms of LTP, *J. Neurophysiol.*, 88, 249, 2002.

101. Kumar, A. and Foster, T.C., Enhanced long-term potentiation during aging is masked by processes involving intracellular calcium stores, *J. Neurophysiol.*, 91, 2437, 2004.

102. Landfield, P.W. and Pitler, T.A., Prolonged Ca^{2+}-dependent afterhyperpolarizations in hippocampal neurons of aged rats, *Science*, 226, 1089, 1984.

103. Shah, M. and Haylett, D.G., Ca^{2+} channels involved in the generation of the slow afterhyperpolarization in cultured rat hippocampal pyramidal neurons, *J. Neurophysiol.*, 83, 2554, 2000.

104. Foster, T.C., Involvement of hippocampal synaptic plasticity in age-related memory decline, *Brain Res. Brain Res. Rev.*, 30, 236, 1999.

105. Rosenzweig, E.S. and Barnes, C.A., Impact of aging on hippocampal function: plasticity, network dynamics, and cognition, *Prog. Neurobiol.*, 69, 143, 2003.

106. Larson, J. et al., Alterations in synaptic transmission and long-term potentiation in hippocampal slices from young and aged PDAPP mice, *Brain Res.*, 840, 23, 1999.

107. Guo, Q. et al., Increased vulnerability of hippocampal neurons to excitotoxic necrosis in presenilin-1 mutant knock-in mice, *Nat. Med.*, Jan. 5, 101, 1999.

108. Leissring, M.A. et al., A physiologic signaling role for the gamma-secretase-derived intracellular fragment of APP, *Proc. Natl. Acad. Sci. U.S.A.*, 99, 4697, 2002.

109. Kagan, B.L. et al., The channel hypothesis of Alzheimer's disease: current status, *Peptides*, 23, 1311, 2002.

110. Mark, R.J. et al., Amyloid beta-peptide impairs ion-motive ATPase activities: evidence for a role in loss of neuronal Ca^{2+} homeostasis and cell death, *J. Neurosci.*, 15, 6239, 1995.

111. Thinakaran, G. and Parent, A.T., Identification of the role of presenilins beyond Alzheimer's disease, *Pharmacol. Res.*, 50, 411, 2004.

112. Schneider, I. et al., Mutant presenilins disturb neuronal calcium homeostasis in the brain of transgenic mice, decreasing the threshold for excitotoxicity and facilitating long-term potentiation, *J. Biol. Chem.*, 276, 11539, 2001.
113. Chan, S.L. et al., Presenilin-1 mutations increase levels of ryanodine receptors and calcium release in PC12 cells and cortical neurons, *J. Biol. Chem.*, 275, 18195, 2000.
114. Stutzmann, G.E. et al., Dysregulated IP3 signaling in cortical neurons of knock-in mice expressing an Alzheimer's-linked mutation in presenilin1 results in exaggerated Ca^{2+} signals and altered membrane excitability, *J. Neurosci.*, 24, 508, 2004.
115. Yang, Y. and Cook, D.G., Presenilin-1 deficiency impairs glutamate-evoked intracellular calcium responses in neurons, *Neuroscience*, 124, 501, 2004.
116. Harman, D., Free radical theory of aging: dietary implications, *Am. J. Clin. Nutr.*, 25, 839, 1972.
117. Miquel, J. et al., Mitochondrial role in cell aging, *Exp. Gerontol.*, 15, 575, 1980.
118. Toescu, E.C., Verkhratsky, A., and Landfield, P.W., Ca^{2+} regulation and gene expression in normal brain aging, *Trends Neurosci.*, 27, 614, 2004.
119. Mattson, M.P. and Kroemer, G., Mitochondria in cell death: novel targets for neuroprotection and cardioprotection, *Trends Mol. Med.*, 9, 196, 2003.
120. Drew, B. and Leeuwenburgh, C., Aging and subcellular distribution of mitochondria: role of mitochondrial DNA deletions and energy production, *Acta Physiol. Scand.*, 182, 333, 2004.
121. Melov, S., Modeling mitochondrial function in aging neurons, *Trends Neurosci.*, 27, 601, 2004.
122. Toescu, E.C. and Verkhratsky, A., Neuronal aging from an intraneuronal perspective: roles of endoplasmic reticulum and mitochondria, *Cell Calcium*, 34, 311, 2003.
123. Kirichok, Y., Krapivinsky, G., and Clapham, D.E., The mitochondrial calcium uniporter is a highly selective ion channel, *Nature*, 427, 360, 2004.
124. Gunter, K. and Gunter, T., Transport of calcium by mitochondria, *J. Bioenerg. Biomembr.*, 26, 471, 1994.
125. Nicholls, D. and Budd, S., Mitochondria and neuronal survival, *Physiol. Rev.*, 80, 315, 2000.
126. Nicholls, D.G. and Scott, I.D., The regulation of brain mitochondrial calcium-ion transport. The role of ATP in the discrimination between kinetic and membrane-potential-dependent calcium-ion efflux mechanisms, *Biochem. J.*, 186, 833, 1980.
127. David, G., Mitochondrial clearance of cytosolic Ca^{2+} in stimulated lizard motor nerve terminals proceeds without progressive elevation of mitochondrial matrix $[Ca(2+)]$, *J. Neurosci.*, 19, 7495, 1999.
128. McCormack, J. and Denton, R., Signal transduction by intramitochondrial Ca^{2+} in mammalian energy metabolism, *News Physiol. Sci.*, 9, 71, 1994.
129. Zoratti, M. and Szabo, I., The mitochondrial permeability transition, *Biochim. Biophys. Acta*, 1241, 139, 1995.
130. Andreyev, A. and Fiskum, G., Calcium induced release of mitochondrial cytochrome c by different mechanisms selective for brain versus liver, *Cell Death Differ.*, 6, 825, 1999.
131. Gunter, T. and Pfeiffer, D., Mechanisms by which mitochondria transport calcium, *Am. J. Physiol.*, 258, C755, 1990.
132. Bezprozvanny, I., Watras, J., and Ehrlich, B.E., Bell-shaped calcium-response curves of Ins(1,4,5)P3- and calcium-gated channels from endoplasmic reticulum of cerebellum, *Nature*, 351, 751, 1991.
133. Jouaville, L. et al., Synchronization of calcium waves by mitochondrial substrates in *Xenopus laevis* oocytes, *Nature*, 377, 438, 1995.

134. Parekh, A.B., Store-operated Ca^{2+} entry: dynamic interplay between endoplasmic reticulum, mitochondria and plasma membrane, *J. Physiol.*, 547, 333, 2003.

135. Putney, J.W., Jr., Capacitative calcium entry in the nervous system, *Cell Calcium*, 34, 339, 2003.

136. Peterson, B.Z. et al., Calmodulin is the Ca^{2+} sensor for Ca^{2+}-dependent inactivation of L-type calcium channels, *Neuron*, 22, 549, 1999.

137. Yang, F. et al., Ca^{2+} influx-independent synaptic potentiation mediated by mitochondrial Na(+)-Ca^{2+} exchanger and protein kinase C, *J. Cell. Biol.*, 163, 511, 2003.

138. Toescu, E. and Verkhratsky, A., Assessment of mitochondrial polarization status in living cells based on analysis of the spatial heterogeneity of rhodamine 123 fluorescence staining., *Pfluegers Archiv.*, 440, 941, 2000.

139. Hagen, T. et al., Mitochondrial decay in hepatocytes from old rats: membrane potential declines, heterogeneity and oxidants increase, *Proc. Natl. Acad. Sci. U.S.A.*, 94, 3064, 1997.

140. Ward, M. et al., Mitochondrial membrane potential and glutamate excitotoxicity in cultured cerebellar granule cells, *J. Neurosci.*, 20, 7208, 2000.

141. Kamo, N. et al., Membrane potential of mitochondria measured with an electrode sensitive to tetraphenyl phosphonium and relationship between proton electrochemical potential and phosphorylation potential in steady state, *J. Membr. Biol.*, 49, 105, 1979.

142. Kokoszka, J.E. et al., Increased mitochondrial oxidative stress in the Sod2 (+/-) mouse results in the age-related decline of mitochondrial function culminating in increased apoptosis, *Proc. Natl. Acad. Sci. U.S.A.*, 98, 2278, 2001.

143. Wilson, P.D. and Franks, L.M., The effect of age on mitochondrial ultrastructure and enzymes, *Adv. Exp. Med. Biol.*, 53, 171, 1975.

144. Harper, M.E. et al., Age-related increase in mitochondrial proton leak and decrease in ATP turnover reactions in mouse hepatocytes, *Am. J. Physiol.*, 275, E197, 1998.

145. Xiong, J., Verkhratsky, A., and Toescu, E.C., Changes in mitochondrial status associated with altered Ca^{2+} homeostasis in aged cerebellar granule neurons in brain slices, *J. Neurosci.*, 22, 10761, 2002.

146. Brocard, J.B., Tassetto, M., and Reynolds, I.J., Quantitative evaluation of mitochondrial calcium content in rat cortical neurons following a glutamate stimulus, *J. Physiol.*, 531, 793, 2001.

147. Duchen, M., Contributions of mitochondria to animal physiology: from homeostatic sensor to calcium signaling and cell death, *J. Physiol.*, 516, 1, 1999.

148. Rego, A., Ward, M., and Nicholls, D., Mitochondria control AMPA/Kainate receptor-induced cytoplasmic calcium deregulation in rat cerebellar granule cells, *J. Neurosci.*, 21, 1893, 2001.

149. Toescu, E.C., Normal brain aging: models and mechanisms, *Philos. Trans. R. Soc. Lond.*, 360, 2347, 2005.

150. Ankarcrona, M. et al., Glutamate-induced neuronal death: a succession of necrosis or apoptosis depending on mitochondrial function, *Neuron*, 15, 961, 1995.

151. Khodorov, B., Glutamate-induced deregulation of calcium homeostasis and mitochondrial dysfunction in mammalian central neurons, *Prog. Biophys. Mol. Biol.*, 86, 279, 2004.

152. White, R. and Reynolds, I., Mitochondrial depolarization in glutamate-stimulated neurons — an early signal specific to excitotoxin exposure, *J. Neurosci.*, 16, 5688, 1996.

153. Budd, S.L. and Nicholls, D.G., Mitochondria, calcium regulation, and acute glutamate excitotoxicity in cultured cerebellar granule cells, *J. Neurochem.*, 67, 2282, 1996.

154. Stout, A.K. et al., Glutamate-induced neuron death requires mitochondrial calcium uptake., *Nat. Neurosci.,* 1, 366, 1998.
155. Crompton, M., Mitochondria and aging: a role for the permeability transition? *Aging Cell,* 3, 3, 2004.
156. Lafon-Cazal, M. et al., Nitric oxide, superoxide and peroxynitrite: putative mediators of NMDA-induced cell death in cerebellar granule cells, *Neuropharmacology,* 32, 1259, 1993.
157. Atlante, A, et al Glutamate neurotoxicity in rat cerebellar granule cells. a major role for xanthine oxidase in oxygen radical formation, *J. Neurochem.,* 68, 2038, 1997.
158. Nicholls, D.G. et al., Interactions between mitochondrial bioenergetics and cytoplasmic calcium in cultured cerebellar granule cells, *Cell Calcium,* 34, 407, 2003.
159. St-Pierre, J. et al., Topology of superoxide production from different sites in the mitochondrial electron transport chain, *J. Biol. Chem.,* 277, 44784, 2002.
160. Skulachev, V.P., Role of uncoupled and non-coupled oxidations in maintenance of safely low levels of oxygen and its one-electron reductants, *Q. Rev. Biophys.,* 29, 169, 1996.
161. Brookes, P.S. et al., Calcium, ATP, and ROS: a mitochondrial love-hate triangle, *Am. J. Physiol. Cell. Physiol.,* 287, C817, 2004.
162. Nicholls, D.G., Mitochondrial membrane potential and aging, *Aging Cell,* 3, 35, 2004.
163. Terry, R.D. and Katzman, R., Life span and synapses: will there be a primary senile dementia? *Neurobiol. Aging,* 22, 347, 2001.
164. Vaillant, G.E. and Mukamal, K., Successful aging, *Am. J. Psychiatry,* 158, 839, 2001.
165. Przedborski, S., Vila, M., and Jackson-Lewis, V., Neurodegeneration: what is it and where are we? *J. Clin. Invest.,* 111, 3, 2003.
166. Anderton, B.H., Aging of the brain, *Mech. Aging Dev.,* 123, 811, 2002.
167. Teter, B. and Finch, C.E., Caliban's heritance and the genetics of neuronal aging, *Trends Neurosci.,* 27, 627, 2004.
168. Verkhratsky, A. and Toescu, E.C., *Integrative Aspects of Calcium Signaling,* Plenum Press, New York, 1998, 408.
169. Xia, Z. and Storm, D.R., The role of calmodulin as a signal integrator for synaptic plasticity, *Nat. Rev. Neurosci.,* 6, 267, 2005.
170. Huang, P.L., Nitric oxide and cerebral ischemic preconditioning, *Cell Calcium,* 36, 323, 2004.
171. Chern, Y., Regulation of adenylyl cyclase in the central nervous system, *Cell Signal.,* 12, 195, 2000.
172. Hudmon, A. and Schulman, H., Neuronal Ca^{2+}/calmodulin-dependent protein kinase II: the role of structure and autoregulation in cellular function, *Annu. Rev. Biochem.,* 71, 473, 2002.
173. Groth, R.D., Dunbar, R.L., and Mermelstein, P.G., Calcineurin regulation of neuronal plasticity, *Biochem. Biophys. Res. Commun.,* 311, 1159, 2003.
174. Sudhof, T.C., The synaptic vesicle cycle, *Annu. Rev. Neurosci.,* 27, 509, 2004.
175. Catterall, W.A., Structure and regulation of voltage-gated Ca^{2+} channels, *Annu. Rev. Cell. Dev. Biol,* 16, 521, 2000.
176. Faber, E.S. and Sah, P., Calcium-activated potassium channels: multiple contributions to neuronal function, *Neuroscientist,* 9, 181, 2003.
177. Berridge, M.J., Lipp, P., and Bootman, M.D., The versatility and universality of calcium signaling, *Nat. Rev. Mol. Cell. Biol.,* 1, 11, 2000.
178. Farooqui, A.A. and Horrocks, L.A., Brain phospholipases A2: a perspective on the history, *Prostaglandins Leukot. Essent. Fatty Acids,* 71, 161, 2004.

179. Chan, S.L. and Mattson, M.P., Caspase and calpain substrates: roles in synaptic plasticity and cell death, *J. Neurosci. Res.*, 58, 167, 1999.
180. Catterall, W., Structure and function of neuronal Ca^{2+} channels and their role in neurotransmitter release, *Cell Calcium*, 25, 1998.
181. Berridge, M.J., Bootman, M.D., and Roderick, H.L., Calcium signaling: dynamics, homeostasis and remodelling, *Nat. Rev. Mol. Cell. Biol.*, 4, 517, 2003.
182. Davare, M.A. et al., A beta2 adrenergic receptor signaling complex assembled with the Ca^{2+} channel Cav1.2, *Science*, 293, 98, 2001.
183. Gubellini, P. et al., Metabotropic glutamate receptors and striatal synaptic plasticity: implications for neurological diseases, *Prog. Neurobiol.*, 74, 271, 2004.
184. Verkhratsky, A., Orkand, R.K., and Kettenmann, H., Glial calcium: homeostasis and signaling function, *Physiol. Rev.*, 78, 99, 1998.
185. Gunter, T. et al., Mitochondrial calcium transport: mechanisms and functions, *Cell Calcium*, 28, 285, 2000.

15 Oxidative Stress and the Aging Brain: From Theory to Prevention

Carmelina Gemma, Jennifer Vila,
Adam Bachstetter, and Paula C. Bickford

CONTENTS

I. INTRODUCTION: THE FREE RADICAL THEORY OF AGING

Aging is characterized by a progressive decline in the efficiency of physiological function and by the increased susceptibility to disease and death. Currently, one of the most plausible and acceptable explanations for the mechanistic basis of aging is the "free radical theory of aging." This theory postulates that aging and its related diseases are the consequence of free radical-induced damage to cellular macromolecules and the inability to counterbalance these changes by endogenous anti-oxidant defenses. The origin of this explanation has a foundation in the "rate of living theory" [1], according to which the lifespan of an individual depends on its rate of energy utilization (metabolic rate) and on a genetically determined amount of energy consumed during adult life. Pearl [1] proposed that the longevity of an organism is inversely correlated to its mass-specific metabolic rate: increasing an organism's metabolic rate will decrease longevity, whereas factors that decrease the metabolic rate will increase longevity. The correlation between metabolic rate and longevity has been questioned due to the exception posed by birds, which have a high metabolic rate yet live much longer than mammals [2]. However, despite their high rate of oxygen consumption, it has been shown that birds have a low rate of free radical production in brain and in other tissues; their mitochondria produce up to 10-fold fewer reactive oxygen species (ROS) *in vitro* [3, 4]. This observation suggests that the mitochondrial rate of free radical production may be more important than the metabolic rate in terms of longevity. Indeed, the mitochondrial rate of free radical production seems to have a much stronger correlation with maximum longevity.

Harman [5] originally proposed the "free-radical theory" of aging in the mid-1950s. He suggested that free radicals produced during aerobic respiration have deleterious effects on cell components and connective tissues, causing cumulative damage over time that ultimately results in aging and death. He initially speculated that free radicals were most likely produced through reactions involving molecular oxygen catalyzed in the cells by the oxidative enzymes and enhanced by trace metals such as iron, cobalt, and manganese. The skepticism first spread around this theory was weakened by the discovery in 1969 of the enzyme superoxide dismutase (SOD) [6]. The existence of an intracellular enzyme whose sole function is to remove superoxide anions ($O_2^{-\bullet}$) has provided strong biological evidence that free radicals are involved in the aging process. In 1972, Harman expanded his original studies to include the involvement of mitochondria in the physiological processes of aging [7]. Harman proposed that mitochondria generate a significant amount of cellular energy and, through consumption of most of the intracellular oxygen, set the limit on the lifespan. Approximately 90% of cellular oxygen is consumed within the mitochondria, mainly in the inner membrane, where oxidative phosphorylation occurs. Since the early 1970s, several studies have emerged to give support to this theory, and the free radical theory of aging has been expanded to the mitochondrial free radical theory of aging. The premise of the mitochondrial free radical theory of aging is that mitochondria are both producers and targets of reactive oxidative species. According to the theory, oxidative stress attacks mitochondria, leading to increased oxidative damage. As a consequence, damaged mitochondria progressively become less efficient, losing their functional integrity and releasing more oxygen molecules, increasing oxidative damage to the mitochondria, and culminating in an accumulation of dysfunctional mitochondria with age.

Although the deleterious effects of free radicals in the aging process have been demonstrated, ROS also are important in maintaining homeostasis. Recent studies have shown that ROS act as an additional class of small molecules that function as cellular messengers. For example, oxidants (nitrous oxide [NO]) act as signaling molecules to promote long-term potentiation (LTP) [8]. Moreover, it has been shown that stimulation of growth factors induces the production of free radicals that are subsequently involved in regulating the proliferative response [9]. The human organism is equipped with very efficient antioxidative defense mechanisms that, among others, include antioxidative enzymes such as SOD, catalase, glutathione peroxidase, and glutathione reductase [10]. When the production of ROS is prolonged, the endogenous reserves of antioxidants become insufficient, leading to cell damage. Similarly, the production of ROS below physiological levels induces a decreased proliferative response.

II. FREE RADICAL GENERATION

Free radicals are chemical species with a single unpaired electron. The unpaired electron is highly reactive as it seeks to pair with another free electron; this results in the production of another free radical. The newly produced free radical is unstable in most cases and, as a result, it can also react with another molecule to produce yet another free radical. Thus, a chain reaction of free radicals can occur, leading to more and more damaging reactions. The majority of free radicals that damage biological systems are oxygen radicals and other reactive oxygen species, which are by-products formed in the cells of aerobic organisms. There are several sites of ROS production: mitochondrial electron transport, peroxisomal fatty acid, cytochrome P-450, and phagocytic cells.

A. ROS Generation in the Mitochondria

Mitochondria are the main source of ROS [11, 12]. The generation of mitochondrial ROS is a consequence of oxidative phosphorylation, a process that occurs in the inner mitochondrial membrane and involves the oxidation of NADH to produce energy. This energy is then used to phosphorylate ADP. Mitochondrial electron transport involves four-electron reduction of O_2 to H_2O: NADH and succinate donate electrons respectively to complex I (NADH dehydrogenase) and complex II (succinate dehydrogenase) of the mitochondrial electron transport chain. Coenzyme Q accepts electrons from Complexes I and II, and next donates electrons to cytochrome b in complex III (ubiquinone-cytochrome c reductase). In complex III, the electrons are donated to cytochrome c1, and so to cytochrome c, to complex IV (cytochrome c oxidase), which finally reduces O_2 to H_2O. However, during mitochondrial electron transport, a one-electron reduction of O_2 results in $O_2^{-\bullet}$. Studies on isolated mitochondria in the presence of a high, nonphysiological concentration of oxygen estimated that mitochondria convert 1 to 2% of the oxygen molecules consumed into $O_2^{-\bullet}$ [13], but subsequent investigations under more physiological conditions reduced this value to 0.2% [14, 15]. Superoxide anion is detoxified by the mitochondrial mangansese (Mn) superoxide dismutase (MnSOD) to yield hydrogen peroxide (H_2O_2), and the H_2O_2 is then converted to H_2O by catalase. H_2O_2 in the presence of reduced transition metals can also be converted to hydroxyl radical (OH^-). Each of these by-products is a potential source of oxidative damage to the mitochondria, cellular proteins, lipids, and nucleic acids.

B.   NONMITOCHONDRIAL GENERATION OF ROS

A second source of oxygen radicals is peroxisomal β-oxidation of fatty acids, which generates H_2O_2 as a by-product. Peroxisomes are organelles responsible for degrading fatty acids as well as other molecules [12]. Peroxisomes possess a high concentration of catalase, so whether or not leakage of H_2O_2 from peroxisomes contributes significantly to cytosolic oxidative stress under normal circumstances is still unclear. Phagocytic cells are another important source of oxidants; these cells defend the central nervous system against invading microorganisms and clear the debris from damaged cells by an oxidative burst of nitric oxide, H_2O_2, and O_2^-. Finally, cytochrome P450 enzymes in animals are one of the first defenses against natural toxic chemicals from plants.

III.   OXIDATIVE STRESS IN THE AGING BRAIN

A.   MITOCHONDRIAL CHANGES

In the aging brain, as well as in the case of several neurodegenerative diseases, there is a decline in the normal antioxidant defense mechanisms, which increases the vulnerability of the brain to the deleterious effects of oxidative damage [16]. The antioxidant enzymes SOD, catalase, glutathione peroxidase and glutathione reductase, for example, display reduced activities in the brains of patients with Alzheimer's disease [17, 18]. It is believed that free radicals of mitochondrial origin are among the primary causes of mitochondrial DNA (mtDNA) damage. Several studies have found increased levels of 8-hydroxy-2'-deoxyguanosine (8-OHdG), a biomarker of oxidative DNA damage, in mtDNA in the aged brain [19, 20]. High levels of 8-OHdG have been found in both nuclear DNA (nDNA) and in mtDNA of the post mortem brains of aged subjects [21]. Other studies have shown that the age-related increase in oxidative damage to mitochondrial DNA is greater than the oxidative damage that occurs to nuclear DNA in rodents [20, 22]. For example, oxidative DNA damage has been detected in human brain mitochondrial DNA and in rat liver at levels more than 10 times higher than in nuclear DNA from the same tissue [19]. This higher susceptibility of mtDNA to oxidative damage may be due to a lack of mtDNA repair mechanisms, a lack of protection by histone proteins, as well as the fact that mtDNA is located close to the inner mitochondrial membrane where reactive oxygen species are generated [21, 23]. In agreement with the mitochondrial free radical theory of aging, an inverse correlation has been shown between the levels of oxidative damage to mtDNA and maximum longevity [24] in both the heart and the brain: slowly aging mammals exhibit lower mtDNA damage than those who age faster. In contrast, this correlation is not associated with nuclear DNA. Mitochondrial DNA has a very high mutation rate; and when a mutation occurs, cells initially contain a combination of wild-type and mutant mtDNAs. During cell division, both types of mtDNA are randomly distributed into the offspring cells. Over many generations, the mtDNA genotype of a cellular lineage can move toward predominantly mutant or wild-type mtDNAs. As the percentage of mutant mtDNA increases, the cellular energy capacity decreases until it falls below the bioenergetic threshold

— the minimum energy output necessary for a cell or tissue to function normally. Damage to mtDNA is often accompanied by an increased level of DNA mutations and deletions [25, 26]. Several studies have shown that oxidative-induced mutations in mtDNA accumulate with age in postmitotic tissues such as the brain [27–29]. Several age-related disorders have been shown to be associated with high levels of mtDNA mutations. For example, elevated levels of cortical mtDNA deletions have been found in patients with Alzheimer's disease [30, 31]. Ikebe et al. [32] found 17 times the level of mtDNA deletion in the striatum of Parkinson's disease patients when compared with control subjects. Increasing evidence indicates that accumulation of oxidation of DNA, lipid, and protein by free radicals is responsible for the functional decrease in the aged brain.

B.   MEMBRANE COMPOSITION AND LIPID DAMAGE

Aging also is accompanied by changes in membrane fatty acid composition, including a decrease in the levels of polyunsaturated fatty acids (PUFAs) and an increase in monosaturated fatty acids. PUFAs, such as arachidonic acid (AA), are abundant in the aging brain and are highly susceptible to free radical attack. A correlation between the concentration of AA and long-term potentiation has been shown [33, 34], suggesting that oxidative depletion of AA levels may relate to a cognitive deficit in rats. For example, levels of AA are decreased in the hippocampus of aged rats with impaired ability to sustain long-term potentiation. Oxidative damage to lipids can also occur indirectly through the production of highly reactive aldehydes. Peroxidation of AA forms malondialdehyde (MDA), which induces DNA damage by reacting with amino acids in protein to form adducts that disrupt DNA base-pairing. Increased levels of MDA have been found in the aged canine brain [35]. In the aged human brain, increased levels of MDA have been found in inferior temporal cortex and in the cytoplasm of neurons and astrocytes [36], as well as in the hippocampus and cerebellum of aged rodents [37, 38]. Peroxidation of linoleic acid forms 4-hydroxy-2-nonenal (HNE). HNE is more stable than free radicals and it is able to migrate to sites that are distant from its formation, resulting in greater damage. The most damaging effect of HNE is its ability to form covalent adducts with histidine, lysine, and cysteine residues in proteins, enabling a modification in their activity [39]. It has been shown that the HNE-modified proteins, along with neurofibrillary tangles, are present in the senile plaques in aged dogs [40]. Increased levels of HNE have also been found in Alzheimer's and Parkinson's disease [41, 42]. These findings support the hypothesis that lipid peroxidation contributes to the deterioration of central nervous system (CNS) function.

C.   PROTEIN OXIDATION

Most of the studies conducted to assess the role of protein oxidation in aging brains conclude that there is an increase in oxidized proteins. An increase in the oxidation of mitochondrial proteins with age has been demonstrated by measuring the levels of protein carbonyl groups in the human cerebral cortex along with age [43]. Carbonyl formation can occur through a variety of mechanisms, including direct oxidation of amino acid side chains and oxidation-induced peptide cleavage. Increasing evidence suggests that protein oxidation may be responsible for the gradual decline in physiological functioning that accompanies aging. Elevated protein carbonyls have been shown to be present in the hippocampus of aged rats with memory impairment [44]. Increased protein carbonyl levels were found in the frontal and occipital cortex of aged humans [43] and rats [45, 46]. Measuring protein 3-nitrotyrosine (3-NT) levels is another way to assess the oxidative modification of proteins. Increased 3-NT levels have been identified in the hippocampus and the cerebral cortex of aged animals as well as in the CSF of aged human and in the white matter of aging monkeys [47–49]. 3-NT immunoreactivity has been observed in the cerebellum in the Purkinje cell layer, the molecular layer, and in the cerebellar nuclei of aged rats [50]. However, contradictory findings of decreased protein 3-NT levels of brain homogenate were reported in aged Wistar rats. Recently, proteomics studies enabled the identification of specific proteins that undergo oxidative stress in AD patients [51, 52].

D.   OXIDATIVE STRESS AND CHRONIC INFLAMMATION

Increasing evidence associates aging and age-related diseases with inflammation [53–55]. The key cellular event signaling ongoing inflammation in the brain is the accumulation of reactive microglia in the degenerative areas [56, 57]. Microglia are the resident immune cells of the central nervous system; they constitutively express surface receptors that trigger or amplify the innate immune response. These include complement receptors, cytokine receptors, chemokine receptors, major histocompatibility complex II, and others [58]. In the case of cellular damage, they respond promptly by inducing a protective immune response, which consists of a transient upregulation of inflammatory molecules as well as neurotrophic factors [59]. This innate immune response usually resolves potential pathogenic conditions. However, when chronic inflammation occurs, prolonged activation of microglia triggers a release of a wide array of neurotoxic products [60] and proinflammatory cytokines such as interleukin-1 (IL-1β), interleukin-6 (IL-6), tumor necrosis factor alpha (TNFα), and many others. Elevated protein levels of IL-1β, TNFα, and IL-6 have been found in the brains of aged animals [37, 61, 62]. Animal studies have shown that increased levels of IL-6 in the hippocampus and cerebral cortex are primarily from microglia [55]. It has been proposed that the increase in brain microglial activation may be one of the early events that leads to oxidative damage. Activated microglia are indeed the most abundant source of free radicals in the brain and release radicals such as superoxide and nitric oxide [63]. Microglia-derived radicals, as well as their reaction products hydrogen peroxide and peroxynitrite, can harm cells and these products have been shown to be involved in oxidative damage and neuronal cell death in neurological diseases [64]. It also should be noted that microglial cells have efficient antioxidative defense mechanisms. These cells contain high concentrations of glutathione, the antioxidative SOD enzymes, catalase, glutathione peroxidase, and glutathione reductase, as well as NADPH-regenerating enzymes [64]. When the production of ROS is prolonged, the endogenous reserves of antioxidants become exhausted and result in cell damage (Figure 15.1).

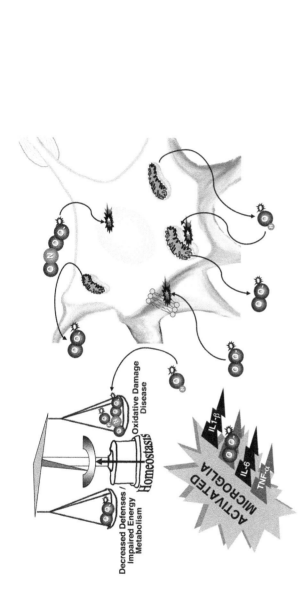

FIGURE 15.1 Oxidative stress and inflammation are two processes that go hand in hand during the aging process and in neurodegeneration and disease. There are at least two major sources for reactive oxygen species (ROS) in the CNS: the mitochondrion and the microglia. ROS are produced as a result of normal production of energy by the mitochondrion and are part of the natural defense system of the microglia to kill invading microorganisms. Under normal conditions, there is a balance of production of ROS, and homeostasis exists where energy metabolism is at the appropriate level in the mitochondrion and the microglia are either at rest, because there is no infection, or are responding normally to an injury or infection. ROS are essential for the normal function of the cell, and underproduction of ROS would lead to a decrease in energy production and a decrease in the ability of microglia to mount a defense against invading organisms. The other end of the spectrum appears to be the situation in the aging brain where increased ROS produced from the mitochondrion and the microglia can lead to damage to lipids, DNA, and proteins. This leads to a functional decline in neurons, such as changes in neurotransmitter receptor signal transduction. The microglia also produce pro-inflammatory cytokines, such as Il-1β, TNFα, and IL-5, that provide positive feedback to keep the inflammation cycle active. The rise in ROS may also act as a stressor that activates redox-sensitive signaling pathways. Thus, once activated, these diverse signaling pathways can continue to have damaging effects, leading the neurodegeneration and disease.

E.   ANTIOXIDANT DEFENSE MECHANISMS

Several antioxidant defense mechanisms have evolved to protect cell components from the attack of oxidative stress and associated oxidative damage. These mechanisms include antioxidant enzymes, such as SOD, superoxide reductases, catalase, glutathione peroxidases (Gpx), and many heat-shock proteins. The enzymes catalase and SOD are the major defenses against ROS. SOD converts superoxide anions into H_2O_2, and catalase converts H_2O_2 to molecular oxygen and water. SOD exists in two forms: Cu/ZnSOD is present primarily in the cytoplasm while MnSOD is present primarily in the mitochondria.

The hypothesis that lifespan can be enhanced by increasing antioxidant defenses has been controversial because of conflicting results in several aging models. For example, many studies have shown that endogenous levels of antioxidant enzymes in the brain and other tissues do not decrease during aging [65, 66]. Moreover, studies in mammals in which levels of antioxidants are experimentally increased have shown that maximum longevity is not affected [67, 68]. Experiments with *Drosophila melanogaster* have shown that overexpression of MnSOD increased lifespan [69], while overexpression of CuZn-SOD had only minor incremental effects on lifespan [70]. Similarly, enhanced levels of catalase (up to 80%) did not prolong the lifespan of flies, nor did it provide improved protection against oxidative stress induced by hyperoxia or paraquat treatment [71]. In contrast, the simultaneous overexpression of CuZn-SOD and catalase was found to extend and slow down various age-related biochemical and functional alterations in *Drosophila* [72]. Similarly, *Drosophila* selected for longevity and *Caenorhabditis elegans* with the *age-1* mutation (a mutation associated with increased lifespan), were found to have increased activity of CuZn-SOD and catalase [73–75]. These conflicting results suggest that an optimal balance between SOD and catalase is important for lowering the levels of oxidative stress and increasing lifespan. The effect of overexpression of SOD on lifespan has also been observed in mice [76]. Although several studies have shown that elevated CuZN-SOD induced protection against oxidative stress, other reports did not find a correlation between such protection and increased lifespan. For example, homozygous transgenic mice with a two to fivefold increase of CuZN-SOD showed only a small increase in lifespan [77].

IV.   EXPERIMENTAL CONTROL OF OXIDATIVE STRESS PATHWAYS

A.   GENETIC MANIPULATIONS

Work with *Drosophila*, yeast cells, *Neurospora* (a type of fungus), and the nematode *Caenorhabditis elegans* has established a genetic link between stress responsiveness and lifespan. For example, when exposed to a low-energy environment, *C. elegans* converts to its dauer state in which reproductive function is arrested. During this state, this organism is more resistant to stress. *C. elegans* mutations have been reported to extend life expectancy by 40% to more than 100%. The first of these mutations to be discovered involved the *age-1* gene; mutations in this gene have been shown to increase longevity by about 100% but do not affect reproduction or movement. Biochemical studies have revealed that strains carrying *age-1* alleles have enhanced oxidative defenses. For example, when the wild-type and *age-1* strains were examined for resistance to H_2O_2 exposure, the 50% effective lethal dose (LD_{50}) of the wild type remained constant over the lifespan whereas the LD_{50} of the *age-1* strain increased with aging [75]. Moreover, the increased resistance to oxidative stress was associated with elevated antioxidant activity, as shown by an increase in the activity of SOD and catalase [78]. A variety of other life-extending mutations that are correlated with enhanced stress tolerance have been described.

There are a number of mutated genes that regulate the insulin/insulin growth factor 1 (IGF-1) signaling pathway. *Age-1, daf-2,* and *daf-16* genes in *C. elegans* are associated with an insulin-like signaling pathway. *Age-1* and *daf-2* suppress the activity of the downstream target *daf-16*, a transcription factor that belongs to the Forkhead family of proteases [79]. Hence, loss of function of either of these upstream regulators enhances *daf-16* function and leads to increased lifespan. Importantly, loss-of-function mutations in *daf-16* not only prevents longevity conferred by the *age-1* and *daf-2 mutations*, but also abolishes stress resistance [80], thereby strengthening the intimate link between longevity and the stress responsiveness associated pathway. These animals are smaller in size, and have a decreased body temperature and a modest increase in antioxidant capacity. Recent studies have shown that knockout mice for the IGF receptor live longer and display greater resistance to oxidative stress [81, 82].

One additional long-lived mutant strain of *C. elegans,* which provides an important link between metabolism, oxidants, and aging, is *clk-1. Clk-1* lacks an enzyme required for the synthesis of ubiquinone, or coenzyme Q [83]. Coenzyme Q is an important electron acceptor for both complex I- and complex II-dependent respiration. Overexpression of *clk-1* leads to a reduction in lifespan [84], probably by increasing the rate of metabolism, which in turn might lead to a faster accumulation of damage resulting from metabolic by-products such as ROS. Another mutant with reduced longevity is *mev-1. Mev-1* encodes a subunit of the enzyme succinate dehydrogenase cytochrome b, a component of complex II of the mitochondrial electron transport chain. These animals show hypersensitivity to hyperoxia, and have compromised mitochondrial function and increased ROS generation [85]. SOD activity is about half that found in the wild type, and the average lifespan is reduced by approximately 35% [86]. These worms also were shown to exhibit increased levels of nuclear DNA damage [87]. Similarly, mice heterozygous for SOD2 have an increased incidence of nDNA as well as a significant increase in tumor formation. Another interesting mutation affecting longevity involves the p66shc gene. The p66shc protein belongs to a family of adaptor proteins that regulate protein-protein interaction for several cell surface receptors. These mice live 30% longer than control mice and also have an increased resistance to oxidative stress [88].

Links between longevity and stress resistance, similar to those demonstrated in *C. elegans,* also exist in *Drosophila melanogaster.* Various strains of flies selected for extended lifespan display increased resistance to oxidative stress that in some cases is correlated with enhanced activity of antioxidant enzymes. Methuselah (*mth*), a long-lived mutant, encodes a G protein-coupled receptor that is thought to play a role in signal transduction [89]. This mutant not only enhances longevity, but also increases resistance to heat stress and paraquat (an intracellular ROS generator). *Mth* exhibits a 35% increase in average lifespan and is resistant to several stressors, such as oxidants, starvation, and heat [89]. Another *Drosophila* mutant, *Indy,* belongs to a family of proteins involved in the Krebs cycle. This mutant shows a 50% increase in lifespan [90].

Several groups have been developing animal models with mitochondria deficiencies [91–93]. These models include the adenine nucleotide translocator (ANT-1), mitochondria superoxide dismutase- (SOD2-) deficient mice, Tfam-deficient mice, and the PolgA. ANT-1- deficient mice are a model for chronic ATP deficiency. These mice have increased production of ROS and hydrogen peroxide and a parallel increase in mtDNA mutations consistent with levels seen in much older mice [94]. SOD2-deficient mice die in the neonatal period from dilated cardiomyopathy or neonatal degeneration in the brain stem [92, 93]. The Tfam-deficient mice exhibit cytochrome *c* oxidase deficiency and die at around 3 weeks of age [95]. PolgA is a more recent mouse model, independently developed by two groups [29, 96], that expresses a deficient version of the nucleus-encoded catalytic subunit of mtDNA polymerase. These mice develop a mtDNA mutator phenotype with a three- to fivefold increase in levels of mtDNA point mutations, as well as an increase in the amount of deleted DNA. This increase in mtDNA is associated with a premature onset of aging-related phenotypes, including osteoporosis, alopecia, kuphosis, and a median survival of 48 weeks of age and a maximum survival of 61 weeks. Interestingly, these mice do not show an increase in oxidative damage markers [96, 97]. One possible explanation for the decreased longevity in these mice is an increase in markers of apoptosis, suggesting a possible decline in regenerative capacity of tissues in these mice [96, 97].

B.   CALORIC RESTRICTION

Caloric restriction is the only reproducible experimental manipulation for extending lifespan in many species. Restriction of food intake by 30 to 50% below *ad libitum* levels during the early growth phase of life has been shown to produce significant increases in the mean lifespan of several species, including insects, mice, fish, and rats [98]. Moreover, calorically restricted rhesus monkeys showed physiological changes similar to those observed in rodents on a calorie-restricted diet. Both calorically restricted monkeys and rats are smaller, mature later, have lower blood glucose and insulin levels, lower body temperature, and increased daytime activity [99]. Although several theories have been proposed to explain the anti-aging effects of caloric restriction, one hypothesis proposes that it acts by decreasing oxidative stress. In support of this hypothesis, it has been shown that caloric restriction can stabilize mitochondrial function and reduce oxidative stress in brain cells [100]. In the same study, the authors showed that the reduction in ROS production is not due to reduced mitochondria oxygen consumption, but rather to a lower percentage release of ROS per total flow in the respiratory chain [100]. It has been shown that caloric restriction decreases H_2O_2 in rat heart mitochondria. On the other hand, contradictory results have been obtained on the effect of caloric restriction on the expression of the antioxidant enzymes SOD, catalase, and GSH-peroxidase. In particular, some reports have shown that caloric restriction did not increase antioxidant defenses, while other studies demonstrated that the activity of SOD, catalase, and GSH was increased in older ages [101, 102]. Caloric restriction also prevents many of the changes in gene expression and transcription-factor activity that normally occur with aging, including basal elevations in expression of heat-shock proteins. Caloric restriction can also induce the expression of neurotrophic factors, such as brain-derived neurotrophic factor (BDNF). Increased levels of BDNF have been found in neurons in the hippocampus and other brain regions of rodents maintained on caloric restriction [103]. Given all the positive effects of caloric restriction, one could assume that this translates to an improvement in cognition in animals with caloric restriction; however, the data are mixed on this aspect of behavior; although some reports have found positive benefits [104–106], others have found either only small benefits or no benefits at all [107, 108]. Mixed benefits have also been reported on motor behaviors; improvements were noted on some motor learning tasks and complex locomotor behaviors [107, 109] but negative effects of caloric restriction were observed when testing some aspects of drug-induced rotational behavior and stereotopy [110].

Although caloric restriction is a reproducible way to increase the functional and maximal lifespan, it is questionable whether humans will choose to adopt this lifestyle change and it is still controversial whether caloric restriction will increase lifespan in nonhuman and human primates [111]. There is now accumulating evidence that selection of appropriate whole foods or the addition of antioxidants into the diet is beneficial to increasing the functional lifespan, if not the maximal lifespan (for a review, see [112]). One could then argue that caloric selection may be as important as caloric restriction.

V.   SUPPLEMENTARY ANTIOXIDANTS AS APPROACHES TO IMPROVE BRAIN HEALTH

A.   VITAMIN E

Vitamin E (Vit E) is the most studied antioxidant supplement and has been shown to increase longevity in short-lived species such as *C. elegans* and the rotifer *Asplanchna brightwelli* [113, 114]. There is little evidence that it increases maximum lifespan in rodents [115, 116] but evidence for an improvement in functional lifespan (i.e., improvements in aspects of physiology and brain health) is more compelling. For example, Vit E administered to rodents can improve age-related impairments in LTP [117] and improve cognitive behaviors [118, 119]. Vit E has also been shown to have actions that can prevent neurodegenerative disease in animal models and in *in vitro* studies. For example, Vit E is neuroprotective in apoE-deficient mice [120] and modifies Aβ toxicity in cultured hippocampal neurons [121]. The prevention of Aβ toxicity *in vivo* has also been observed [122]. In that study, Vit E prevented the onset of behavioral deficits induced by infusions of Aβ into the cerebroventricles. However, the data in humans are less convincing; clinical prevention trials using Vit E did not demonstrate improvements in cognition in AD patients, although some improvement in living performance was noted [123, 124]. Epidemiological studies have not always shown a positive link between increased intake of Vit E and decreased incidence of AD, Parkinson's disease or cerebrovascular disease [125,126]. Some studies have noted a correlation between dietary intake of foods high in Vitamin E, such as nuts, or diets high in fruits and vegetables and a decreased incidence of these diseases [127], suggesting that perhaps whole food sources of antioxidants and other phytochemicals may be of benefit.

B.   PHYTOCHEMICALS AND POLYPHENOLIC COMPOUNDS

Fruits, vegetables, nuts, and other whole foods, such as blue-green algae, contain thousands of phytochemicals, including polyphenolic compounds that express antioxidant activity and anti-inflammatory compounds [106, 128–130]. Some of these foods, such as the blue-green algae, also contain omega fatty acids, including gamma-linolenic acid (GLA), that can act to reduce lipid peroxidation and also reduce inflammation. Nature has packaged a wide array of phytochemicals that likely act in synergy to promote health. The area of nutritional neuroscience is growing quickly and there are many studies on the effects of whole foods and herbs as neuroprotective agents.

Green tea has been widely studied, with particular interest in one of the polyphenolic components, (−)-epigallocatechin-3 gallate (EGCG). EGCG has been extensively researched for its anticarcinogenic effects [131, 132]; however, it has also been shown to have actions that inhibit pro-inflammatory cytokines [133, 134]. The green tea catechin EGCG has been examined for activity in Alzheimer's disease. EGCG has been shown to reduce amyloid precursor protein cleavage that produces Aβ in primary neurons derived from Swedish mutant APP-overexpressing mice. When EGCG is given to these Tg APP$_{sw}$2576 mice, there is a reduction in amyloid load in the brain [133]. EGCG also protects against Aβ toxicity in cell cultures, an action that is likely related to its antioxidant activity [136]. Other phytochemicals that have been studied for potential activity in Alzheimer's disease include curcumin and other related flavones, as well as flavonoids such as quercitin [137–139]. Further, blueberries have also been shown to reduce amyloid load in an animal model of AD [140].

Foods such as blueberries, spinach, and spirulina, a blue-green algae with high oxygen radical absorbance capacity (ORAC = 320; [141]), have also been studied extensively for neuroprotective actions. For example, in the cerebellum there is a correlation between the loss of function of β-adrenergic receptors in the aged brain and a loss in the ability to learn complex motor skills [142]. Feeding aged F344 rats a diet rich in spinach improves cerebellar β-adrenergic receptor function and improves motor learning that is associated with a decrease in oxidized glutathione and the pro-inflammatory cytokine TNFα [143, 144]. Further studies have attempted to correlate the ability to improve cerebellar β-adrenergic receptor function with the *in vitro* antioxidant capacity of the foods added into the diet. For example, cucumber is very low in polyphenolic compounds and, when added to the diets of aged rats, produced no improvement in cerebellar β-adrenergic receptor function and no reduction in malondialdehyde or TNFα [141]. On the other hand, the addition of spirulina to the normal rat diet (0.1% w/w) significantly improved β-adrenergic receptor function, decreased malondialdehyde, and reduced pro-inflammatory cytokine levels [141]. Although correlations between reduced markers of oxidative stress and inflammation do not guarantee a causative relationship, there is increasing evidence from many studies supporting this hypothesis.

Blueberries and spirulina have also been shown to be neuroprotective in animal models of Parkinson's disease. In one study by Strömberg et al. [145], blueberries and spirulina both improved the recovery from a neurotoxic 6-hydroxydopamine (6-OHDA) lesion of dopamine projections to the striatum. In this study, there was a reduced lesion area 1 month following 6-OHDA administration; however, the lesion was similar in size to controls at 1 week following the neurotoxic insult, suggesting that what the dietary supplementation was doing was to improve the recovery and regeneration of the dopamine terminals in the striatum following the lesion, rather than preventing the initial damage. One mechanism by which this might occur is through an interaction with microglial activation in response to the injury. This study reports that 1 week following the injury, there was an increased microglial response to the injury. In this early period, the microglia are phagocytotic and aid in repairing the damage caused by the neurotoxic insult; the increased microglial response at this time may help to prepare the brain for regeneration of the dopamine fibers into the lesioned area (Figure 15.2). A second finding of this study was that microglial reaction to the injury continued to increase over time in the lesioned rats fed a control diet but was reduced at during later time points in rats fed the supplemented diet. This chronic phase of the microglial response may actually be detrimental; reducing this later phase of inflammation correlated with the smaller lesion size in the rats that consumed the supplemented diet. Green tea catechins have also been studied for their potential actions in Parkinson's disease. For example, EGCG attenuates 6-hydroxydopamine-induced cell death in neuronal cultures [146, 147].

Neuroprotection from ischemic brain damage is another area where nutritional and herbal approaches have been examined. Multiple epidemiological studies have shown a correlation between diets high in fruits and vegetables, and specifically, the Mediterranean diet, and a decreased risk of cardiovascular disease and stroke [148, 149]. This has also been examined in animal models. For example, a study by Wang and colleagues [150] reported that dietary supplementation with either blueberries, spinach, or spirulina for 1 month prior to a middle cerebral artery inclusion reduced the size of the damage. The most effective supplement in this study was spirulina, which reduced the infarction size by 70% when incorporated into the diet at 0.1% w/w. Blueberries and spinach reduced the infarct size by 50% when incorporated into the rat diet at 2% w/w (Figure 15.3). A study by Sweeney et al. [151] had shown that a much higher dose of blueberries prevented cell loss in the hippocampus following an ischemic event. It must be recognized, however, that all of these studies, when converted to human equivalents, are on the high side if converted to a nutraceutical dosage for optimal health. Perhaps a more interesting approach is to examine the synergy of nutrients to determine if there may be combinations of whole foods that will synergize to produce even more potent effects at maintaining optimal brain health and preventing neurodegenerative disease.

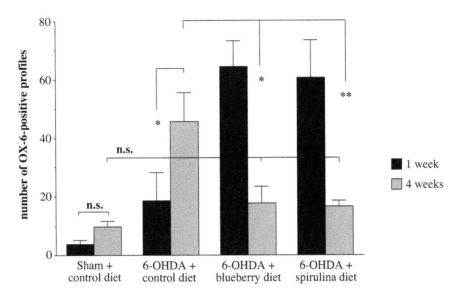

FIGURE 15.2 Bar graph depicting the number of OX-6 positive microglia in the striatum of rats following either sham of 6-hydroxydopamine (6-OHDA) lesions into the corpus striatum. This quantification of MHC class II receptors on microglia demonstrates that in rats treated with 6-OHDA and fed the control diet with normal levels of vitamins and minerals the inflammatory process continues to increase over the 4 weeks following the 6-OHDA insult. In rats that were fed the blueberry or spirulina diet prior to the insult, there was initially a much larger response to the 6-OHDA at 1 week; however, at 1 month following the insult, there was a significant reduction in the numbers of OX-6 positive microglia observed in the striatum. * = $p < 0.05$, $p < 0.01$, one-way ANOVA (see [143] for a full description).

VI. SUMMARY AND CONCLUSIONS

In closing, this chapter has summarized some of the literature that supports a role for oxidative stress as one aspect of age and disease that contributes to declines in function of the central nervous system. The free radical theory as proposed by Harmon in the mid-1950s was the catalyst for many studies into aspects of free radical metabolism and mitochondrial function that have shown links between oxidative stress, brain aging, and neurodegenerative disease. Interestingly, in recent years, the oxidative stress theory of aging has also come to include a role for inflammation. These two processes are interlinked and have many feedback loops such that separating the two processes is difficult. Many studies are now defining the critical mitochondrial and inflammatory pathway changes that underlie this increase in oxidative stress and inflammation with age. Genetic manipulations of many species have assisted in delineating the critical aspects of free radical metabolism that either induce premature aging or increase longevity. These genetic manipulations are not, however, applicable as interventions to improve brain health with age. There are two interventional strategies discussed in this chapter: (1) caloric restriction and (2) nutritional intervention. Caloric restriction is the most

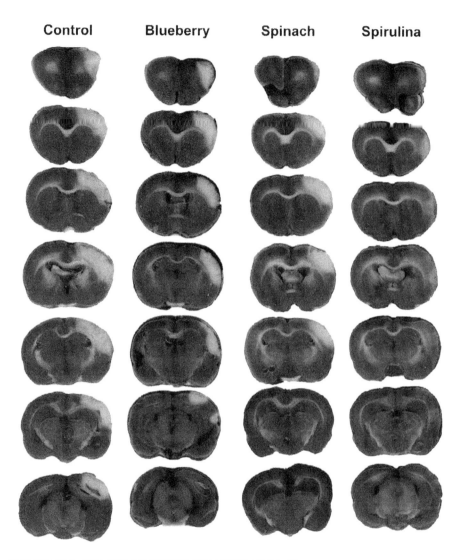

FIGURE 15.3 (SEE COLOR INSERT FOLLOWING PAGE 204) Pretreatment with either blueberry, spinach, or spirulina enriched diets significantly reduced the cortical infarction induced by middle cerebral artery occlusion/reperfusion. The right middle cerebral artery was ligated for 60 minutes. Animals were euthanized for TTC staining 48 hours after ischemia/reperfusion. Marked infarction (white areas) in the right cerebral cortex was found in animals receiving the control diet. Pretreatment with either blueberry, spinach, or spirulina significantly reduced the amount of infarction.

reproducible way to increase lifespan among many species and reduces many diseases associated with aging. But how many humans will comply with this rigorous lifestyle change? Antioxidants and polyphenolic compounds from fruits, vegetables, nuts, and grains decrease markers of oxidative damage, such as malondialdehyde and protein carbonyls, and decrease levels of pro-inflammatory cytokines either directly or indirectly by reducing oxidative damage. Epidemiological evidence supports that a diet high in fruits and vegetables may help prevent certain diseases of aging, including stroke, diabetes, Parkinson's disease, and Alzheimer's disease. So, your mother was right when she told you to eat your fruits and vegetables!

REFERENCES

1. Pearl, R., *The Rate of Living: Being an Account of Some Experimental Studies on the Biology of Life Duration*, A.A. Knopf, New York, 1928.
2. Holliday, R., *Understanding Ageing*, Cambridge University Press, New York, 1995.
3. Barja, G., Mitochondrial free radical production and aging in mammals and birds, *Ann. N.Y. Acad. Sci.*, 854, 224, 1998.
4. Barja, G., The quantitative measurement of H_2O_2 generation in isolated mitochondria, *J. Bioenerg. Biomembr.*, 34, 227, 2002.
5. Harman, D., Aging: a theory based on free radical and radiation chemistry, *J. Geront.*, 11, 289, 1956.
6. McCord, J.M. and Fridovich, I., Superoxide dismutase. An enzymic function for erythrocuprein (hemocuprein), *J. Biol. Chem.*, 244, 6049, 1969.
7. Harman, D., The biologic clock: the mitochondria? *J. Am. Geriatr. Soc.*, 20, 145, 1972.
8. Knapp, L.T. and Klann, E., Role of reactive oxygen species in hippocampal long-term potentiation: contributory or inhibitory? *J. Neurosci. Res.*, 70, 1, 2002.
9. Finkel, T., Oxygen radicals and signaling, *Curr. Opin. Cell Biol.*, 10, 248, 1998.
10. Poon, H.F. et al., Free radicals and brain aging, *Clin. Geriatr. Med.*, 20, 329, 2004.
11. Balaban, R.S., Nemoto, S., and Finkel, T., Mitochondria, oxidants, and aging, *Cell*, 120, 483, 2005.
12. Beckman, K.B. and Ames, B.N., The free radical theory of aging matures, *Physiol. Rev.*, 78, 547, 1998.
13. Chance, B., Sies, H., and Boveris, A., Hydroperoxide metabolism in mammalian organs, *Physiol. Rev.*, 59, 527, 1979.
14. Staniek, K. and Nohl, H., Are mitochondria a permanent source of reactive oxygen species? *Biochim. Biophys. Acta*, 1460, 268, 2000.
15. Aguilaniu, H. et al., Asymmetric inheritance of oxidatively damaged proteins during cytokinesis, *Science*, 299, 1751, 2003.
16. Finkel, T. and Holbrook, N.J., Oxidants, oxidative stress and the biology of ageing, *Nature*, 408, 239, 2000.
17. Zemlan, F.P., Thienhaus, O.J., and Bosmann, H.B., Superoxide dismutase activity in Alzheimer's disease: possible mechanism for paired helical filament formation, *Brain Res.*, 470, 160, 1989.
18. Pappolla, M.A. et al., Immunohistochemical evidence of oxidative stress in Alzheimer's disease, *Am. J. Pathol.*, 140, 621, 1992.
19. Richter, C., Park, J.W., and Ames, B.N., Normal oxidative damage to mitochondrial and nuclear DNA is extensive, *Proc. Natl. Acad. Sci. U.S.A.*, 85, 6465, 1988.
20. Agarwal, S. and Sohal, R.S., Aging and protein oxidative damage, *Mech. Ageing Dev.*, 75, 11, 1994.
21. Mecocci, P. et al., Oxidative damage to mitochondrial DNA shows marked age-dependent increases in human brain, *Ann. Neurol.*, 34, 609, 1993.

22. Ames, B.N., Shigenaga, M.K., and Hagen, T.M., Oxidants, antioxidants, and the degenerative diseases of aging, *Proc. Natl. Acad. Sci. U.S.A.,* 90, 7915, 1993.

23. Barja, G., Free radicals and aging, *Trends Neurosci.,* 27, 595, 2004.

24. Barja, G. and Herrero, A., Oxidative damage to mitochondrial DNA is inversely related to maximum life span in the heart and brain of mammals, *FASEB J.,* 14, 312, 2000.

25. Shigenaga, M.K. and Ames, B.N., Assays for 8-hydroxy-2'-deoxyguanosine: a biomarker of *in vivo* oxidative DNA damage, *Free Radic. Biol. Med.,* 10, 211, 1991.

26. Yoneda, M. et al., Oxygen stress induces an apoptotic cell death associated with fragmentation of mitochondrial genome, *Biochem. Biophys. Res. Commun.,* 209, 723, 1995.

27. Chomyn, A. and Attardi, G., MtDNA mutations in aging and apoptosis, *Biochem. Biophys. Res. Commun.,* 304, 519, 2003.

28. Kraytsberg, Y. et al., Mutation and intracellular clonal expansion of mitochondrial genomes: two synergistic components of the aging process? *Mech. Ageing Dev.,* 124, 49, 2003.

29. Trifunovic, A. et al., Premature ageing in mice expressing defective mitochondrial DNA polymerase, *Nature,* 429, 417, 2004.

30. Corral-Debrinski, M. et al., Marked changes in mitochondrial DNA deletion levels in Alzheimer brains, *Genomics,* 23, 471, 1994.

31. Horton, T.M. et al., Marked increase in mitochondrial DNA deletion levels in the cerebral cortex of Huntington's disease patients, *Neurology,* 45, 1879, 1995.

32. Ikebe, S. et al., Increase of deleted mitochondrial DNA in the striatum in Parkinson's disease and senescence, *Biochem. Biophys. Res. Commun.,* 170, 1044, 1990.

33. Lynch, M.A., Analysis of the mechanisms underlying the age-related impairment in long-term potentiation in the rat, *Rev. Neurosci.,* 9, 169, 1998.

34. Ulmann, L. et al., Brain and hippocampus fatty acid composition in phospholipid classes of aged-relative cognitive deficit rats, *Prostaglandins Leukot. Essent. Fatty Acids,* 64, 189, 2001.

35. Head, E. et al., Oxidative damage increases with age in a canine model of human brain aging, *J. Neurochem.,* 82, 375, 2002.

36. Dei, R. et al., Lipid peroxidation and advanced glycation end products in the brain in normal aging and in Alzheimer's disease, *Acta Neuropathol. (Berl.),* 104, 113, 2002.

37. Gemma, C. et al., Diets enriched in foods with high antioxidant activity reverse age-induced decreases in cerebellar beta-adrenergic function and increases in proinflammatory cytokines, *J. Neurosci.,* 22, 6114, 2002.

38. Cini, M. and Moretti, A., Studies on lipid peroxidation and protein oxidation in the aging brain, *Neurobiol. Aging,* 16, 53, 1995.

39. Butterfield, D.A. et al., Oxidatively induced structural alteration of glutamine synthetase assessed by analysis of spin label incorporation kinetics: relevance to Alzheimer's disease, *J. Neurochem.,* 68, 2451, 1997.

40. Papaioannou, N. et al., Immunohistochemical investigation of the brain of aged dogs. I. Detection of neurofibrillary tangles and of 4-hydroxynonenal protein, an oxidative damage product, in senile plaques, *Amyloid,* 8, 11, 2001.

41. Zarkovic, K., 4-Hydroxynonenal and neurodegenerative diseases, *Mol. Aspects Med.,* 24, 293, 2003.

42. Yoritaka, A. et al., Immunohistochemical detection of 4-hydroxynonenal protein adducts in Parkinson disease, *Proc. Natl. Acad. Sci. U.S.A.,* 93, 2696, 1996.

43. Smith, C.D. et al., Excess brain protein oxidation and enzyme dysfunction in normal aging and in Alzheimer disease, *Proc. Natl. Acad. Sci. U.S.A.,* 88, 10540, 1991.

44. Nicolle, M. M. et al., Signatures of hippocampal oxidative stress in aged spatial learning-impaired rodents, *Neuroscience*, 107, 415, 2001.

45. Aksenova, M.V. et al., Protein oxidation and enzyme activity decline in old brown Norway rats are reduced by dietary restriction, *Mech. Ageing Dev.*, 100, 157, 1998.

46. Cakatay, U. et al., Relation of oxidative protein damage and nitrotyrosine levels in the aging rat brain, *Exp. Gerontol.*, 36, 221, 2001.

47. Shin, C.M. et al., Age-related changes in the distribution of nitrotyrosine in the cerebral cortex and hippocampus of rats, *Brain Res.*, 931, 194, 2002.

48. Sloane, J.A. et al., Increased microglial activation and protein nitration in white matter of the aging monkey, *Neurobiol. Aging*, 20, 395, 1999.

49. Tohgi, H. et al., Remarkable increase in cerebrospinal fluid 3-nitrotyrosine in patients with sporadic amyotrophic lateral sclerosis, *Ann. Neurol.*, 46, 129, 1999.

50. Chung, Y.H. et al., Immunohistochemical study on the distribution of nitrotyrosine and neuronal nitric oxide synthase in aged rat cerebellum, *Brain Res.*, 951, 316, 2002.

51. Butterfield, D.A., Proteomics: a new approach to investigate oxidative stress in Alzheimer's disease brain, *Brain Res.*, 1000, 1, 2004.

52. Aldred, S., Grant, M.M., and Griffiths, H.R., The use of proteomics for the assessment of clinical samples in research, *Clin. Biochem.*, 37, 943, 2004.

53. Bodles, A.M. and Barger, S.W., Cytokines and the aging brain — what we don't know might help us, *Trends Neurosci.*, 27, 621, 2004.

54. Forsey, R.J. et al., Plasma cytokine profiles in elderly humans, *Mech. Ageing Dev.*, 124, 487, 2003.

55. Ye, S.M. and Johnson, R.W., Increased interleukin-6 expression by microglia from brain of aged mice, *J. Neuroimmunol.*, 93, 139, 1999.

56. David, J.P. et al., Glial reaction in the hippocampal formation is highly correlated with aging in human brain, *Neurosci. Lett.*, 235, 53, 1997.

57. Streit, W.J., Walter, S.A., and Pennell, N.A., Reactive microgliosis, *Prog. Neurobiol.*, 57, 563, 1999.

58. Aloisi, F., Immune function of microglia, *Glia*, 36, 165, 2001.

59. Batchelor, P.E. et al., Activated macrophages and microglia induce dopaminergic sprouting in the injured striatum and express brain-derived neurotrophic factor and glial cell line-derived neurotrophic factor, *J. Neurosci.*, 19, 1708, 1999.

60. Colton, C.A. and Gilbert, D.L., Production of superoxide anions by a CNS macrophage, the microglia, *FEBS Lett.*, 223, 284, 1987.

61. Terao, A. et al., Immune response gene expression increases in the aging murine hippocampus, *J. Neuroimmunol.*, 132, 99, 2002.

62. Weindruch, R. and Prolla, T.A., Gene expression profile of the aging brain, *Arch. Neurol.*, 59, 1712, 2002.

63. Chang, J.Y. and Liu, L.Z., Manganese potentiates nitric oxide production by microglia, *Brain Res. Mol. Brain Res.*, 68, 22, 1999.

64. Dringen, R., Oxidative and antioxidative potential of brain microglial cells, *Antioxid. Redox. Signal.*, 7, 1223, 2005.

65. Benzi, G. and Moretti, A., Age- and peroxidative stress-related modifications of the cerebral enzymatic activities linked to mitochondria and the glutathione system, *Free Radic. Biol. Med.*, 19, 77, 1995.

66. Barja, G., Aging in vertebrates, and the effect of caloric restriction: a mitochondrial free radical production-DNA damage mechanism?, *Biol. Rev. Camb. Philos. Soc.*, 79, 235, 2004.

67. Harris, S.B. et al., Dietary restriction alone and in combination with oral ethoxyquin/2-mercaptoethylamine in mice, *J. Gerontol.*, 45, B141, 1990.

68. Orr, W.C. et al., Effects of overexpression of copper-zinc and manganese superoxide dismutases, catalase, and thioredoxin reductase genes on longevity in *Drosophila melanogaster, J. Biol. Chem.,* 278, 26418, 2003.
69. Sun, J. et al., Induced overexpression of mitochondrial Mn-superoxide dismutase extends the life span of adult *Drosophila melanogaster, Genetics,* 161, 661, 2002.
70. Orr, W.C. and Sohal, R.S., Effects of Cu-Zn superoxide dismutase overexpression of life span and resistance to oxidative stress in transgenic *Drosophila melanogaster, Arch. Biochem. Biophys.,* 301, 34, 1993.
71. Orr, W.C. and Sohal, R.S., The effects of catalase gene overexpression on life span and resistance to oxidative stress in transgenic *Drosophila melanogaster, Arch. Biochem. Biophys.,* 297, 35, 1992.
72. Orr, W.C. and Sohal, R.S., Extension of life-span by overexpression of superoxide dismutase and catalase in *Drosophila melanogaster, Science,* 263, 1128, 1994.
73. Dudas, S.P. and Arking, R., A coordinate upregulation of antioxidant gene activities is associated with the delayed onset of senescence in a long-lived strain of *Drosophila, J. Gerontol. A Biol. Sci. Med. Sci.,* 50, B117, 1995.
74. Hari, R., Burde, V., and Arking, R., Immunological confirmation of elevated levels of CuZn superoxide dismutase protein in an artificially selected long-lived strain of *Drosophila melanogaster, Exp. Gerontol.,* 33, 227, 1998.
75. Larsen, P.L., Aging and resistance to oxidative damage in *Caenorhabditis elegans, Proc. Natl. Acad. Sci. U.S.A.,* 90, 8905, 1993.
76. Li, Y. et al., Dilated cardiomyopathy and neonatal lethality in mutant mice lacking manganese superoxide dismutase, *Nat. Genet.,* 11, 376, 1995.
77. Huang, T.T. et al., Ubiquitous overexpression of CuZn superoxide dismutase does not extend life span in mice, *J. Gerontol. A Biol. Sci. Med. Sci.,* 55, B5, 2000.
78. Vanfleteren, J.R., Oxidative stress and ageing in *Caenorhabditis elegans, Biochem. J.,* 292, 605, 1993.
79. Lin, K. et al., daf-16: an HNF-3/forkhead family member that can function to double the life-span of *Caenorhabditis elegans, Science,* 278, 1319, 1997.
80. Murakami, S. and Johnson, T.E., A genetic pathway conferring life extension and resistance to UV stress in *Caenorhabditis elegans, Genetics,* 143, 1207, 1996.
81. Tatar, M. et al., A mutant *Drosophila* insulin receptor homolog that extends life-span and impairs neuroendocrine function, *Science,* 292, 107, 2001.
82. Holzenberger, M. et al., IGF-1 receptor regulates lifespan and resistance to oxidative stress in mice, *Nature,* 421, 182, 2003.
83. Ewbank, J.J. et al., Structural and functional conservation of the *Caenorhabditis elegans* timing gene clk-1, *Science,* 275, 980, 1997.
84. Branicky, R., Benard, C., and Hekimi, S., clk-1, mitochondria, and physiological rates, *Bioessays,* 22, 48, 2000.
85. Senoo-Matsuda, N. et al., A defect in the cytochrome b large subunit in complex II causes both superoxide anion overproduction and abnormal energy metabolism in *Caenorhabditis elegans, J. Biol. Chem.,* 276, 41553, 2001.
86. Ishii, N. et al., A methyl viologen-sensitive mutant of the nematode *Caenorhabditis elegans, Mutat. Res.,* 237, 165, 1990.
87. Hartman, P. et al., Mitochondrial oxidative stress can lead to nuclear hypermutability, *Mech. Ageing Dev.,* 125, 417, 2004.
88. Migliaccio, E. et al., The p66shc adaptor protein controls oxidative stress response and life span in mammals, *Nature,* 402, 309, 1999.
89. Lin, Y.J., Scroude, L., and Benzer, S., Extended life-span and stress resistance in the *Drosophila* mutant *methuselah, Science,* 282, 943, 1998.

90. Rogina, B. et al., Extended life-span conferred by cotransporter gene mutations in *Drosophila, Science,* 290, 2137, 2000.
91. Wallace, D.C., Mitochondrial diseases in man and mouse, *Science,* 283, 1482, 1999.
92. Esposito, L.A. et al., Mitochondrial disease in mouse results in increased oxidative stress, *Proc. Natl. Acad. Sci. U.S.A.,* 96, 4820, 1999.
93. Melov, S., Coskun, P.E., and Wallace, D.C., Mouse models of mitochondrial disease, oxidative stress, and senescence, *Mutat. Res.,* 434, 233, 1999.
94. Bauer, M.K. et al., Adenine nucleotide translocase-1, a component of the permeability transition pore, can dominantly induce apoptosis, *J. Cell Biol.,* 147, 1493, 1999.
95. Silva, J.P. and Larsson, N.G., Manipulation of mitochondrial DNA gene expression in the mouse, *Biochim. Biophys. Acta,* 1555, 106, 2002.
96. Kujoth, G.C. et al., Mitochondrial DNA mutations, oxidative stress, and apoptosis in mammalian aging, *Science,* 309, 481, 2005.
97. Trifunovic A. et al., Somatic mtDNA mutations cause aging phenotypes without affecting reactive oxygen species production, *Proc. Natl. Acad. Sci. U.S.A.,* 102, 17993, 2005.
98. Masoro, E.J., Caloric restriction and aging: an update, *Exp. Gerontol.,* 35, 299, 2000.
99. Bodkin, N.L. et al., Mortality and morbidity in laboratory-maintained Rhesus monkeys and effects of long-term dietary restriction, *J. Gerontol. A Biol. Sci. Med. Sci.,* 58, 212, 2003.
100. Gredilla, R. et al., Caloric restriction decreases mitochondrial free radical generation at complex I and lowers oxidative damage to mitochondrial DNA in the rat heart, *FASEB J.,* 15, 1589, 2001.
101. Sohal, R.S. et al., Oxidative damage, mitochondrial oxidant generation and antioxidant defenses during aging and in response to food restriction in the mouse, *Mech. Ageing Dev.,* 74, 121, 1994.
102. Weindruch, R. et al., Microarray profiling of gene expression in aging and its alteration by caloric restriction in mice, *J. Nutr.,* 131, 918S, 2001.
103. Duan W., Guo Z., and Mattson M.P., Brain-derived neurotrophic factor mediates an excitoprotective effect of dietary restriction in mice, *J. Neurochem.,* 76, 629, 2001.
104. Beatty, W.W., Clouse, B.A., and Bierley, R.A., Effects of long-term restricted feeding on radial maze performance by aged rats, *Neurobiol. Aging,* 8, 325, 1987.
105. Stewart, J., Mitchell, J., and Kalant, N., The effects of life-long food restriction on spatial memory in young and aged Fischer 344 rats measured in the eight arm radial and the Morris water mazes, *Neurobiol. Aging,* 10, 669, 1989.
106. Macheix, J.-J, Fleuriet, A., and Billot, J., *Fruit Polyphenolics,* CRC Press, Boca Raton, FL, 1990.
107. Gould, T.J. et al., Effects of dietary restriction on motor learning and cerebellar noradrenergic dysfunction in aged F344 rats, *Brain Res.,* 684, 150, 1995.
108. Markowska, A.L., Life-long diet restriction failed to retard cognitive aging in Fischer-344 rats, *Neurobiol. Aging,* 20, 177, 1999.
109. Ingram, D.K. et al., Dietary restriction benefits learning and motor performance of aged mice, *J. Gerontol.,* 42, 78, 1987.
110. Joseph, J.A. et al., Life-long dietary restriction affects striatally-mediated behavioral responses in aged rats, *Neurobiol. Aging,* 4, 191, 1983.
111. Lane, M.A. et al., Effects of long-term diet restriction on aging and longevity in primates remain uncertain, *J. Gerontol. A Biol. Sci. Med. Sci.,* 59, 405, 2004.
112. Casadesus, G., Shukitt-Hale, B., and Joseph, J.A., Qualitative versus quantitative caloric intake: are they equivalent paths to successful aging? *Neurobiol. Aging,* 23, 747, 2002.

113. Harrington, L.A. and Harley, C.B., Effect of vitamin E on lifespan and reproduction in *Caenorhabditis elegans*, *Mech. Ageing Dev.*, 43, 71, 1988.

114. Sawada, M. and Enesco, H.E., Vitamin E extends lifespan in the short-lived rotifer *Asplanchna brightwelli*, *Exp. Gerontol.*, 19, 179, 1984.

115. Morley, A.A. and Trainor, K.J., Lack of an effect of vitamin E on lifespan of mice, *Biogerontology*, 2, 109, 2001.

116. Blackett, A.D. and Hall, D.A., Vitamin E — its significance in mouse ageing, *Age. Ageing*, 10, 191, 1981.

117. Murray, C.A. and Lynch, M.A., Dietary supplementation with vitamin E reverses the age-related deficit in long term potentiation in dentate gyrus, *J. Biol. Chem.*, 273, 12161, 1998.

118. Joseph, J.A. et al., Reversals of age-related declines in neuronal signal transduction, cognitive, and motor behavioral deficits with blueberry, spinach, or strawberry dietary supplementation, *J. Neurosci.*, 19, 8114, 1999.

119. Joseph, J.A. et al., Long-term dietary strawberry, spinach, or vitamin E supplementation retards the onset of age-related neuronal signal-transduction and cognitive behavioral deficits, *J. Neurosci.*, 18, 8047, 1998.

120. Veinbergs, I. et al., Role of apolipoprotein E receptors in regulating the differential *in vivo* neurotrophic effects of apolipoprotein E, *Exp. Neurol.*, 170, 15, 2001.

121. Butterfield, D.A. et al., Vitamin E as an antioxidant/free radical scavenger against amyloid beta-peptide-induced oxidative stress in neocortical synaptosomal membranes and hippocampal neurons in culture: insights into Alzheimer's disease, *Rev. Neurosci.*, 10, 141, 1999.

122. Yamada, K. et al., Protective effects of idebenone and alpha-tocopherol on beta-amyloid-(1-42)-induced learning and memory deficits in rats: implication of oxidative stress in beta-amyloid-induced neurotoxicity *in vivo*, *Eur. J. Neurosci.*, 11, 83, 1999.

123. Sano, M. et al., A controlled trial of selegiline, alpha-tocopherol, or both as treatment for Alzheimer's disease. The Alzheimer's Disease Cooperative Study [see comments], *N. Engl. J. Med.*, 336, 1216, 1997.

124. Sano, M. et al., Rationale and design of a multicenter study of selegiline and alpha-tocopherol in the treatment of Alzheimer disease using novel clinical outcomes. Alzheimer's Disease Cooperative Study., *Alzheimer Dis. Assoc. Disord.*, 10, 132, 1996.

125. Lonn, E. et al., Effects of long-term vitamin E supplementation on cardiovascular events and cancer: a randomized controlled trial, *JAMA*, 293, 1338, 2005.

126. Lee, I.M. et al., Vitamin E in the primary prevention of cardiovascular disease and cancer: the Women's Health Study: a randomized controlled trial, *JAMA*, 294, 56, 2005.

127. Zhang, S.M. et al., Intakes of vitamins E and C, carotenoids, vitamin supplements, and PD risk, *Neurology*, 59, 1161, 2002.

128. Annapurna, V.V., Deosthale, Y.G., and Bamji, M.S., Spirulina as a source of vitamin A, *Plant Foods Hum. Nutr.*, 41, 125, 1991.

129. Careri, M. et al., Supercritical fluid extraction for liquid chromatographic determination of carotenoids in *Spirulina Pacifica* algae: a chemometric approach, *J. Chromatogr. A*, 912, 61, 2001.

130. Reddy, M.C. et al., C-phycocyanin, a selective cyclooxygenase-2 inhibitor, induces apoptosis in lipopolysaccharide-stimulated RAW 264.7 macrophages, *Biochem. Biophys. Res. Commun.*, 304, 385, 2003.

131. Lin, J.K. and Liang, Y.C., Cancer chemoprevention by tea polyphenols, *Proc. Natl. Sci. Counc. Repub. China B*, 24, 1, 2000.

132. Moyers, S.B. and Kumar, N.B., Green tea polyphenols and cancer chemoprevention: multiple mechanisms and endpoints for phase II trials, *Nutr. Rev.*, 62, 204, 2004.

133. Ahmed, S. et al., Green tea polyphenol epigallocatechin-3-gallate inhibits the IL-1 beta-induced activity and expression of cyclooxygenase-2 and nitric oxide synthase-2 in human chondrocytes, *Free Radic. Biol. Med.*, 33, 1097, 2002.

134. Han, M.K., Epigallocatechin gallate, a constituent of green tea, suppresses cytokine-induced pancreatic beta-cell damage, *Exp. Mol. Med.*, 35, 136, 2003.

135. Rezai-Zadeh, K. et al., Green tea epigallocatechin-3-gallate (EGCG) modulates amyloid precursor protein cleavage and reduces cerebral amyloidosis in Alzheimer transgenic mice, *J. Neurosci.*, 25, 8807, 2005.

136. Levites, Y. et al., Neuroprotection and neurorescue against Abeta toxicity and PKC-dependent release of nonamyloidogenic soluble precursor protein by green tea polyphenol (–)-epigallocatechin-3-gallate, *FASEB J.*, 17, 952, 2003.

137. Kim, H. et al., Effects of naturally occurring compounds on fibril formation and oxidative stress of beta-amyloid, *J. Agric. Food Chem.*, 53, 8537, 2005.

138. Ringman, J.M. et al., A potential role of the curry spice curcumin in Alzheimer's disease, *Curr. Alzheimer Res.*, 2, 131, 2005.

139. Frautschy, S.A. et al., Phenolic anti-inflammatory antioxidant reversal of Abeta-induced cognitive deficits and neuropathology, *Neurobiol. Aging*, 22, 993, 2001.

140. Joseph, J.A. et al., Blueberry supplementation enhances signaling and prevents behavioral deficits in an Alzheimer disease model, *Nutr. Neurosci.*, 6, 153, 2003.

141. Gemma, C. et al., Diets enriched in foods with high antioxidant activity reverse age-induced decreases in cerebellar beta-adrenergic function and increases in proinflammatory cytokines, *J. Neurosci.*, 22, 6114, 2002.

142. Bickford, P., Motor learning deficits in aged rats are correlated with loss of cerebellar noradrenergic function, *Brain Res.*, 620, 133, 1993.

143. Bickford, P.C. et al., Antioxidant-rich diets improve cerebellar physiology and motor learning in aged rats, *Brain Res.*, 866, 211, 2000.

144. Cartford, M. C., Gemma, C., and Bickford, P.C., Eighteen-month-old Fischer 344 rats fed a spinach-enriched diet show improved delay classical eyeblink conditioning and reduced expression of tumor necrosis factor alpha (TNFalpha) and TNFbeta in the cerebellum, *J. Neurosci.*, 22, 5813, 2002.

145. Strömberg, I. et al., Blueberry- and spirulina-enriched diets enhance striatal dopamine recovery and induce a rapid, transient microglia activation after injury of the rat nigrostriatal dopamine system, *Exp. Neurol.*, 196, 298, 2005.

146. Levites, Y. et al., Attenuation of 6-hydroxydopamine (6-OHDA)-induced nuclear factor-kappaB (NF-kappaB) activation and cell death by tea extracts in neuronal cultures, *Biochem. Pharmacol.*, 63, 21, 2002.

147. Levites, Y. et al., Involvement of protein kinase C activation and cell survival/cell cycle genes in green tea polyphenol ()-epigallocatechin 3-gallate neuroprotective action, *J. Biol. Chem.*, 277, 30574, 2002.

148. Willett, W. C., The Mediterranean diet: science and practice, *Public Health Nutr.*, 9, 105, 2006.

149. He, F.J., Nowson, C.A., and MacGregor, G.A., Fruit and vegetable consumption and stroke: meta-analysis of cohort studies, *Lancet*, 367, 320, 2006.

150. Wang, Y. et al., Dietary supplementation with blueberries, spinach, or spirulina reduces ischemic brain damage, *Exp. Neurol.*, 193, 75, 2005.

151. Sweeney, M.I. et al., Feeding rats diets enriched in lowbush blueberries for six weeks decreases ischemia-induced brain damage, *Nutr. Neurosci.*, 5, 427, 2002.

Index

Printed and bound by CPI Group (UK) Ltd, Croydon, CR0 4YY

23/10/2024

01778227-0018